PEDIATRIC NURSING CARE PLANS FOR THE HOSPITALIZED CHILD

THIRD EDITION

Sharon Axton, RN, MS, PNP–BC

Adjunct Associate Clinical Professor
Texas Woman's University
Nelda C. Stark College of Nursing
Houston Center
Houston, Texas

Terry Fugate, RN, MSN

Pediatric Nurse Consultant

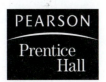

PEARSON
Prentice
Hall

Upper Saddle River, New Jersey

Library of Congress Cataloging-in-Publication Data

Axton, Sharon Ennis.
    Pediatric nursing care plans for the hospitalized child/Sharon Ennis Axton, Terry Fugate.—3rd ed.
        p. ; cm.
    Rev. ed. of: Pediatric nursing care plans. 2nd ed. c2003.
    Includes bibliographical references and index.
    ISBN-13: 978-0-13-503592-4 (alk. paper)
    ISBN-10: 0-13-503592-9 (alk. paper)
    1. Pediatric nursing—Handbooks, manuals, etc. 2. Nursing care plans—Handbooks, manuals, etc.
I. Fugate, Terry. II. Axton, Sharon Ennis. Pediatric nursing care plans. III. Title.
    [DNLM: 1. Pediatric Nursing—Handbooks. 2. Patient Care Planning—Handbooks.
    WY 49 A9721p 2009]
    RJ245.A885 2009
    618.92'00231—dc22   2008016765

Publisher: Julie Levin Alexander
Publisher's Assistant: Regina Bruno
Editor-in-Chief: Maura Connor
Assistant to Editor-in-Chief: Marion Gottlieb
Executive Editor: Pamela Lappies
Editorial Assistant: Sarah Wrocklage
Director of Marketing: Karen Allman
Marketing Manager: Francisco Del Castillo
Marketing Specialist: Michael Sirinides
Managing Editor: Patrick Walsh
Production Liaison: Anne Garcia

Operations Manager: Ilene Sanford
Creative Director: Christy Mahon
Senior Art Director: Maria Guglielmo-Walsh
Interior Design: S4Carlisle
Cover Design: Cheryl Asherman
Composition: S4Carlisle Publishing Services
Full-Service Project Management: Lynn Steines, S4Carlisle
Publishing Services
Cover Printer: R.R. Donnelley & Sons, Harrisonburg, VA
Printer/Binder: R.R. Donnelley & Sons, Harrisonburg, VA

Notice: Care has been taken to confirm the accuracy of information presented in this book. The authors, editors, and the publisher, however, cannot accept any responsibility for errors or omissions or for consequences from application of the information in this book and make no warranty, express or implied, with respect to its contents.

The authors and publisher have exerted every effort to ensure that drug selections and dosages set forth in this text are in accord with current recommendations and practice at time of publication. However, in view of ongoing research, changes in government regulations, and the constant flow of information relating to drug therapy and reactions, the reader is urged to check the package inserts of all drugs for any change in indications or dosage and for added warning and precautions. This is particularly important when the recommended agent is a new and/or infrequently employed drug.

Pearson Education Ltd., London
Pearson Education Singapore, Pte. Ltd
Pearson Education, Canada, Ltd., Toronto
Pearson Education–Japan

Pearson Education Australia PTY, Limited
Pearson Education North Asia Ltd., Hong Kong
Pearson Educación de Mexico, S.A. de C.V.
Pearson Education Malaysia, Pte. Ltd.
Pearson Education, Inc., Upper Saddle River, New Jersey

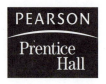

10 9 8 7 6 5 4 3 2 1
ISBN-13: 978-0-13-503592-4
ISBN-10:   0-13-503592-9

CONTENTS

PREFACE

The goal of this book is to assist practicing nurses, nurse educators, and students in implementing the nursing process for pediatric patients. This book provides a quick reference for correlating frequently encountered pediatric medical diagnoses with nursing diagnoses. These care plans are designed for children who are on a general pediatric floor (for a routine admission, after emergency care has been provided, or after the child is stable enough to be transferred out of the intensive care unit).

There are several special features of this book. The first feature is that teaching goals are incorporated into each care plan. Secondly, the Nursing Interventions, Rationale, and Evaluation for Charting columns of each care plan correspond to each other. It is expected that the nurse will individualize each care plan, making each section as specific as possible for the child's growth and development and physical condition.

Most of the nursing diagnoses are those accepted by the North American Nursing Diagnosis Association (NANDA). On a few occasions, it was necessary to use nursing diagnoses that are not on the NANDA list. These are identified by asterisks. Each diagnostic entry has a standard set of components:

Medical Diagnosis

Pathophysiology. This is a basic and brief overview of the pathophysiology of the medical diagnosis.

Primary Nursing Diagnosis. This can be stated as either actual or at risk for occurring. The nurse writing the care plan makes the determination.

Definition. This refers only to the nursing diagnosis and not to the medical diagnosis.

Possibly Related to. The rationale for the selection of each nursing diagnosis is inherent in this statement.

Assessment/Defining Characteristics. These are assessment findings and characteristics of the selected nursing diagnosis and of the identified medical diagnosis. The list presents possible signs and symptoms specific to the identified nursing and medical diagnoses.

Expected Outcomes. Listing expected outcomes is the next step in the nursing process after identification of the nursing diagnosis. Expected outcomes may be listed on a nursing care plan as patient goals or objectives. Outcomes are written as specifically as possible so that they can be measured and easily evaluated. Directions are sometimes included to help individualize the expected outcomes for each infant/child. For example, Expected Outcomes might read as follows:

> Child will have adequate cardiac output as evidenced by heart rate within acceptable range (state specific range).

To individualize this statement, the nurse needs to include the range of acceptable heart rates for each child. The range will vary depending upon the child's age and disease state. The expected outcome for a 1-month-old infant with normal cardiac function would read:

> Infant will have adequate cardiac output as evidenced by heart rate of 100 to 160 beats/minute.

Distinguishing which expected outcomes are short-term and which are long-term can further assist the nurse in individualizing the outcomes for each infant/child. Teaching goals have been incorporated into each care plan. These should also be made specific for each child and family.

Possible Nursing Interventions. These are ways in which the nurse can assist the infant/child and/or family to achieve the expected outcomes. Some of these interventions are *independent* nursing actions, whereas others are *collaborative* (the nurse implements the physician's orders). For example, a nursing intervention to "elevate head of bed at 30° angle" could be instituted for an infant or child with increased intracranial pressure without a specific order from the physician. This would be an independent nursing intervention. A nursing intervention to "administer antibiotic on schedule" depends upon the physician's order.

Since hospital policies and protocols vary, the words "when indicated" or "as indicated" have been used to identify actions which some hospitals may allow the nurse to perform independently, while other hospitals may require a physician's order. Also included in this section is information for which the nurse is responsible. For example, "Check and record urine specific gravity every 4 hours or as indicated" means that the nurse should be aware of this value, even if the laboratory performs urine specific gravity testing. As with the implementation of all nursing interventions, the nurse is encouraged to follow the policies and protocols of each specific institution.

Nursing interventions addressing teaching goals have been incorporated into each care plan.

Rationale. This section provides specific rationale (the reason "why") for the corresponding nursing intervention.

Evaluation for Charting. This section, which deals with the final step in the nursing process, evaluates the expected outcomes and, to some extent, the identified nursing interventions. Statements made here direct the reader to describe or document results. For example, the reader may be directed to "describe breath sounds." This would be correlated with the expected outcome "infant/child will have clear and equal breath sounds" and with a nursing intervention such as "assess and record breath sounds every 4 hours and PRN."

Evaluation is an ongoing process; the evaluation statement may need to be changed frequently. For this reason, the nurse may wish to include this part of the nursing process in the daily charting, noting on the nursing care plan under the evaluation column "see nurses' notes," documenting the date and time, and initialing the note. This section includes documentation for all appropriate forms, such as flowsheets, graphic sheets, medication records, or nurses' notes.

Nursing Diagnoses. Following the primary nursing diagnosis are one to two associated nursing diagnoses that are prioritized and carried through the nursing process. The nurse writing the care plan decides if these are actual nursing diagnoses or if the patient is at risk for the selected nursing diagnoses.

Related Nursing Diagnoses. These are nursing diagnoses that are most likely to be included in a nursing care plan for an infant or child with the stated medical diagnosis. Many of these nursing diagnoses are actual; the patient is at risk for others. The nurse determines which. The related nursing diagnoses are in priority order for an infant/child with the stated medical diagnosis. However, the needs and condition of the infant or child will determine whether the nurse must reorder the priorities. All related nursing diagnoses are completely developed through the nursing process and can be found in the text; refer to the index for location.

To use this book most efficiently, scan the Table of Contents for the applicable medical diagnosis. After finding it in the text, read the pathophysiology, review the accompanying nursing care plan and related nursing diagnoses and select the appropriate expected outcomes and nursing interventions. Write those on the nursing care plan and then implement them. Later, at intervals that you designate when writing the care plan, evaluate the infant's or child's response to your nursing interventions and record your findings.

REVIEWERS

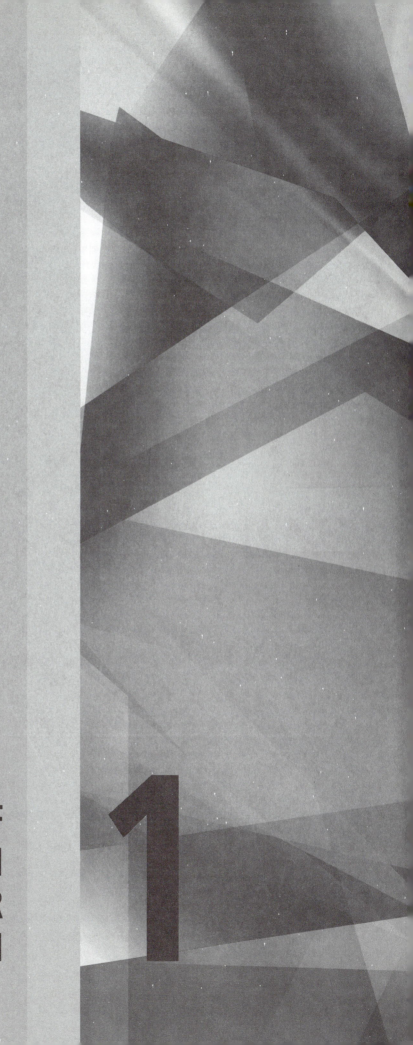

CARE OF
CHILDREN WITH
CARDIOVASCULAR
DYSFUNCTION

1

CARDIAC CATHETERIZATION
PROCEDURE

DESCRIPTION Cardiac catheterization is an invasive procedure of the heart that is used for diagnostic purposes, therapeutic interventions, and electrophysiologic evaluation and treatment. Objectives for diagnostic cardiac catheterization include measurement of oxygen saturation and pressures within the heart chambers and great vessels, measurement of cardiac output and function, visualization of the structures of the heart, and evaluation of the blood flow through the heart. During interventional cardiac catheterization, certain cardiac defects may be corrected without surgical intervention. Procedures that may be performed during interventional catheterization include the creation or closure of atrial septal defects, device closure of ventricular septal defects, transcatheter closure using coils to occlude patent ductus arteriosus, balloon dilatation for coarctation, balloon valvuloplasty for aortic stenosis, stent placement for pulmonary artery stenosis, the insertion of pacer wires, and the assessment of a child's hemodynamic response to certain medications. During electrophysiologic cardiac catheterization, dysrhythmias are evaluated and treated. Radio frequency ablation is used during interventional electrophysiologic catheterization to destroy accessory pathways, which may be causing tachydysrhythmias.

During cardiac catheterization, the physician inserts a thin, flexible, radiopaque catheter through an artery and/or vein and into the chambers of the heart. One of the femoral vessels is most often used, but vessels in the jugular, axillary, and antecubital fossa areas are other possibilities. To gain access to the vessels, the physician uses percutaneous entry or, if necessary, a cutdown procedure may be performed. Fluoroscopy is used, allowing for visualization of the catheter's movement and location. Both right-sided and left-sided catheterizations can be performed. To enter the right side of the heart, the physician usually inserts a catheter into a vein, then passes it into the superior or inferior vena cava and advances it into the right atrium, the right ventricle, and the pulmonary artery. The left side of the heart can be entered by passing the catheter through the former foramen ovale to the left atrium and ventricle, or by passing the catheter retrograde through the femoral artery, through the aorta, and across the aortic valve. At the end of the procedure, the catheter is removed. Pressure is applied to the insertion site.

The injection of contrast material (angiography) into the great vessels or chambers of the heart during catheterization can facilitate their visualization. The contrast medium may cause nausea, vomiting, a generalized burning sensation, allergic rashes, central nervous system symptoms (such as headache or restlessness), tachycardia, hypotension, and/or anaphylactic shock. Complications other than contrast medium reactions include arrhythmias, bleeding, perforation, cardiac tamponade, cardiac perforation, cerebrovascular accident, thrombosis, hematoma, and/or cardiopulmonary arrest.

The child undergoing a cardiac catheterization is not allowed to eat or drink prior to the procedure. Preoperative medications vary among institutions but usually include an analgesic and a sedative/anxiolytic drug combination. In many institutions, cardiac catheterizations are performed on an outpatient basis if the child is in stable condition.

Precardiac Catheterization Nursing Care Plan

Primary Nursing Diagnosis   Anxiety: Child/Family

Definition   Feeling of apprehension resulting from a known or unknown cause

Possibly Related to
- Cardiac catheterization
- Unknown specific heart defect of child
- Unknown prognosis for child
- Fear of undesirable outcome for child

Primary Nursing Diagnosis: Anxiety: child/family related to cardiac catheterization, unknown specific heart diagnosis of child, unknown prognosis for child, and fear of undesirable outcome for child.

Assessment/Defining Characteristics of Child and/or Family (Subjective & Objective Data):

- Verbalization of apprehension or nervousness
- Inability to relax
- Anticipation of misfortune for child during the cardiac catheterization
- Inappropriate or hostile behavior toward health care team
- Inability to concentrate
- Report of somatic discomfort

Expected Outcomes	Possible Nursing Interventions	Rationale	Evaluation for Charting
Child/family will demonstrate decreased anxiety as evidenced by • verbalization of decreased anxiety • ability to relax • lack of statements indicating anticipated misfortune for child during the cardiac catheterization • lack of inappropriate or hostile behavior toward health care team • ability to concentrate • decreased reports of somatic discomfort	Listen to child's/family's concerns and complaints. Encourage expressions of feelings to health care team, other family members, or friends regarding the procedure and its implications.	Allows child/family to express feelings and concerns and provides them with a way to gain knowledge and decrease anxiety about the procedure.	Describe child's/family's behavior, concerns and complaints. Describe any successful measures used to encourage family to express their feelings and/or decrease their anxiety.
	Remove excess stimulation from the environment.	This will help child and/or family to concentrate on information being taught.	Describe successful measures used to decrease stimulation in the environment.
	Record interactions with child/family.	Allows health care team to tailor the best way to provide care for family and child.	Describe interactions with child and/or family and any successful measures that decreased anxiety.
	Allow family to stay with child as much as possible.	Allowing the family and child to stay together assists child/family in their ability to cope.	Document when family stayed with child. Describe child's/family's behavior.
	Allow child to keep a familiar item with him/her.	A familiar item may comfort the child and ease the family's concern.	Document whether child had a familiar item for comfort and describe effectiveness.
	Explain the cardiac catheterization procedure. Instruct the child/family in post-procedural and home care. Explain potential changes in the child's behavior after the procedure and upon returning home. Keep explanations simple and concise; use illustrations. Repeat explanations as necessary.	Increased knowledge will increase understanding and acceptance in the child and/or family.	Document whether child and/or family was able to verbalize an understanding of explanations regarding the procedure, child's care, and child's condition.

(continued)

Primary Nursing Diagnosis: Anxiety: Child/Family *(continued)*			
Expected Outcomes	**Possible Nursing Interventions**	**Rationale**	**Evaluation for Charting**
	Answer any questions the child and/or family may have regarding the procedure, child's care, or child's condition.	Allowing child and/or family to ask questions provides an opportunity to make sure information is correctly understood.	Document whether child and/or family had questions and if the questions were sufficiently answered.
	Dispel any misinformation.	Provides an opportunity for health care team to correct any misinformation.	Document any misinformation stated by child and/or family and measures used to dispel misinformation.
TEACHING GOALS Child and/or family will be able to verbalize at least 4 characteristics of increased anxiety such as • inability to relax • inappropriate or hostile behavior toward health care team • inability to concentrate • reports of somatic discomfort • asking the same questions repeatedly	Teach child/family about characteristics of anxiety. Assess and record results.	Increased knowledge will assist the child/family in recognizing and reporting changes in their anxiety.	Document whether teaching was done and describe results.
Child and/or family will be able to verbalize knowledge of care such as • identification of any signs/symptoms of anxiety (such as those listed under Assessment) • when to contact health care provider	Teach child/family about care. Assess and record child's/family's knowledge of and participation in care regarding identification of any signs/symptoms of anxiety, etc.	Education of child/family will allow for accurate care.	Document whether teaching was done and describe results.

Nursing Diagnosis   Deficient Knowledge: Child/Family

Definition   Lack of information concerning the child's disease and care

Possibly Related to   Misconceptions or inaccurate information concerning cardiac catheterization, possibly caused by
- fear of cardiac catheterization procedure
- fear of cardiac catheterization outcome
- sensory overload

Cognitive or cultural-language limitations

Nursing Diagnosis: Deficient knowledge: child/family related to misconceptions, inaccurate information, fear of procedure, fear of outcome of procedure, sensory overload, cognitive or cultural-language limitations.

Assessment/Defining Characteristics of Child and/or Family (Subjective & Objective Data):

- Verbalization by child and or family indicating lack of knowledge
- Relation of incorrect information to members of the health care team
- Requests for information

Expected Outcomes	Possible Nursing Interventions	Rationale	Evaluation for Charting
TEACHING GOALS Child and/or family will have an adequate knowledge base concerning the child's cardiac catheterization and care as evidenced by • ability to correctly state information previously taught regarding the cardiac catheterization procedure and home care • ability to relate appropriate information to the health care team • ability to request additional information and/or clarification of information	Listen to child's/family's concerns and fears. Document findings.	Allows child/family to express feelings and concerns and provides them with a way to gain knowledge.	Describe child's/family's concerns and fears and any successful measures used to encourage family to express their feelings.
	Assess and record child's/family's knowledge concerning the cardiac catheterization. Encourage questions.	Generates a baseline of knowledge, which allows for teaching of accurate information and dispelling of incorrect knowledge.	Document whether teaching was done and describe results.
	Provide child/family with information about the cardiac catheterization, including • preoperative medications • preparation of the insertion site • equipment • monitoring of child during the procedure • X-ray films • any diversional activities available for the child (e.g., cassette tapes) should the child awake during the procedure • time frame for the procedure • condition of child (sleepiness) after the procedure • care of child after the procedure (assessment of vital signs, cardiovascular assessment, site assessment, initial diet of clear liquids)	Education of child/family will allow for accurate care and increase coping ability of child/family.	Document whether teaching was done and describe results.

(continued)

Nursing Diagnosis: Deficient Knowledge: Child/Family *(continued)*			
Expected Outcomes	**Possible Nursing Interventions**	**Rationale**	**Evaluation for Charting**
	Use pictures as necessary to facilitate teaching.	Facilitates understanding and reinforces learning.	Document whether pictures were used and effectiveness of teaching.
	Provide child/family with any available literature or booklets concerning cardiac catheterization.	Facilitates understanding and reinforces learning.	Document whether literature or booklets were used and describe effectiveness of teaching.
	Arrange a preliminary visit to the catheterization laboratory.	Facilitates understanding, reinforces learning, and helps child's/family's coping ability.	Document whether visit was done and describe effectiveness of the experience.
	Assign primary nurse as usual spokesperson to child/family.	Promotes trust and communication and enhances learning.	Document if primary nurse was assigned and effectiveness that this method had in enhancing child/family learning.
	When indicated, obtain an interpreter.	To ensure accurate communication of information.	Document whether an interpreter was necessary and effectiveness in enhancing learning for child/family.
	Dispel any misinformation.	Provides an opportunity for health care team to correct any misinformation.	Document any misinformation stated by child and/or family and measures used to dispel misinformation.
	Instruct child/family in home care: • observation of the catheterization site for bleeding, swelling, redness, drainage • observation of the extremity for paleness, pain • site care • monitoring of child's temperature • monitoring of child's extremity for any numbness • diet • hygiene	Education and instruction of child/family will allow for accurate care.	Document whether teaching was done and describe results.
	Identify resources (for support or for information) that the parents may contact for assistance after the child's discharge.	Facilitates understanding, reinforces learning, and assists child/family in their ability to cope.	Document whether teaching was done and describe results.

Related Nursing Diagnoses

Decreased Cardiac Output	*related to* congenital heart defect
Fear: Child/Family	*related to* a. invasive procedure b. outcome of cardiac catheterization
Compromised Family Coping	*related to* a. child's hospitalization b. invasive procedure c. potential for child to have a fatal or chronic disease

Postcardiac Catheterization Nursing Care Plan

Primary Nursing Diagnosis   Decreased Cardiac Output

Definition	Decrease in the amount of blood that leaves the left ventricle
Possibly Related to	• Dysrhythmias secondary to catheter irritation • Septal perforation • Hemorrhage • Shock • Reaction to contrast medium • Reaction to sedation • Cardiopulmonary arrest

Primary Nursing Diagnosis: Decreased cardiac output related to dysrhythmias secondary to catheter irritation, septal perforation, hemorrhage, shock, reaction to contrast medium, reaction to sedation, cardiopulmonary arrest

Assessment/Defining Characteristics of Child and/or Family (Subjective & Objective Data):

- Tachycardia
- Tachypnea
- Hypotension
- Unequal, decreased, or absent peripheral pulses
- Excessive bleeding from catheter insertion site
- Cool, clammy extremities
- Prolonged capillary refill, longer than 2 to 3 seconds
- Decreased urine output
- Hematoma
- Cardiopulmonary arrest

Expected Outcomes	Possible Nursing Interventions	Rationale	Evaluation for Charting
Child will have adequate cardiac output as evidenced by • heart rate within acceptable range (state specific range)	Assess and record HR, RR, and BP every 15 minutes until stable, then every 30 minutes for two times, then every 4 hours, or as otherwise indicated.	If child experiences decreased cardiac output (CO) the HR and RR will increase and the BP will decrease.	Document range of HR, RR, and BP.

(continued)

Primary Nursing Diagnosis: Decreased Cardiac Output *(continued)*			
Expected Outcomes	**Possible Nursing Interventions**	**Rationale**	**Evaluation for Charting**
• respiratory rate within acceptable range (state specific range) • blood pressure within acceptable range (state specific range) • strong and equal peripheral pulses • minimal bleeding from catheterization site • brisk capillary refill, within 2 to 3 seconds • skin warm to touch • regular heart rate and rhythm • adequate urinary output (state specific range; 1 to 2 ml/kg/hr) • lack of signs/symptoms of decreased cardiac output (such as those listed under Assessment)	Assess and record the following with vital signs or per postcatheterization protocol • condition of catheter site or dressing. Notify physician of excessive drainage. • peripheral pluses. If indicated, use a Doppler device to locate pulses. • capillary refill • skin temperature and color • signs/symptoms of decreased cardiac output (such as those listed under Assessment)	Site assessment is necessary to detect bleeding. Assessment of peripheral pulses, capillary refill, skin temperature and color are needed to detect vascular flow problems. Assessment of signs/symptoms of decreased cardiac output is necessary for early detection of problems.	Describe condition of catheter site or dressing. Describe quality of peripheral pulses, capillary refill, and skin temperature and color. Describe any signs/symptoms of decreased cardiac output noted (such as those listed under assessment).
	When indicated, initiate use of cardiac monitor. Evaluate and record results of EKG strips.	Cardiac monitor can reveal changes in cardiac rhythm. Changes in EKG may indicate decreased CO.	Describe results of cardiac monitor or EKG when indicated.
	Keep accurate record of intake and output.	Decreased output may indicate decreased CO possibly due to a shift of the intravascular fluid into the interstitial space.	Document intake and output.
	Have emergency medications and equipment ready.	Emergency medications and equipment need to be available in the event of an emergency.	Describe if any emergency interventions were necessary. State their effectiveness.
TEACHING GOALS Child and/or family will be able to verbalize at least 4 characteristics of decreased cardiac output such as • rapid heart rate • excessive bleeding from catheter insertion site • cool, clammy extremities • decreased urinary output	Teach child/family about characteristics of decreased cardiac output. Assess and record results.	Increased knowledge will assist the child/family in recognizing and reporting changes in the child's condition.	Document whether teaching was done and describe results.

Primary Nursing Diagnosis: Decreased Cardiac Output *(continued)*

Expected Outcomes	Possible Nursing Interventions	Rationale	Evaluation for Charting
Child and/or family will be able to verbalize knowledge of care such as • catheter site care • medication administration (if indicated) • sufficient rest period following procedure • identification of any signs/symptoms of decreased cardiac output (such as those listed under Assessment) • when to contact health care provider	Teach child/family about care. Assess and record child's/family's knowledge of and participation in care regarding catheter site care, etc.	Education of child/family will allow for accurate care.	Document whether teaching was done and describe results.

Nursing Diagnosis   Ineffective Tissue Perfusion: Peripheral

Definition   Inadequate amount of blood and oxygen being delivered to the tissues in the body

Possibly Related to
- Hemorrhage from catheterization site
- Arterial or venous clots obstructing blood flow
- Decreased cardiac output

Nursing Diagnosis: Ineffective tissue perfusion: peripheral related to hemorrhage from catheterization site, arterial or venous clots obstructing blood flow, decreased cardiac output

Assessment/Defining Characteristics of Child and/or Family (Subjective & Objective Data):

Catheterized extremity may have the following characteristics

- cool, clammy skin
- pale or mottled color
- decreased intensity of pulses
- spasms of artery
- thrombus
- prolonged capillary refill, longer than 2 to 3 seconds
- excessive bleeding at catheterization site
- hematoma
- edema
- decreased movement or sensation of limb

(continued)

Nursing Diagnosis: Ineffective Tissue Perfusion: Peripheral *(continued)*

Expected Outcomes	Possible Nursing Interventions	Rationale	Evaluation for Charting
Child's catheterized extremity will have adequate tissue perfusion as evidenced by • skin warm to touch • pink color • strong, equal peripheral pulses • brisk capillary refill, within 2 to 3 seconds • adequate movement and sensation as compared to other extremities • lack of signs/ symptoms of ineffective peripheral tissue perfusion (such as those listed under Assessment)	Assess and record the following with vital signs or per postcatheterization protocol • condition of catheterization site or dressing. Notify physician of excessive drainage. • peripheral pulses. If indicated, use a Doppler device to locate pulses. • capillary refill • skin temperature and color • signs/symptoms of ineffective peripheral tissue perfusion (such as those listed under Assessment). Notify physician of any abnormalities.	Site assessment is necessary to detect bleeding. Assessment of peripheral pulses, capillary refill, skin temperature and color are needed to detect vascular flow problems. Assessment of signs/symptoms of ineffective peripheral tissue perfusion is necessary for early detection of problems.	Describe condition of insertion site and/or dressing. Describe quality of peripheral pulses, capillary refill, and skin temperature and color. Describe any signs/ symptoms of ineffective peripheral tissue perfusion noted.
	Minimize movement and attempt to prevent flexion of catheterized extremity.	This is done in order to prevent mobilization of any clots that may form.	Document whether movement and flexion were minimized. Describe effectiveness.
	Maintain bed rest for child as indicated.	Bed rest is necessary in order to help decrease bleeding and strain at the insertion site.	Document whether bed rest was indicated and if it was maintained.
	When indicated, • elevate extremity to facilitate venous return (specify if extremity is edematous) • apply additional direct pressure or reinforce dressing at the catheterization site	Elevation of the extremity facilitates venous return, and pressure or reinforcement of the dressing is necessary to reduce excess bleeding.	Describe any therapeutic measures used to improve peripheral perfusion. State their effectiveness.

Nursing Diagnosis: Ineffective Tissue Perfusion: Peripheral *(continued)*

Expected Outcomes	Possible Nursing Interventions	Rationale	Evaluation for Charting
TEACHING GOALS Child and/or family will be able to verbalize at least 4 characteristics of ineffective peripheral tissue perfusion to catheterized limb such as • cool, clammy skin • pale or mottled skin • decreased movement or sensation • excessive bleeding at catheterization site	Teach child/family about characteristics of ineffective peripheral tissue perfusion. Assess and record results.	Increased knowledge will assist the child/family in recognizing and reporting changes in the child's condition.	Document whether teaching was done and describe results.
Child and/or family will be able to verbalize knowledge of care such as • catheter site care • medication administration (if indicated) • sufficient rest period following procedure • identification of any signs/symptoms of ineffective peripheral tissue perfusion (such as those listed under Assessment) • when to contact health care provider	Teach child/family about care. Assess and record child's/family's knowledge of and participation in care regarding catheter site care, etc.	Education of child/family will allow for accurate care.	Document whether teaching was done and describe results.

Related Nursing Diagnoses

Acute Pain   *related to* catheter insertion site

Risk for Infection   *related to* invasive procedure

Deficient Fluid Volume   *related to*
a. vomiting secondary to medications
b. diuresis caused by contrast medium

Compromised Family Coping   *related to* outcome of procedure

TWO

CONGENITAL HEART DISEASE
MEDICAL DIAGNOSIS

PATHOPHYSIOLOGY Congenital heart disease (CHD) occurs in approximately 8 out of 1,000 live births. In most cases, the specific cause is unknown. Inheritance, genetic predisposition, and environmental influences (such as viruses, alcohol, and drugs) have been associated with CHD. Certain chromosomal aberrations, such as trisomies 13, 18, and 21, also increase the risk of CHD.

Congenital heart defects can be categorized as either acyanotic or cyanotic lesions. Acyanotic cardiac defects can be further divided into lesions with increased pulmonary blood flow (such as ventricular septal defect) and lesions with obstruction to blood flow from the ventricles (such as coarctation of the aorta). Cyanotic defects can be further divided into lesions with decreased pulmonary blood flow (such as tetrology of Fallot) and lesions with mixed defects (such as transposition of the great arteries). Cardiovascular surgery can be performed for palliation and/or correction of many cardiac defects.

The basic pathophysiologies of 12 congenital heart defects are presented here. The postoperative nursing care plan that follows applies to children who have been moved out of the intensive care unit setting. For immediate postoperative care, consult a pediatric critical care nursing care plan book.

Acyanotic Heart Defects/Lesions with Increased Pulmonary Flow

Atrial Septal Defect (ASD) An atrial septal defect is an opening between the right and left atrium. It can vary in size and location in the septum and can be associated with other cardiac defects. Some of the oxygenated blood going to the higher-pressure left atrium is shunted through the ASD to the lower-pressure right atrium; thus, an ASD is a left-to-right shunt. From the right atrium, the blood passes through the tricuspid valve to the right ventricle; it then recirculates through the lungs, increasing the blood flow to the lungs. Pulmonary vascular changes occur very slowly, and increased pulmonary vascular resistance usually does not occur until early adulthood. Small ASDs may close spontaneously. Surgical intervention to close the ASD is recommended by school age. Earlier closure is recommended if the

child is experiencing problems. Nonsurgical closure is also possible using transcatheter devices during cardiac catheterization. Most children with an ASD are asymptomatic. ASD occurs in approximately 6 to 10% of all congenital cardiac defects.

Atrioventricular (AV) Canal Defect Atrioventricular canal defect, also called endocardial cushion defect, refers to a combination of defects in the atrial and ventricular septa and portions of the mitral and tricuspid valves allowing free communication of blood flow between all four chambers of the heart. In the most complex of these malformations a large central atrioventricular valve is created by clefts of the mitral and tricuspid valves with the presence of a low atrial septal defect and a high ventricular septal defect. A left-to-right shunt (most common), right-to-left shunt, and/or bidirectional shunt may exist. Oxygenated blood is recirculated to the lungs. Increased blood flow going under increased pressure to the lungs can lead to increased pulmonary vascular resistance and pulmonary hypertension, which can ultimately result in congestive heart failure. Surgical repair is usually performed in infancy. Prior to surgical repair, medical management of congestive heart failure is initiated and weight gain is emphasized. Clinical manifestations include symptoms of congestive heart failure, and the infant appears small and undernourished. Cyanosis, which worsens with crying, is also present. AV canal defect occurs in 3 to 4% of children with congenital cardiac defects, and it is the most common cardiac defect in children with Down syndrome.

Patent Ductus Arteriosus (PDA) The ductus arteriosus, a connection between the pulmonary artery and the descending aorta, is a normal pathway in fetal circulation that usually closes permanently during the first few weeks of life. Failure of the ductus arteriosus to close results in a left-to-right shunt. Oxygenated blood flows from the higher-pressure aorta into the lower-pressure pulmonary artery and is recirculated through the lungs. The lungs then receive increased blood flow under increased pressure. If the patent ductus arteriosus is not corrected, irreversible pulmonary vascular disease can result. Some PDAs may close spontaneously. Surgical treatment, either by ligation (tying off) or division (cutting) is recommended for closure. The use of prostaglandin inhibitor (indomethacin) is often used for closure of PDAs in preterm infants who are symptomatic. Older infants and children who have not had spontaneous closure will also require closure by surgical intervention or by transcatheter closure done during cardiac catheterization. Clinical manifestations may include a machinery-like murmur associated with a thrill, widened pulse pressure, frequent respiratory infections, failure to thrive, and signs/symptoms of congestive heart failure. This defect accounts for 9 to 12% of all congenital cardiac defects.

Ventricular Septal Defect (VSD)   A ventricular septal defect is an abnormal opening between the left and right ventricles. It can vary in size, location in the septum, and number (there can be multiple VSDs). A VSD is often associated with other, more complex defects. It causes a left-to-right shunt that results in increased blood flow going to the lungs under increased pressure. This increased blood flow has already been oxygenated and is recirculating through the lungs. Irreversible pulmonary vascular changes can result (usually when the child is around 2 years of age) if the condition is not corrected. Approximately 60% of all VSDs close spontaneously sometime during the first 2 years of life. Surgical intervention for closure of the VSD is required when the child is symptomatic and the defect does not close spontaneously. Nonsurgical treatment using device closure may also be used. Clinical manifestations may include a loud, harsh, pansystolic murmur, frequent respiratory infections, failure to thrive, and signs/symptoms of congestive heart failure. VSD is the most common heart lesion occurring in approximately 20% of all children with congenital cardiac defects.

Acyanotic Heart Defects/Lesions with Obstruction to Blood Flow

Aortic Stenosis (AS)   Aortic stenosis is a narrowing of the aortic outflow tract obstructing blood flow to the systemic circulation. It can be supravalvular, valvular, or subvalvular, with valvular being the most common. Pressure builds on the left side of the heart, due to the resistance to ejection of blood from the left ventricle, and causes left ventricular hypertrophy. Left atrial pressure then increases, causing increased pressure in the pulmonary veins. The increased pulmonary vascular pressure causes fluid to leak into the interstitial spaces, which results in pulmonary edema. Newborns with severe AS need their ductus arteriosus to remain patent (with the use of Prostaglandin E1) until the aortic valve can be dilated. When necessary balloon dilatation of the aortic valve may be done during cardiac

catheterization or surgically. If the condition is severe, the aortic valve is surgically replaced. Often, the child will require more than one procedure during his/her lifetime. There is a lifelong risk of endocarditis. Infants with AS can manifest symptoms of left ventricular failure and low cardiac output such as respiratory distress, faint peripheral pulses, decreased urine output, and poor feeding. If AS is not severe, it may go undiagnosed until preadolescence, when the child may manifest symptoms such as fainting, dizziness, epigastric pain, or exercise intolerance. Acute dysrhythmias may develop and result in sudden death following exertion in some individuals. AS occurs in approximately 3 to 6% of all cases of congenital cardiac defects.

Coarctation of the Aorta (COA)   Coarctation of the aorta is a narrowing of the aorta that can vary from mild constriction to total occlusion. The most common location is juxtaductal (at the junction of the ductus arteriosus on the aortic arch). The degree of narrowing determines the severity of the symptoms. In juxtaductal coarctation, blood flow to the lower part of the body is decreased, manifested by diminished pulses in the lower extremities. Pressure builds proximal to the obstruction and results in upper extremity hypertension. Elective surgical correction is recommended within the first 2 years of life to prevent hypertension. Nonsurgical treatment using balloon dilatation during cardiac catheterization may be used as a primary intervention or for recoarctation. Clinical manifestations of congestive heart failure may be present in symptomatic infants with COA. Children with COA may be asymptomatic, and the defect is first detected during a routine physical examination when upper extremity systemic hypertension, weak or absent femoral pulses, and a heart murmur are present. It occurs in about 5 to 8% of all cases of congenital cardiac defects.

Pulmonary Stenosis (PS)   Pulmonary stenosis is a narrowing at the area around the pulmonary valve, resulting in an obstruction that interferes with blood flow out of the right ventricle. The narrowing can vary in degree from mild to severe and can be supravalvular, valvular, or subvalvular. Pressure builds in the right ventricle and can result in right ventricular hypertrophy. In young infants, this increase in pressure may cause the foramen ovale to reopen, resulting in right-to-left shunting of unoxygenated blood. If pulmonary stenosis is severe, systemic venous engorgement results and can lead to congestive heart failure. Balloon dilatation during cardiac catheterization or surgical intervention may be required to correct the defect. Clinical manifestations may include a systolic ejection murmur, dyspnea, cyanosis, fatigue, and signs/symptoms of congestive heart failure. PS occurs in approximately 8 to 12% of all cases of congenital cardiac defects.

Cyanotic Heart Defects/Lesions with Decreased Pulmonary Blood Flow

Tetralogy of Fallot (TOF) Classic tetralogy of Fallot has four components: pulmonary stenosis, ventricular septal defect, an overriding aorta, and right ventricular hypertrophy (creating a boot-shaped heart as seen on X-ray). A fifth defect, either an open foramen ovale or an atrial septal defect may also be present in some children. The pattern of blood flow in this defect is determined by the degree of pulmonary stenosis. If pulmonary stenosis is severe, pressure builds in the right ventricle and unoxygenated blood passes through the VSD into the overriding aorta (right-to-left shunt), producing cyanosis. If the pulmonary stenosis is mild and the pressure in the right ventricle is not increased, the blood shunts left to right through the VSD and the child is acyanotic. In time, the pulmonary stenosis becomes more severe and the child becomes more cyanotic as less blood flows to the lungs. Hypoxic, or "tet," spells occur in some children with TOF. These spells are thought to occur as a result of a transient increase in obstruction of the right ventricle outflow tract causing cyanosis and a decreased level of consciousness. Tet spells can be treated by placing the child in the knee-chest position, which is thought to increase venous return to the heart and dilate the right ventricle and should decrease the pulmonary outflow obstruction effect. Surgical correction involves closing the VSD and resectioning the infundibular stenosis and enlarging the right ventricular outflow tract. Elective surgery is usually performed prior to 1 year of age. If surgical correction needs to be delayed, a palliative procedure may be done prior to total correction in order to increase pulmonary blood flow. Clinical manifestations may include cyanosis, hypoxemia, increased hemoglobin and hematocrit, and a pansystolic murmur. Since surgical repair is usually done early (before the child is 1 year of age), squatting, once common, is rarely seen now. There is a lifelong risk for endocarditis. Tetralogy of Fallot accounts for anywhere between 4 to 10% of all cases of congenital cardiac defects. It is the most common cyanotic congenital heart defect.

Tricuspid Atresia Tricuspid atresia is total occlusion of the tricuspid valve. There is no communication between the right atrium and the right ventricle. Other anomalies, such as atrial septal defect (ASD), ventricular septal defect (VSD), or patent ductus arteriosus (PDA) are commonly present, and a mandatory right-to-left atrial shunt exists. The right ventricle is usually small, and the pulmonary arteries may also be small. Blood returning from the body empties into the right atrium and cannot pass into the right ventricle; therefore, the blood goes through the ASD to the left atrium. From the left atrium, blood flows to the left ventricle, and a portion of this blood goes to the lungs via a VSD. If a VSD is not present, the blood can flow to the lungs via a PDA. In infants with a PDA, prostaglandin E1 can be given to maintain the patency of the ductus arteriosus. Palliative surgery designed to increase blood flow to the lungs may also be done prior to total correction. Total repair involves creating communication between the right atrium (or right ventricle) and the pulmonary artery. There is a lifelong risk for endocarditis. The most consistent clinical manifestation is cyanosis in conjunction with tachypnea and dyspnea. Tricuspid atresia is an uncommon defect, occurring in 2.7% of all cases of congenital cardiac defects.

Cyanotic Heart Defects/Lesions with Mixed Blood Flow

Total Anomalous Pulmonary Venous Connection (TAPVC) Total anomalous pulmonary venous connection, also called total anomalous pulmonary venous return (TAPVR), occurs when the pulmonary veins do not connect to the left atrium; instead, they connect to the right atrium or to one of the systemic veins draining toward the right atrium (such as the superior vena cava or the inferior vena cava). The blood flow pattern in the heart depends on where the pulmonary veins connect (above or below the diaphragm) and on the presence or absence of pulmonary venous obstruction. In all types of TAPVC, the right atrium ultimately receives systemic blood as well as the blood returning from the lungs. This increased blood flow to the right atrium results in hypertrophy of the right side of the heart. The only way for blood flow to reach the left atrium is through an associated atrial septal defect or a patent foramen ovale. When there is no pulmonary venous obstruction, excessive blood flow to the lungs occurs, which can result in congestive heart failure. If pulmonary venous congestion is present, blood flow to the lungs is decreased and cyanosis can be marked. Pulmonary venous pressure rises proximal to the obstruction, resulting in pulmonary edema.

Surgical correction is required to repair TAPVC. Clinical manifestations include cyanosis, a blowing systolic murmur, a venous hum, tachypnea, feeding difficulties, repeated upper respiratory infections, and signs/symptoms of congestive heart failure. TAPVC occurs in approximately 1% of all cases of congenital heart defects.

Transposition of the Great Arteries (TGA) In transposition of the great arteries, the aorta arises from the right ventricle and the pulmonary artery arises from the left ventricle. This results in two separate circulatory systems and can be life threatening at birth without the presence of a patent foramen ovale and ductus arteriosus. Blood from the systemic circulation enters the right atrium and passes to the right ventricle and out the aorta back to the rest of the body without going to the lungs for oxygenation. The pulmonary veins empty into the left atrium. The oxygenated blood goes to the left ventricle, out the pulmonary artery, and back to the lungs. Associated lesions (atrial septal defect, ventricular septal defect, and patent ductus arteriosus) are usually present and account for any mixing of oxygenated and unoxygenated blood. Corrective surgery is usually performed before one week of life. Surgeries for total correction involve an arterial switch procedure (preferred) or intraatrial redirection of blood flow. Balloon septostomy can be performed as a palliative procedure during cardiac catheterization in order to enlarge the interatrial communication and mixing of blood, resulting in a dramatic increase in arterial oxygenation. There is a lifelong risk for endocarditis. Clinical manifestations may include cyanosis and signs/symptoms of congestive heart failure. The defect occurs in about 5% of all cases of congenital cardiac defects.

Truncus Arteriosus Truncus arteriosus is characterized by a single vessel that arises from the left and right ventricles and overrides a ventricular septal defect (VSD). This single vessel gives rise to pulmonary, systemic, and coronary circulations. Blood from both ventricles enters the single vessel and flows to the lung and to the rest of the body. Blood flow to the lungs is usually under systemic pressure, depending on the type of truncus present. The type of truncus is determined by the existence and location of the main pulmonary artery and the pulmonary artery branches. Infants with truncus arteriosus are usually at high risk for early pulmonary vascular disease because the blood flows under increased pressure to the lungs. Corrective surgery is usually performed in the first few months of life. Palliative surgery may be done prior to corrective surgery and is aimed at decreasing pulmonary blood flow. There is a lifelong risk for endocarditis. Clinical manifestations include cyanosis and signs/symptoms of congestive heart failure. Truncus arteriosus accounts for 1% of all cases of congenital cardiac defects.

Postoperative, Postpediatric ICU Nursing Care Plan

Primary Nursing Diagnosis   Decreased Cardiac Output

Definition   Decrease in the amount of blood that leaves the left ventricle

Possibly Related to   • Surgical complications:
  • thrombus
  • ineffective circulation
  • interference with electrical conduction of the heart
  • dysrhythmias
  • tachycardia or bradycardia

Primary Nursing Diagnosis: Decreased cardiac output related to thrombus, ineffective circulation, interference with electrical conduction of the heart, dysrhythmias, tachycardia or bradycardia

Assessment/Defining Characteristics of Child and/or Family (Subjective & Objective Data):

- Tachycardia/bradycardia
- Dysrhythmias
- Hypotension/hypertension
- Unequal, decreased, or absent peripheral pulses
- Cyanosis
- Prolonged capillary refill, longer than 2 to 3 seconds
- Murmur, gallop, rub, click
- Cool, pale skin
- Fever
- Activity intolerance
- Fatigue
- Decreased urine output

Expected Outcomes	Possible Nursing Interventions	Rationale	Evaluation for Charting
Child will have adequate cardiac output as evidenced by • heart rate, respiratory rate, and blood pressure within acceptable range (state specific range for each) • strong and equal peripheral pulses • brisk capillary refill within 2 to 3 seconds • skin warm to touch • strong and equal peripheral pulses • lack of murmur, gallop, rub, click, cyanosis, fatigue, activity intolerance • adequate urine output (state specific range; 1 to 2 ml/kg/hr)	Assess and record the following every 4 hours and PRN • HR, RR, and BP • peripheral pulses • capillary refill • any signs/symptoms of decreased cardiac output (such as those listed under Assessment)	If child experiences decreased cardiac output (CO) the HR, RR will increase and BP will decrease. Peripheral pulses will be weak and unequal. Capillary refill will be longer than 2 to 3 seconds.	Document range of HR, RR, and BP. Describe quality of peripheral pulses and capillary refill. Describe any signs/symptoms of decreased cardiac output noted.
	Assess and record condition of dressing and/or incision site every shift and PRN. Notify physician of excessive drainage.	Excessive drainage or bleeding could result in decreased cardiac output.	Describe condition of dressing and/or incision site.
	Administer cardiac drugs (such as digoxin) on schedule. Assess and record any side effects or any signs/symptoms of toxicity (such as vomiting with digoxin). Follow hospital protocol for administration, such as 2 RNs checking the dosage prior to administration and documenting the HR or BP at the time of medication administration.	Cardiac drugs are given to increase the strength of cardiac contractions and/or increase return of blood flow to the heart, thereby increasing CO.	Document whether cardiac medications were administered on schedule. Describe effectiveness and any side effects noted.

Primary Nursing Diagnosis: Decreased Cardiac Output *(continued)*			
Expected Outcomes	**Possible Nursing Interventions**	**Rationale**	**Evaluation for Charting**
	If indicated, monitor and record digoxin levels. Notify physician if levels are out of the acceptable range. (A decreased potassium level increases the risk for digoxin toxicity.)	Digoxin is a potent medication that needs careful monitoring. If digoxin levels are high, the child will experience signs/symptoms of toxicity (such as vomiting).	Document digoxin levels. If levels are out of the acceptable range, describe any corrective measures implemented.
	Ensure that chest physiotherapy is done on schedule. Record effectiveness and child's response to treatment.	Chest percussion loosens secretions and positioning can help to assist the flow of secretions out of the lungs by gravity.	Document whether chest physiotherapy was done on schedule. Describe effectiveness and child's response to treatment.
	Elevate head of bed at a 30° angle.	Elevating the head of the bed to a 30° angle causes a shift of the abdominal contents downward and this will allow for increased lung expansion. This will aid in reducing workload on the heart.	Document whether head of bed was elevated.
	Keep accurate record of intake and output.	Decreased output may indicate decreased CO possibly due to a shift of the intravascular fluid into the interstitial space.	Document intake and output.
TEACHING GOALS Child and/or family will be able to verbalize at least 4 characteristics of decreased cardiac output such as • rapid heart rate • unequal pulses • cold extremities • decreased urine output (for infants less than six wet diapers/day)	Teach child/family about characteristics of decreased cardiac output. Assess and record results.	Increased knowledge will assist the child/family in recognizing and reporting changes in the child's condition.	Document whether teaching was done and describe results.

(continued)

	Primary Nursing Diagnosis: Decreased Cardiac Output *(continued)*		
Expected Outcomes	**Possible Nursing Interventions**	**Rationale**	**Evaluation for Charting**
Child and/or family will be able to verbalize knowledge of care such as • medication administration • chest physiotherapy, if indicated • monitoring intake and output • identification of any signs/symptoms of decreased cardiac output (such as those listed under Assessment) • when to contact health care provider	Teach child/family about care. Assess and record child's/family's knowledge of and participation in care regarding medication administration, etc.	Education of child/family will allow for accurate care.	Document whether teaching was done and describe results.

Nursing Diagnosis   Acute Pain

Definition   Condition in which an individual experiences acute mild to severe pain

Possibly Related to   • Incision site
                               • Treatments and procedures

	Nursing Diagnosis: Acute pain related to incision site, treatments, and procedures		
Assessment/Defining Characteristics of Child and/or Family (Subjective & Objective Data):			
• Verbal communication of pain or tenderness • Crying unrelieved by usual comfort measures • Facial grimacing • Restlessness		• Rating of pain on pain-assessment tool • Physical signs/symptoms (tachycardia, tachypnea/bradypnea, increased blood pressure, diaphoresis)	
Expected Outcomes	**Possible Nursing Interventions**	**Rationale**	**Evaluation for Charting**
Child will be free of severe and/or constant pain as evidenced by • verbal communication of comfort • lack of constant crying	Assess and record HR, RR, BP, and any signs/symptoms of pain (such as those listed under Assessment) every 2 to 4 hours and PRN. Use an appropriate pain-assessment tool.	Provides data regarding the level of pain child is experiencing.	Document range of HR, RR, BP, and degree of pain child was experiencing. Describe any successful measures used to decrease pain.

Nursing Diagnosis: Acute Pain *(continued)*

Expected Outcomes	Possible Nursing Interventions	Rationale	Evaluation for Charting
• lack of extreme restlessness • heart rate within acceptable range (state specific range) • respiratory rate within acceptable range (state specific range) • rating of decreased pain or no pain on pain-assessment tool • lack of signs/symptoms of acute pain (such as those listed under Assessment) • lack of diaphoresis • lack of signs/symptoms of acute pain (such as those listed under Assessment)	Handle child gently.	Helps to minimize pain and promote comfort.	Document if child was handled gently and effectiveness of measure.
	When indicated, administer analgesics on schedule. Assess and record effectiveness.	Analgesics are administered to decrease pain.	Document whether analgesics were administered on schedule. Describe effectiveness and any side effects noted.
	Encourage family members to stay and comfort child when possible.	Helps to comfort and support the child.	Document whether family was able to remain with child and describe effectiveness of their presence.
	Use diversional activities (e.g., music, television, playing games, relaxation) when appropriate.	Diversional activities can distract child and may help to decrease pain.	Document whether diversional activities were successful in helping to manage pain.
TEACHING GOALS Child and/or family will be able to verbalize at least 4 characteristics of pain such as • verbal communication of pain or tenderness • crying unrelieved by usual comfort measures • facial grimacing • rapid heart rate	Teach child/family about characteristics of pain. Assess and record results.	Increased knowledge will assist the child/family in recognizing and reporting changes in the child's condition.	Document whether teaching was done and describe results.
Child and/or family will be able to verbalize knowledge of care such as • medication administration • appropriate diversional activities • identification of any signs/symptoms of pain (such as those listed under Assessment) • when to contact health care provider	Teach child/family about care. Assess and record child's/family's knowledge of and participation in care regarding medication administration, etc.	Education of child/family will allow for accurate care.	Document whether teaching was done and describe results.

(continued)

Nursing Diagnosis   Fear: Child/Family

Definition   Feeling of apprehension resulting from a known cause

Possibly Related to
- Outcome of surgical procedure
- Pain and discomfort following surgery
- Unfamiliar surroundings
- Forced contact with strangers
- Treatments and procedures

Nursing Diagnosis: Fear: child/family related to outcome of surgical procedure, postoperative pain, unfamiliar surroundings, forced contact with strangers, treatments and procedures

Assessment/Defining Characteristics of Child and/or Family (Subjective & Objective Data):

- Uncooperativeness
- Regressed behavior
- Hostile behavior
- Restlessness

- Inability to recall previously taught information
- Decreased communication
- Decreased attention span

Expected Outcomes	Possible Nursing Interventions	Rationale	Evaluation for Charting
Child/family will exhibit only a minimal amount of fear as evidenced by • ability to relate appropriately to family members and members of the health care team • lack of regressed or hostile behavior • ability to rest and sleep when indicated • ability to restate information previously taught • ability to participate in care	Assess and record level of child's/family's fear and the source of the fear.	Provides information about the level of fear and possibly the source of the fear.	Document level of fear and any identified sources of the fear.
	Decrease child's/family's fears when possible by • encouraging family members to stay with child • encouraging child/family members to participate in care • assigning same staff members to provide care for child • spending extra time with child when family members are unable to be present • encouraging family members to bring in familiar articles and toys from home • explain to child/family what to expect during this recovery phase	These measures will help make the child and family members more comfortable and can help to decrease fear.	Document any measures used to help alleviate fear. State effectiveness of measures.

Nursing Diagnosis: Fear: Child/Family *(continued)*

Expected Outcomes	Possible Nursing Interventions	Rationale	Evaluation for Charting
	Initiate age-appropriate therapeutic play when indicated. Document effectiveness.	Play can be a useful distraction or outlet to help decrease fears.	Document whether therapeutic play was used and describe its effectiveness.
	Encourage child/family to express fears to members of the health care team.	Expression and identification of fears can help the child/family to find ways to manage these fears.	Document any identified fears.
	Encourage child/family to meet basic needs, such as eating and resting appropriately. Assist them as needed.	Assist child/family in decreasing stress, which can help to identify and alleviate fears.	Document whether child/family were able to separate for short periods so that family members could meet their own basic needs.
TEACHING GOALS Child and/or family will be able to verbalize at least 4 characteristics of fear such as • uncooperativeness • regressed behavior • hostile behavior • decreased communication • verbal communication of fear	Teach child/family about characteristics of fear. Assess and record results.	Increased knowledge will assist the child/family in recognizing and reporting changes in the child's condition.	Document whether teaching was done and describe results.
Child and/or family will be able to verbalize knowledge of care such as • medication administration • appropriate diversional activities • identification of any signs/symptoms of fear (such as those listed under Assessment) • when to contact health care provider	Teach child/family about care. Assess and record child's/family's knowledge of and participation in care regarding appropriate diversional activities, etc.	Education of child/family will allow for accurate care.	Document whether teaching was done and describe results.

Related Nursing Diagnoses

Risk for Infection   *related to* compromised immunity secondary to surgical procedure

Compromised Family Coping   *related to*
     a. child's surgery
     b. child's hospitalization
     c. lack of support systems
     d. financial considerations

Activity Intolerance   *related to* postoperative status

Delayed Growth and Development   *related to* underlying disease process

THREE

CONGESTIVE HEART FAILURE
MEDICAL DIAGNOSIS

PATHOPHYSIOLOGY Congestive heart failure (CHF) is a group of signs and symptoms that reflect the heart's inability to effectively pump blood to meet the metabolic requirements of the body. The name congestive heart failure is misleading; the heart does not actually have to fail. Congestive heart failure can result from increased pulmonary blood flow, increased blood volume, obstruction to outflow from the ventricles, decreased contractility, blood volume overload, and/or high cardiac output demands. The most common cause of CHF in children is altered hemodynamics secondary to congenital heart defects.

By the time CHF is present, the body has already made some acute adjustments in an attempt to maintain and improve cardiac output. The sympathetic nervous system responds to decreased blood pressure detected by vascular stretch receptors and baroreceptors. This response leads to the release of catecholamines. Catecholamines increase venous tone in order to improve blood return to the heart. Blood supply to the heart, lungs, and brain is maximized by decreasing circulation to the skin, extremities, stomach, intestines, and kidneys. Decreased blood flow to the kidneys stimulates the release of renin, angiotensin, and aldosterone. As a result, the kidneys retain fluid and sodium, which initially aids in cardiac output. However, hypervolemia ultimately occurs and increases the workload on the already stressed cardiac musculature.

It is difficult to clinically separate right-sided and left-sided heart failure in children; the two usually occur together. If one chamber fails, failure in the opposite chamber is only a matter of time. Right-sided heart failure causes increased central venous pressure, resulting in systemic congestion and edema. Elevated pressure in the inferior vena cava causes hepatomegaly. With left-sided heart failure, the pressure in the left atrium rises, and blood returning from the lungs via the pulmonary veins has difficulty entering the left atrium. Pressure then begins to rise in the pulmonary vasculature. Fluid leaks out of the pulmonary capillaries into the interstitial spaces, resulting in pulmonary edema.

Therapeutic management includes measures to decrease the workload on the heart and increase its efficiency. Management usually includes diuretics, such as furosemide (Lasix). Digoxin (Lanoxin) is given to increase myocardial contractility. Angiotensin-converting inhibitors (ACE), such as captopril (Capoten), can be used to decrease afterload.

Primary Nursing Diagnosis   Decreased Cardiac Output

Definition   Decrease in the amount of blood that leaves the left ventricle

Possibly Related to
- Increased volume
- Obstruction to outflow
- Decreased contractility
- High cardiac output demands
- These four conditions can result from
  - hypervolemia
  - fluid volume overload
  - increased volume of blood circulating through the heart
  - increased flow of blood to the lungs
  - congenital heart defect
  - acquired heart defect
  - dysrhythmias
  - myocarditis
  - myopathies
  - anemia
- Noncardiovascular disease (e.g., respiratory disease, anemia, metabolic disorders, renal disorders, endocrine disorders)

Primary Nursing Diagnosis: Decreased cardiac output related to increased blood volume, obstruction to outflow, decreased contractility, high cardiac output demands
These four conditions can result from

- hypervolemia
- fluid volume overload
- increased volume of blood circulating through the heart
- increased flow of blood to the lungs
- congenital heart defect

- acquired heart defect
- dysrhythmias
- myocarditis
- myopathies
- anemia

Noncardiovascular diseases (e.g., respiratory disease, anemia, metabolic disorders, renal disorders, endocrine disorders)

Assessment/Defining Characteristics of Child and/or Family (Subjective & Objective Data):

- Tachycardia
- Tachypnea
- Dyspnea at rest
- Costal retractions
- Nasal flaring
- Crackles
- Cough
- Decreased peripheral circulation, cold extremities
- Pallor and mottling of skin
- Transient duskiness of skin
- Cyanosis
- Diaphoresis (especially over head and neck)
- Hypotension
- Rapid, weak peripheral pulses
- Prolonged capillary refill, longer than 2 to 3 seconds

- Narrow pulse pressure
- Distended neck veins in older children
- Cardiomegaly revealed on chest X-ray
- Gallop rhythm
- Edema (periorbital, sacral, scrotal, peripheral in older children)
- Rapid weight gain
- Hepatosplenomegaly
- Feeding difficulty
- Decreased urine output (less than 0.5 to 1 ml/kg/hr)
- Weakness
- Exercise intolerance
- Fatigue
- Growth rate lower than normal
- Irritability

Expected Outcomes	Possible Nursing Interventions	Rationale	Evaluation for Charting
Child will have adequate cardiac output as evidenced by - heart rate within acceptable range (state specific range) - respiratory rate within acceptable range (state specific range) - blood pressure within acceptable range (state specific range) - skin warm to touch - strong and equal peripheral pulses - pulse pressure within acceptable limits of 20 to 50 mm/Hg - brisk capillary refill within 2 to 3 seconds	Assess and record HR, RR, BP, and any signs/symptoms of decreased cardiac output (such as those listed under Assessment) every 2 to 4 hours and PRN.	If child experiences decreased cardiac output (CO) the HR and RR will increase and BP will decrease.	Document range of HR, RR, and BP. Describe any signs/symptoms of decreased cardiac output noted.
	Keep accurate record of intake and output.	Decreased output may indicate decreased CO possibly due to a shift of the intravascular fluid into the interstitial space.	Document intake and output.
	Evaluate and record results of EKG strips.	Changes in EKG may indicate decreased CO.	Describe results of EKG when indicated.
	Weigh child daily on same scale at same time of day. Document results and compare to previous weight.	Sudden increase in weight gain may indicate extravascular fluid overload and may result in decreased CO.	Document weight and determine if it was an increase or decrease from the previous weight.

Primary Nursing Diagnosis: Decreased Cardiac Output *(continued)*

Expected Outcomes	Possible Nursing Interventions	Rationale	Evaluation for Charting
• lack of distended neck veins • appropriate heart size on chest X-ray • normal sinus rhythm • lack of edema • adequate urine output (state specific range; 1 to 2 ml/kg/hr) • steady progress on growth curve • lack of irritability • lack of signs/ symptoms of decreased cardiac output (such as those listed under Assessment)	Administer cardiac drugs on schedule. Assess and record any side effects or any signs/symptoms of toxicity (such as vomiting with digoxin). Follow hospital protocol for administration, such as 2 RNs checking the dosage prior to administration and documenting the HR or BP at the time of medication administration.	Cardiac drugs are given to increase the strength of cardiac contractions and/or increase return of blood flow to the heart, thereby increasing CO.	Document whether cardiac medications were administered on schedule. Describe effectiveness and any side effects noted.
	If indicated, monitor and record digoxin levels. Notify physician if levels are out of the acceptable range. (A decreased potassium level increases the risk for digoxin toxicity.)	Digoxin is a potent medication that needs careful monitoring. If digoxin levels are high, the child will experience signs/ symptoms of toxicity (such as vomiting).	Document digoxin levels. If levels are out of the acceptable range, describe any corrective measures implemented.
	Administer diuretics on schedule. Assess and record effectiveness and any side effects noted (e.g., hypokalemia or dehydration).	Diuretics are given in order to decrease excess intravascular fluid through increased urine output, which will decrease the workload on the heart.	Document whether diuretics were administered on schedule. Describe effectiveness and any side effects noted.
	Elevate head of bed at a 30° angle.	Elevating the head of the bed to a 30° angle causes a shift of the abdominal contents downward and this will allow for increased lung expansion.	Document whether head of bed was elevated.
	Organize nursing care to allow child uninterrupted rest.	Proper rest will help to decrease workload on the heart.	Document whether child was able to have uninterrupted rest periods.
	Check and record results of chest X-ray when indicated.	Changes in chest X-ray results may indicate need for a change in therapy.	Document results of chest X-ray when indicated.
TEACHING GOALS Child and/or family will be able to verbalize at least 4 characteristics of	Teach child/family about characteristics of decreased cardiac output. Assess and record results.	Increased knowledge will assist the child/ family in recognizing and reporting changes in the child's condition.	Document whether teaching was done and describe results.

(continued)

Primary Nursing Diagnosis: Decreased Cardiac Output *(continued)*			
Expected Outcomes	**Possible Nursing Interventions**	**Rationale**	**Evaluation for Charting**
decreased cardiac output such as • rapid heart rate • cold extremities • weakness • irritability • decreased appetite			
Child and/or family will be able to verbalize knowledge of care such as • medication administration • head elevated position • sufficient rest periods • monitoring intake and output • identification of any signs/symptoms of decreased cardiac output (such as those listed under Assessment) • when to contact health care provider	Teach child/family about care. Assess and record child's/family's knowledge of and participation in care regarding medication administration, etc.	Education of child/family will allow for accurate care.	Document whether teaching was done and describe results.

Nursing Diagnosis   Ineffective Breathing Pattern

Definition   Breathing pattern that results in inadequate oxygen consumption (failure to meet the cellular requirements of the body)

Possibly Related to   • Decreased cardiac output

• Pulmonary hypertension

• Increased flow of blood to the lungs

• Pulmonary edema

Nursing Diagnosis: Ineffective breathing pattern related to pulmonary congestion, pulmonary hypertension, increased blood flow to the lungs, pulmonary edema, decreased cardiac output
Assessment/Defining Characteristics of Child and/or Family (Subjective & Objective Data):

• Tachypnea
• Dyspnea
• Retractions (type, location)
• Nasal flaring
• Grunting
• Fatigue
• Pallor, mottling
• Cyanosis

• Crackles
• Use of accessory muscles
• Head bobbing (for an infant)
• Dry, hacking cough
• Orthopnea
• Shortness of breath
• Activity intolerance

Nursing Diagnosis: Ineffective Breathing Pattern *(continued)*

Expected Outcomes	Possible Nursing Interventions	Rationale	Evaluation for Charting

Child will have effective breathing pattern as evidenced by
 	
• respiratory rate within acceptable range (state specific range)
• clear and equal breath sounds bilaterally A & P
• absence of
  1. nasal flaring
  2. grunting
  3. retractions
  4. cough
  5. head bobbing
  6. cyanosis
• lack of signs/ symptoms of ineffective breathing pattern (such as those listed under Assessment)
	Assess and record RR, breath sounds and any signs/symptoms of ineffective breathing pattern (such as those listed under Assessment) every 2 to 4 hours and PRN.	If child experiences ineffective breathing pattern the RR will increase and the child will work harder to breathe, exhibiting some of the characteristics of ineffective breathing pattern.	Document range of RR. Describe breath sounds and any signs/ symptoms of ineffective breathing pattern noted.

	Administer humidified oxygen in correct amount and route of delivery. Record percent of oxygen and route of delivery. Assess and record effectiveness of therapy.	Humidified oxygen will dilate the pulmonary vasculature, which increases surface area available for gas exchange. Extra source oxygen will also allow for better oxygenation to body tissues and thus help combat ineffective breathing pattern.	Document amount and route of oxygen delivery. Describe effectiveness.
	Keep head of bed elevated at a 30° angle.	Elevating the head of the bed to a 30° angle causes a shift of the abdominal contents downward and this in turn will allow for increased lung expansion in order to help improve breathing pattern.	Document whether head of bed was kept elevated.
	Ensure that chest physiotherapy is done on schedule. Record effectiveness and child's response to treatment. Modification of procedure may be necessary if child becomes stressed.	Chest percussion loosens secretions and positioning can help to assist the flow of secretions out of the lungs by gravity. This will aid in effective breathing pattern.	Document whether chest physiotherapy was done on schedule. Describe effectiveness and child's response to treatment.
	Suction if child is unable to cough up secretions. Assess and record amount and characteristics of secretions.	Suctioning assists in removing excess secretions and this in turn helps to improve breathing pattern.	Document frequency and type of suctioning if indicated. Describe amount and characteristics of secretions.
	Assess and record oxygen saturation every 2 to 4 hours and PRN.	Pulse oximetry detects the oxygen saturation in the bloodstream. It is important to detect small changes in oxygen saturation before the child starts displaying overt characteristics of ineffective breathing pattern.	Document range of oxygen saturation.

(continued)

Nursing Diagnosis: Ineffective Breathing Pattern *(continued)*			
Expected Outcomes	**Possible Nursing Interventions**	**Rationale**	**Evaluation for Charting**
TEACHING GOALS Child and/or family will be able to verbalize at least 4 characteristics of ineffective breathing pattern such as • color change from pink/tan to gray or blue • cough • nasal flaring • rapid respirations • head bobbing • intolerance of normal activities	Teach child/family about characteristics of ineffective breathing pattern. Assess and record results.	Increased knowledge will assist the child/family in recognizing and reporting changes in the child's condition.	Document whether teaching was done and describe results.
Child and/or family will be able to verbalize knowledge of care such as • treatments such as chest physiotherapy • head elevated positioning • oxygen administration • identification of any signs/symptoms of ineffective breathing pattern (such as those listed under Assessment) • when to contact health care provider	Teach child/family about care. Assess and record child's/family's knowledge of and participation in care regarding chest physiotherapy treatments, etc.	Education of child/family will allow for accurate care.	Document whether teaching was done and describe results.

Related Nursing Diagnoses

Excess Fluid Volume	*related to* a. edema secondary to decreased cardiac output b. decreased urinary output
Risk for Infection	*related to* a. reduced body defenses b. pulmonary congestion
Imbalanced Nutrition: Less than Body Requirements	*related to* a. respiratory distress b. feeding difficulties c. fatigue d. increased metabolic demands
Activity Intolerance	*related to* decreased cardiac output

FOUR

HYPERTENSION
MEDICAL DIAGNOSIS

PATHOPHYSIOLOGY Systemic arterial hypertension is becoming an increasingly common health problem in children and adolescents, although it is still more prevalent in adults. Hypertension is usually defined as an elevation of the systolic and/or diastolic blood pressures above the acceptable range for a given age and sex. Blood pressure readings above the 95th percentile for age and sex on three separate occasions over a 6 to 12 month period is one criterion for diagnosing hypertension in children.

Hypertension can be either primary or secondary. Primary hypertension, also called essential hypertension, has no known cause, although genetic and environmental factors may play a role in its development. This is the most common form of hypertension in the adult population and may at times have its origin in childhood. An increased incidence of primary hypertension has recently been noted in older children. Identified environmental factors that may contribute to this condition include stress, increased sodium intake, and obesity. Secondary hypertension results from an existing pathological process, such as renal disease,

endocrine disorders, and cardiovascular disease. It can also occur as a side effect of steroid therapy for chronic illness and ingestion of over-the-counter medications (caffeine, ephedrine), prescription medications (oral contraceptives), and other agents (cocaine, tobacco).

Research has led to speculation that primary hypertension may be a result of both genetic and environmental factors. In younger children, however, hypertension is most often due to secondary causes such as renal disease. When renal ischemia is present, renin is released. Renin in turn causes the eventual formation of angiotensin II, a pressor agent that constricts the arterioles, thus elevating blood pressure. Angiotensin II decreases the glomerular filtration rate by its vasoconstrictive action and causes the release of aldosterone from the adrenal cortex. Aldosterone promotes sodium and water retention, resulting in increased blood volume and increased blood pressure. Children with primary hypertension may be asymptomatic. Blood pressure should be checked routinely for all children 3 years of age and older.

Primary Nursing Diagnosis   Decreased Cardiac Output

Definition   Decrease in the amount of blood that leaves the left ventricle

Possibly Related to
- Increased systemic vascular resistance
- Fluid volume overload
- Underlying disease process (specify)
- Impaired elasticity of the vessels

Primary Nursing Diagnosis: Decreased cardiac output related to increased vascular resistance, fluid volume overload, underlying disease process (specify), impaired elasticity of the vessels

Assessment/Defining Characteristics of Child and/or Family (Subjective & Objective Data):

- Tachycardia
- Tachypnea
- Hypertension
- Palpitations
- Bounding carotid and radial pulses
- Delayed femoral pulse compared to radial pulse
- Absent or diminished lower extremity pulses
- Flushing of skin
- Headache
- Visual disturbance
- Epistaxis
- Chest pain
- Fatigue

Expected Outcomes	Possible Nursing Interventions	Rationale	Evaluation for Charting
Child will have adequate cardiac output as evidenced by • heart rate within acceptable range (state specific range) • respiratory rate within acceptable range (state specific range) • blood pressure within acceptable range (state specific range) • strong and equal peripheral pulses • absence of flushing, headache, epistaxis, visual disturbance, chest pain, and fatigue • adequate urine output (state specific range; 1 to 2 ml/kg/hr) • lack of signs/ symptoms of decreased cardiac output (such as those listed under Assessment)	Assess and record HR, RR, BP, and any signs/symptoms of decreased cardiac output (such as those listed under Assessment) every 2 to 4 hours and PRN.	If child experiences decreased cardiac output (CO) the HR and RR will increase and BP will decrease.	Document range of HR, RR, and BP. Describe any signs/symptoms of decreased cardiac output noted.
	Administer diuretics on schedule. Assess and record effectiveness and any side effects noted (e.g., hypokalemia, dehydration).	Diuretics are given to decrease excess intravascular fluid through increased urine output, which will decrease the workload on the heart.	Document whether diuretics were administered on schedule. Describe effectiveness and any side effects noted.
	Administer antihypertensives on schedule. Assess and record effectiveness and any side effects noted (e.g., dizziness, hypotension, GI disturbance).	Antihypertensive drugs work in various ways to lower BP in order to reach the ultimate goal of decreasing workload on the heart.	Document whether antihypertensive drugs were administered on schedule. Describe effectiveness and any side effects noted.
	Weigh child daily on same scale at same time each day. Record results and compare to previous weight.	Sudden increase in weight gain may indicate extravascular fluid overload and may result in decreased CO.	Document weight and determine if it was an increase or decrease from the previous weight.
	Keep accurate record of intake and output.	Decreased output may indicate decreased CO possibly due to a shift of the intravascular fluid into the interstitial space.	Document intake and output.

Primary Nursing Diagnosis: Decreased Cardiac Output (*continued*)			
Expected Outcomes	**Possible Nursing Interventions**	**Rationale**	**Evaluation for Charting**
TEACHING GOALS Child and/or family will be able to verbalize at least 4 characteristics of decreased cardiac output such as • flushing • headache • decreased urinary output (for infants less than 6 wet diapers/ day) • irritability • visual disturbance	Teach child/family about characteristics of decreased cardiac output. Assess and record results.	Increased knowledge will assist the child/ family in recognizing and reporting changes in the child's condition.	Document whether teaching was done and describe results.
Child and/or family will be able to verbalize knowledge of care such as • accurate procedure for obtaining blood pressure • dietary considerations (sodium reduction) • weight reduction • medication adminis-tration • exercise program • identification of any signs/symptoms of decreased cardiac output (such as those listed under Assessment) • when to contact health care provider	Teach child/family about care. Assess and record child's/family's knowl-edge of and participation in care regarding accurate procedure for obtaining blood pressure, etc.	Education of child/ family will allow for accurate care.	Document whether teaching was done and describe results.

Nursing Diagnosis   Noncompliance

Definition

Inability or unwillingness of an individual or individual's caregiver to adhere to therapeutic recommendations

Possibly Related to

• Asymptomatic condition
• Side effects of medication
• Dietary restrictions
• Forgetfulness in taking medications
• Lack of family support
• Developmental stage of life

Nursing Diagnosis: Noncompliance related to asymptomatic condition, side effect of medication, dietary restrictions, forgetfulness in taking medications, lack of family support, developmental stage of life

Assessment/Defining Characteristics of Child and/or Family (Subjective & Objective Data):

- Evidence of increase in or return of symptoms
- Hypertension
- Weight gain
- Edema
- Inability to attain set goals
- Verbalization of difficulty in maintaining set goals
- Failure to keep appointments

Expected Outcomes	Possible Nursing Interventions	Rationale	Evaluation for Charting
Child/family will comply with therapeutic recommendations as evidenced by • blood pressure within acceptable range (state specific range)	Assess and record BP and any signs/symptoms of noncompliance (such as those listed under Assessment) every 2 to 4 hours and PRN.	If BP increases above the desired level, this will decrease cardiac output.	Document range of BP. Describe any characteristics of decreased compliance in taking BP on schedule.
• lack of sudden weight gain and edema • evidence of weight loss, if appropriate • taking prescribed medications on schedule • ability to follow food plan (reduced sodium) • keeping clinical appointment after discharge • following exercise program (if indicated) • lack of signs/symptoms of noncompliance (such as those listed under Assessment)	Weigh child daily on same scale at same time each day. Record results and compare to previous weight.	Sudden increase in weight gain may indicate extravascular fluid overload and may result in increased blood pressure and decreased CO.	Document weight and determine if it was an increase or decrease from the previous weight.
TEACHING GOALS Child and/or family will be able to verbalize at least 4 characteristics of noncompliant behavior such as failure to • take and record BP measurements as suggested • attain set weight goals (if needed) • administer medications as prescribed • comply with food plan	Teach child/family about characteristics of noncompliant behavior. Assess and record results.	Increased knowledge will assist the child/family in recognizing and reporting changes in the child's condition.	Document whether teaching was done and describe any successful measures used to help child/family comply with therapeutic recommendations.

Nursing Diagnosis: Noncompliance *(continued)*

Expected Outcomes	Possible Nursing Interventions	Rationale	Evaluation for Charting
Child and/or family will be able to verbalize knowledge of care such as • accurate procedure for obtaining blood pressure • weight goals • medication administration • food plan • exercise program • identification of any signs/symptoms of noncompliance (such as those listed under Assessment) • when to contact health care provider • keeping follow-up appointments	Teach child/family about care. Assess and record child's/family's knowledge of and participation in care regarding accurate procedure for obtaining blood pressure, etc.	Education of child/family will allow for accurate care.	Document whether teaching was done and describe results.

Related Nursing Diagnoses

Ineffective Tissue Perfusion	*related to* increased vascular resistance
Deficient Knowledge: Child/Family	*related to* a. disease process b. continuing home management (including diet, exercise, medications)
Activity Intolerance	*related to* a. fatigue b. side effects of medication
Acute Pain	*related to* a. headache b. chest pain
Compromised Family Coping	*related to* needed changes in lifestyle

FIVE

INFECTIVE ENDOCARDITIS
MEDICAL DIAGNOSIS

PATHOPHYSIOLOGY Infective endocarditis (IE) is an infection of the heart valves, endothelium, and endocardium. It includes both bacterial and nonbacterial endocarditis. Bacterial endocarditis is most often caused by gram-positive cocci, with *Streptococcus viridans,* and *Staphylococcus aureus* being the most common of these pathogens. Gram-negative cocci less commonly cause endocarditis. Fungal organisms (e.g., *Candida albicans*) may cause nonbacterial endocarditis.

Although children who do not have a cardiac malformation can develop infective endocarditis, congenital heart disease is the overwhelming predisposing factor for this condition. Children with cardiac lesions associated with a high velocity of blood being injected into a chamber or vessel are most susceptible to infective endocarditis. At the highest risk are children with ventricular septal defects, left-sided valvular disease, and systemic pulmonary arterial communications. Other children at risk include those with prosthetic valves, those with rheumatic heart disease involving the valves, and children having had recent cardiac surgery involving invasive lines. Endocarditis associated with drug abuse is also seen.

Infective endocarditis occurs when bacteremia, resulting from the invading organism, exists in the presence of damaged cardiac or vascular endothelium. The damaged cardiac or vascualar endothelium often results from congenital cardiac defects, which have caused changes in the endocardium and predisposed it to the growth of invading organisms. The damage to the endocardium can be caused by the turbulent blood flow that occurs with abnormal pressure gradients or by the abnormal jet of blood hitting the opposing endocardium (causing thickening). At these areas of damaged endocardium, fibrin is deposited and platelet thrombi form, entrapping circulating microorganisms. Vegetations (verrucae) grow, which can then invade and destroy adjacent tissue such as valves or they can break off, and embolize elsewhere. The bacteria can also cause abscesses by infiltrating the deeper tissues of the heart or arteries.

Infectious agents may be introduced into the child's circulation from any site of localized infection. Surgical or dental procedures can be implicated in most cases of infective endocarditis. Children who have undergone cardiac surgery for a systemic-to-pulmonary artery shunt, valve replacement, or valve conduit repair are at high risk, as are children with cyanotic heart disease who have poor dental hygiene. Other portals of entry include the urinary tract and the bloodstream.

The early signs and symptoms of infective endocarditis can be vague. The child may experience unexplained fevers, headaches, malaise, chills, nausea, joint pain, and/or myalgia. Commonly, there is a history of anorexia and weight loss. A murmur is almost always present. Depending on the virulence of the infectious organism, a variety of cardiovascular changes can follow. The children often have a low-grade bacteremia making effective blood culture technique essential to diagnosing infective endocarditis. The classic signs of Roth spots (retinal hemorrhages), Janeway lesions (painless hemorrhagic areas on the palms and soles), and Osler nodes (painful lesions at fingertips) are rare in children.

Prior to antibiotics, infective endocarditis was fatal. Complications continue to occur in approximately 50% of children with this disease. The most common complication is cardiac failure due to vegetations involving the aortic or mitral valves. Other complications include congestive heart failure, sequelae of pulmonary or neurologic emboli, mycotic aneurysms, acquired ventricular septal defect, and heart block. Fungal endocarditis, which often occurs in immunosuppressed or debilitated children, is difficult to manage and still has a poor prognosis.

Treatment of infective endocarditis involves intravenous antibiotics for approximately 4 to 6 weeks. Infection of prosthetic valves and tissue may require longer treatment. Surgical removal of vegetations, replacement of infected valves, drainage of myocardial abscesses, and excision of areas of infection may be indicated when antibiotic therapy is unsuccessful.

The incidence of infective endocarditis can be reduced in susceptible children by using antimicrobial prophylaxis, which is individualized for each child and depends on the procedure being performed. Proper oral hygiene and routine dental care remain important to reduce the chance of infection.

Primary Nursing Diagnosis   Decreased Cardiac Output

Definition   Decrease in the amount of blood that leaves the left ventricle

Possibly Related to
- Invasion of the endocardium by bacterial or nonbacterial agents secondary to
  - congenital heart defect
  - dental procedures
  - surgical procedures
  - immunosuppression

Primary Nursing Diagnosis: Decreased cardiac output related to invasion of the endocardium by bacterial or nonbacterial agents secondary to congenital heart defect, dental procedures, surgical procedures, immunosuppresion

Assessment/Defining Characteristics of Child and/or Family (Subjective & Objective Data):

- Fatigue
- Activity intolerance
- Tachycardia
- Tachypnea
- Hypotension
- Decreased urine output
- Abdominal pain
- Cough
- Dyspnea
- Orthopnea
- Crackles
- Edema
- Cardiomegaly revealed on chest X-ray
- Gallop rhythm
- Hepatomegaly
- Anorexia
- Fever

Expected Outcomes	Possible Nursing Interventions	Rationale	Evaluation for Charting
Child will have adequate cardiac output as evidenced by • heart rate within acceptable range (state specific range) • respiratory rate within acceptable range (state specific range) • blood pressure within acceptable range (state specific range) • temperature within acceptable range of 36.5°C to 37.2°C	Assess and record T, HR, RR, BP, and any signs/symptoms of decreased cardiac output (such as those listed under Assessment) every 2 to 4 hours and PRN.	If child experiences decreased cardiac output (CO) the HR and RR will increase and BP will decrease. If T increases it will increase HR.	Document range of T, HR, RR, and BP. Describe any signs/symptoms of decreased cardiac output noted.
	Assess and record breath sounds and respiratory effort every 2 to 4 hours and PRN.	Abnormal breath sounds (such as those listed under Assessment) and increased respiratory effort can be a sign of decreased cardiac output.	Describe breath sounds and respiratory effort. If these assessment findings were abnormal, describe any corrective measures implemented.
	Organize nursing care to allow child uninterrupted rest periods.	Proper rest will help to decrease workload on the heart.	Document whether child was able to have uninterrupted rest periods.

(continued)

Primary Nursing Diagnosis: Decreased Cardiac Output *(continued)*

Expected Outcomes	Possible Nursing Interventions	Rationale	Evaluation for Charting
• clear and equal breath sounds bilaterally A & P • appropriate heart size on chest X-ray • adequate urine output (state specific range; 1 to 2 ml/kg/hr) • lack of signs/symptoms of decreased cardiac output (such as those listed under Assessment)	Keep accurate record of intake and output.	Decreased output may indicate decreased CO possibly due to a shift of the intravascular fluid into the interstitial space.	Document intake and output.
	Check and record results of chest X-ray, when indicated.	Changes in chest X-ray results may indicate need for a change in therapy.	Document results of chest X-ray when indicated.
	Elevate head of bed at a 30°angle.	Elevating the head of the bed to a 30° angle causes a shift of the abdominal contents downward and this will allow for increased lung expansion.	Document whether head of bed was elevated.
	Administer cardiac drugs on schedule. Assess and record any side effects or any signs/symptoms of toxicity (such as vomiting with digoxin). Follow hospital protocol for administration, such as 2 RNs checking the dosage prior to administration and documenting the HR or BP at the time of medication administration.	Cardiac drugs are given to increase the strength of cardiac contractions and/or increase return of blood flow to the heart, thereby increasing CO.	Document whether cardiac medications were administered on schedule. Describe effectiveness and any side effects noted.
	If indicated, monitor and record digoxin levels. Notify physician if levels are out of the acceptable range. (A decreased potassium level increases the risk for digoxin toxicity.)	Digoxin is a potent medication that needs careful monitoring. If digoxin levels are high, the child will experience signs/symptoms of toxicity (such as vomiting).	Document digoxin levels. If levels are out of the acceptable range, describe any corrective measures implemented.
	Administer diuretics on schedule. Assess and record effectiveness and any side effects noted (e.g., hypokalemia or dehydration).	Diuretics are given in order to decrease excess intravascular fluid through increased urine output, which will decrease the workload on the heart.	Document whether diuretics were administered on schedule. Describe effectiveness and any side effects noted.
	Administer antibiotics on schedule. Assess and record any side effects (e.g., rash, diarrhea).	Antibiotics combat invading bacterial organisms.	Document whether antibiotics were administered on schedule. Describe any side effects noted.

Primary Nursing Diagnosis: Decreased Cardiac Output (*continued*)

Expected Outcomes	Possible Nursing Interventions	Rationale	Evaluation for Charting
	Administer antifungals on schedule. Assess and record any side effects (e.g., rash, vomiting).	Antifungals combat invading fungal organisms.	Document whether antifungals were administered on schedule. Describe any side effects noted.
	If indicated, administer antipyretics on schedule. Assess and record effectiveness.	Antipyretics are given to decrease temperature to the normal range.	Document whether antipyretics were administered on schedule and describe their effectiveness.
TEACHING GOALS Child and/or family will be able to verbalize at least 4 characteristics of decreased cardiac output such as • fatigue • activity intolerance • rapid heart rate • abdominal pain • cough • puffiness (edema)	Teach child/family about characteristics of decreased cardiac output. Assess and record results.	Increased knowledge will assist the child/family in recognizing and reporting changes in the child's condition.	Document whether teaching was done and describe results.
Child and/or family will be able to verbalize knowledge of care such as • medication administration • head elevated position • sufficient rest periods • monitoring intake and output • identification of any signs/symptoms of decreased cardiac output (such as those listed under Assessment) • when to contact health care provider	Teach child/family about care. Assess and record child's/family's knowledge of and participation in care regarding medication administration, etc.	Education of child/family will allow for accurate care.	Document whether teaching was done and describe results.

Nursing Diagnosis   Activity Intolerance

Definition   Insufficient psychosocial, emotional, or physiological ability to perform required or desired activities

Possibly Related to
- Hypermetabolic state secondary to persistent fever
- Insufficient oxygenation secondary to decreased cardiac output
- Myalgia
- Arthralgia

Nursing Diagnosis: Activity intolerance related to hypermetabolic state secondary to persistent fever, insufficient oxygenation secondary to decreased cardiac output, myalgia, arthralgia

Assessment/Defining Characteristics of Child and/or Family (Subjective & Objective Data):

- Fatigue
- Weakness
- Dyspnea
- Tachypnea
- Tachycardia
- Hypotension
- Headache

- Fever
- Verbalization of weakness or fatigue
- Inability to perform age-appropriate activities of daily living
- Inability to play
- Impaired ability to ambulate

Expected Outcomes	Possible Nursing Interventions	Rationale	Evaluation for Charting
Child will have appropriate activity for age as evidenced by • heart rate within acceptable range (state specific range) • respiratory rate within acceptable range (state specific range) • blood pressure within acceptable range (state specific range) • temperature within acceptable range (state specific range) • ability to ambulate (if not on bed rest) • ability to perform activities of daily living (age appropriate) • ability to play (age appropriate) • lack of signs/symptoms of activity intolerance (such as those listed under Assessment)	Assess and record T, HR, RR, BP, and any signs/symptoms of activity intolerance (such as those listed under Assessment) every 2 to 4 hours and PRN.	If child experiences activity intolerance the HR and RR will increase and BP will decrease. If T increases it will increase HR.	Document range of T, HR, RR, BP. Describe any signs/symptoms of activity intolerance noted.
	Assess and record child's baseline activity tolerance.	Establishing a baseline of the child's activity tolerance will alert the nurse to changes in activity that may indicate decreased cardiac output.	Document range of activities that child tolerated.
	Organize nursing care to allow child uninterrupted rest.	Proper rest will help to decrease workload on the heart.	Document whether child was able to have uninterrupted rest periods.
	Assist with activities of daily living, ambulation (if allowed), and repositioning as needed.	Assisting the child will increase the child's comfort level and help to decrease the workload on the heart.	Document whether assistance was needed, child's tolerance of assistance, and effectiveness of assistance.
	If indicated, administer antipyretics on schedule. Assess and record effectiveness.	Antipyretics are given to decrease temperature to the normal range.	Document whether antipyretics were administered on schedule and describe their effectiveness.

Nursing Diagnosis: Activity Intolerance *(continued)*

Expected Outcomes	Possible Nursing Interventions	Rationale	Evaluation for Charting
	If indicated, administer analgesics on schedule. Assess and record effectiveness and any side effects (e.g., constipation, nausea).	Analgesics are given to decrease pain or discomfort.	Document whether analgesics were administered on schedule. Describe effectiveness and any side effects noted.
TEACHING GOALS Child and/or family will be able to verbalize at least 4 characteristics of activity intolerance such as • fatigue • weakness • trouble breathing • headache • verbalization of weakness or fatigue • inability to perform age appropriate activities of daily living • inability to play • impaired ability to ambulate	Teach child/family about characteristics of activity intolerance. Assess and record results.	Increased knowledge will assist the child/family in recognizing and reporting changes in the child's condition.	Document whether teaching was done and describe results.
Child and/or family will be able to verbalize knowledge of care such as • alterations in activities of daily living, ambulation, repositioning, and play to correspond to child's activity level • medication administration • identification of any signs/symptoms of activity intolerance (such as those listed under Assessment) • when to contact health care provider	Teach child/family about care. Assess and record child's/family's knowledge of and participation in care regarding alterations in child's activity level, etc.	Education of child/family will allow for accurate care.	Document whether teaching was done and describe results.

Related Nursing Diagnoses

Actual Infection*	*related to* invasion of the endocardium by bacterial or nonbacterial agents
Ineffective Breathing Pattern	*related to* a. decreased cardiac output b. congenital heart defect
Altered Level of Consciousness*	*related to* a. cerebral abscesses b. emboli
Anxiety: Parental	*related to* a. lengthy hospitalization of child b. activity intolerance of child c. uncertain prognosis for child d. potential serious complications

*Non-NANDA diagnosis.

SIX

RHEUMATIC FEVER
MEDICAL DIAGNOSIS

PATHOPHYSIOLOGY Acute rheumatic fever (ARF) is a systemic inflammatory disease that follows an acute group A beta-hemolytic streptococcus (GAS) pharyngeal infection. ARF occurs after an asymptomatic latent period of 2 to 6 weeks (following the initial GAS infections) and appears to be an autoimmune response to the GAS antigens. *Streptococci* and normal connective tissues, such as those found in the myocardium, have similar antigen-determinant sites. The body's immune system produces antibodies that begin to destroy the invading *Streptococci* but also destroy the normal cells found in connective tissue. This results in a proliferative inflammation at the site of tissue destruction. The inflammatory process causes lymphocytes and plasma cells to infiltrate cardiac tissue and joints. Inflammatory hemorrhagic bullous lesions, called Aschoff's bodies, form and produce swelling and alterations in the connective tissue, especially in the heart. Aschoff's bodies may also be found in the brain, blood vessels, and serous surfaces of the joints and pleura.

Carditis is a major manifestation of ARF and may include any or all of the myocardium, endocardium, and pericardium. When carditis is present, a murmur is almost always found, resulting from valvulitis. The most commonly affected valves are the mitral and aortic valves. Signs and symptoms of congestive heart failure may be exhibited. Children who develop carditis during the initial attack may sustain sequelae, depending on the severity of the carditis. The child is said to have rheumatic heart disease if cardiac damage occurs.

Another major manifestation is polyarthritis. Inflamed joints—large joints, such as the knees, elbows, hips, shoulders, and wrists—become red, warm, and extremely painful. This joint inflammation (arthritis) is reversible and migratory in nature.

Two other major manifestations, erythema marginatum and subcutaneous nodules, are both rare in children. Erythema marginatum is a macular, nonpruritic, transitory rash, most often found on the trunk and proximal portions of the extremities. The subcutaneous nodules are very small and found in groups over bony prominences, such as the hands, feet, and elbows.

The last major manifestation is chorea, manifested by incoordination, uncontrolled movements, involuntary facial grimacing, speech disturbances, emotional liability, and muscle weakness. These symptoms are exacerbated by stress and anxiety, and relieved by rest and sleep. This chorea is often referred to as Sydenham chorea or St. Vitus' dance.

Minor manifestations of ARF include fever, arthralgia, previous history of ARF, prolonged P-R interval on EKG, leukocytosis, elevated erythrocyte sedimentation rate, and positive C-reactive protein. A laboratory test for antistreptolysin-O (ASO antibiotic titer) may be done. A recent streptococcal infection would be evidenced by an elevated ASO titer. Diagnosis is usually based on a set of guidelines established by the American Heart Association, which include the revised Jones criteria. Acute rheumatic fever is suspected if a child has supporting evidence of an antecedent GAS infection and exhibits two major or one major and two minor manifestations.

Treatment includes antibiotics to eradicate the streptococcal infection and salicylates to reduce the joint inflammation. For patients with valve damage, steroids may be indicated. Streptococcal prophylaxis with antibiotics may be used to decrease further valve damage from repeat infections.

Acute rheumatic fever can occur in children of all ages, but it primarily affects those between 5 and 15 years of age. Adequate treatment of group A beta-hemolytic streptococcal upper respiratory infections with antibiotics will prevent ARF.

Primary Nursing Diagnosis   Decreased Cardiac Output

Definition   Decrease in the amount of blood that leaves the left ventricle

Possibly Related to
- Inflammation and destruction of the connective tissue in the myocardium
- Scarring and stenosis of heart valves (usually mitral and/or aortic)
- Backflow or regurgitation of blood through heart valves (mitral or aortic insufficiency)

Primary Nursing Diagnosis: Decreased cardiac output related to inflammation and destruction of the connective tissue in the myocardium, scarring and stenosis of heart valves (usually mitral and/or aortic), backflow or regurgitation of blood through heart valves (mitral or aortic insufficiency)

Assessment/Defining Characteristics of Child and/or Family (Subjective & Objective Data):

- Tachycardia
- Tachypnea
- Hypotension
- Murmurs
- Fever
- EKG changes, prolonged P-R interval
- Signs of right heart failure (e.g., hepatomegaly, edema, distended neck veins)
- Cardiomegaly revealed on chest X-ray
- Chest pain
- Pericardial friction rub

Expected Outcomes	Possible Nursing Interventions	Rationale	Evaluation for Charting
Child will have adequate cardiac output as evidenced by • heart rate within acceptable range (state specific range) • respiratory rate within acceptable range (state specific range) • blood pressure within acceptable range (state specific range) • temperature within acceptable range of 36.5°C to 37.2°C • normal sinus rhythm • appropriate heart size on chest X-ray • absence of chest pain pericardial friction rub edema hepatomegaly distended neck veins • lack of signs/symptoms of decreased cardiac output (such as those listed under Assessment)	Assess and record HR, RR, BP, T, and any signs/symptoms of decreased cardiac output (such as those listed under Assessment) every 2 to 4 hours and PRN.	If child experiences decreased cardiac output (CO) the HR and RR will increase and BP will decrease. If T increases it will increase HR.	Document range of HR, RR, BP, and T. Describe any signs/symptoms of decreased cardiac output noted.
	Evaluate and record results of EKG strips.	Changes in EKG may indicate decreased CO.	Describe results of EKG when indicated.
	Check and record results of chest X-ray when indicated.	Changes in chest X-ray results may indicate need for a change in therapy.	Document results of chest X-ray when indicated.
	Organize nursing care to allow child uninterrupted rest.	Proper rest will help to decrease workload on the heart.	Document whether child was able to have uninterrupted rest periods.
	Administer salicylates (aspirin) on schedule. Assess and record effectiveness and any signs/symptoms of toxicity (e.g., tinnitus, GI disturbance, headache, irritability, ketosis, bleeding).	Salicylates are administered to decrease inflammation.	Document whether salicylates were administered on schedule. Describe effectiveness and any side effects noted.

Primary Nursing Diagnosis: Decreased Cardiac Output *(continued)*

Expected Outcomes	Possible Nursing Interventions	Rationale	Evaluation for Charting
	If indicated, monitor and record salicylate level. Notify physician if levels are out of the acceptable range.	Salicylate levels need to be carefully monitored in order to prevent bleeding tendencies and organ damage (liver, renal).	Document salicylate levels. If levels are out of the acceptable range, describe any corrective measures implemented.
	If indicated, administer steroids (prednisone) on schedule. Assess and record effectiveness and any side effects (e.g., sodium retention, fluid retention, potassium loss).	Steroids are administered to help decrease the autoimmune response.	Document whether steroids were administered on schedule. Describe effectiveness and any side effects noted.
	If indicated, administer antibiotics on schedule. Assess and record any side effects (e.g., rash, diarrhea).	Antibiotics are administered to eradicate the streptococcal infection.	Document whether antibiotics were administered on schedule. Describe any side effects noted.
TEACHING GOALS Child and/or family will be able to verbalize at least 4 characteristics of decreased cardiac output such as • rapid heart rate • fever • chest pain • activity intolerance • swelling	Teach child/family about characteristics of decreased cardiac output. Assess and record results.	Increased knowledge will assist the child/family in recognizing and reporting changes in the child's condition.	Document whether teaching was done and describe results.
Child and/or family will be able to verbalize knowledge of care such as • medication administration • sufficient rest periods • monitoring intake and output • identification of any signs/symptoms of decreased cardiac output (such as those listed under Assessment) • when to contact health care provider	Teach child/family about care. Assess and record child's/family's knowledge of and participation in care regarding medication administration, etc.	Education of child/family will allow for accurate care.	Document whether teaching was done and describe results.

Nursing Diagnosis   Acute Pain

Definition   Condition in which an individual experiences acute mild to severe pain

Possibly Related to
- Joint tenderness
- Chest pain
- Dyspnea

Nursing Diagnosis: Acute pain related to joint tenderness, inflammation, arthralgia, chest pain, dyspnea			

Assessment/Defining Characteristics of Child and/or Family (Subjective & Objective Data):
• Swollen, red, warm joints
• Verbal communication of pain or tenderness
• Rating of pain on pain-assessment tool
• Crying unrelieved by usual comfort measures
• Moaning
    • Facial grimacing
    • Physical signs/symptoms (tachycardia, tachypnea/bradypnea, increased blood pressure, diaphoresis, restlessness)			

Expected Outcomes	**Possible Nursing Interventions**	**Rationale**	**Evaluation for Charting**
Child will be free of severe and/or constant pain as evidenced by • decrease in swelling, redness, and warmness of joints • verbal communication of comfort • rating of decreased pain or no pain on pain-assessment tool • lack of constant crying or moaning • lack of facial expression of discomfort • heart rate within acceptable range (state specific range) • respiratory rate within acceptable range (state specific range) • blood pressure within acceptable range (state specific range) • lack of diaphoresis and extreme restlessness	Assess and record HR, RR, BP, T, and any signs/symptoms of pain (such as those listed under Assessment) every 2 to 4 hours and PRN. Use age-appropriate pain-assessment tool.	Provides data regarding the level of pain child is experiencing.	Document range of HR, RR, BP, T, and degree of pain child was experiencing. Describe any successful measures used to decrease pain.
	Handle child gently.	Helps to minimize pain and promote comfort.	Document if child was handled gently and effectiveness of measure.
	Administer salicylates (aspirin) on schedule. Assess and record effectiveness and any signs/symptoms of toxicity (e.g., tinnitus, GI disturbance, headache, irritability, ketosis, bleeding).	Salicylates are administered to decrease joint inflammation.	Document whether salicylates were administered on schedule. Describe effectiveness and any side effects noted.
	If indicated, monitor and record salicylate level. Notify physician if levels are out of the acceptable range.	Salicylate levels need to be carefully monitored in order to prevent bleeding tendencies and organ damage (e.g., liver, renal).	Document salicylate levels. If levels are out of the acceptable range, describe any corrective measures implemented.
	Encourage family members to stay and comfort child when possible.	Helps to comfort and support the child.	Document whether family was able to remain with child and describe effectiveness of their presence.

Nursing Diagnosis: Acute Pain *(continued)*

Expected Outcomes	Possible Nursing Interventions	Rationale	Evaluation for Charting
	If indicated, perform limited passive range-of-motion exercises to help increase comfort. Record results.	Helps to decrease joint pain.	When indicated, document effectiveness of range-of-motion exercises.
	Use diversional activities (e.g., music, television, playing games, relaxation) when appropriate.	Diversional activities can distract child and may help to decrease pain.	Document whether diversional activities were successful in helping to manage pain.
TEACHING GOALS Child and/or family will be able to verbalize at least 4 characteristics of pain such as • swollen, red, warm joints • verbal communication of pain or tenderness • crying unrelieved by usual comfort measures • facial grimacing • rapid heart rate	Teach child/family about characteristics of pain. Assess and record results.	Increased knowledge will assist the child/family in recognizing and reporting changes in the child's condition.	Document whether teaching was done and describe results.
Child and/or family will be able to verbalize knowledge of care such as • medication administration • passive range-of-motion exercises • appropriate diversional activities • identification of any signs/symptoms of decreased cardiac output (such as those listed under Assessment) • when to contact health care provider	Teach child/family about care. Assess and record child's/family's knowledge of and participation in care regarding medication administration, etc.	Education of child/family will allow for accurate care.	Document whether teaching was done and describe results.

Related Nursing Diagnoses

Activity Intolerance	*related to* a. joint inflammation b. cardiac inflammation
Risk for Infection	*related to* decreased resistance
Risk for Injury	*related to* involuntary movements of the muscles in the extremities
Deficient Knowledge: Child/Family	*related to* a. disease process b. continuing home management (including medications and limited activity)
Disturbed Body Image	*related to* side effects of steroids

CARE OF
CHILDREN WITH
ENDOCRINE
DYSFUNCTION

2

ONE

DIABETES INSIPIDUS
MEDICAL DIAGNOSIS

PATHOPHYSIOLOGY Children with diabetes insipidus either have central or neurogenic diabetes insipidus where they lack antidiuretic hormone (ADH), or they have nephrogenic diabetes insipidus with decreased renal responsiveness to ADH. Central or neurogenic diabetes insipidus results from decreased production of ADH (vasopressin) usually due to a familial or idiopathic cause. Secondary causes can include incomplete formation of the pituitary gland, central nervous system insults, including head trauma, infections, intracranial lesions, and brain surgery. Neurogenic diabetes insipidus can be transient. Less common is nephrogenic diabetes insipidus in which the renal tubules are unresponsive to ADH. There are various forms of nephrogenic diabetes insipidus: X-linked recessive, autosomal recessive, autosomal dominant, or acquired form. The acquired form of nephrogenic diabetes insipidus may result from adverse drug reactions, electrolyte disorders, or systemic disorders.

Antidiuretic hormone, which is produced in the hypothalamus, is stored and released from the posterior pituitary gland. Normally the body is able to conserve water when the distal renal tubules respond to ADH stimulation. When circulating ADH levels are low or when the kidneys are not responsive to normal levels of ADH, collecting tubules do not reabsorb free water; instead, the water is lost in the urine. Interstitial and intracellular water is pulled into the intravascular space and lost in the urine as well. This water loss occurs even in the presence of increased serum osmolality and hypovolemia, resulting in hypernatremia.

Children with diabetes insipidus experience polyuria and polydipsia, usually preferring water to quench their excessive thirst. Significant dehydration and hypernatremia can occur if the child is unable to maintain adequate fluid intake. The main treatment goal for a child with neurogenic diabetes insipidus is to correct the dehydration. This is done by the administration of appropriate fluids and hormone replacement with vasopressin. Diuretics and sodium restriction are effective adjunct therapies that correct the hypernatremia (this should be done slowly to prevent cerebral edema) and control free water loss by the kidneys. Nephrogenic diabetes insipidus is difficult to treat. Therapy for nephrogenic diabetes insipidus may include thiazide diuretics, a high fluid intake, and a low-osmolar, low-sodium, low-protein diet.

Nursing Care Plan for a Child with Neurogenic Diabetes Insipidus

Primary Nursing Diagnosis   Deficient Fluid Volume

Definition   Decrease in the amount of circulating fluid volume

Possibly Related to   • Polyuria secondary to lack of ADH

Primary Nursing Diagnosis: Deficient fluid volume related to polyuria secondary to lack of ADH

Assessment/Defining Characteristics of Child and/or Family (Subjective & Objective Data):

- Polyuria
- Polydipsia
- Nocturia
- Enuresis
- Intense thirst and preference for water
- Dilute urine, specific gravity less than 1.008
- Weight loss
- Decreased skin turgor (skin recoil greater than 2 to 3 seconds)
- Dry mucous membranes
- Sunken fontanel
- Decreased urine osmolality (less than 280 mOsm/L)

- Increased serum sodium (greater than 145 mEq/L, usually 160 to 200 mEq/L)
- Increased serum osmolality (less than 300 mOsm/L)
- Decreased urine sodium (less than 130 mEq/24 hr)
- Tachycardia
- Tachypnea
- Hypotension
- Cool extremities
- Weak peripheral pulses
- Prolonged capillary refill (longer than 2 to 3 seconds)
- Irritability

Expected Outcomes	Possible Nursing Interventions	Rationale	Evaluation for Charting
Child will have adequate fluid volume as evidenced by • adequate fluid intake, IV and oral (state specific amount of intake needed for each child) • adequate urine output (state specific range; 1 to 2 ml/kg/hr) • urine specific gravity from 1.008 to 1.020 • urine osmolality from 500 to 800 mOsm/L • serum osmolality from 280 to 295 mOsm/L • urine sodium from 130 to 200 mEq/24 hr • serum sodium from 138 to 145 mEq/L • moist mucous membranes • rapid skin recoil (less than 2 to 3 seconds) • heart rate, respiratory rate, and blood pressure within acceptable range (state specific range for each) • lack of signs/symptoms of deficient fluid volume (such as those listed under Assessment)	Keep accurate record of intake and output. When indicated, encourage oral fluids.	Increased urinary output may indicate low levels of circulating ADH and increased water loss in the urine.	Document intake and output.
	Administer oral and IV fluids as ordered, including urine output replacement. Intravenous fluids with low sodium (1/16 to 1/8 normal saline) and low glucose (2.5%) concentrations may be used.	Fluids are needed to counteract the polyuria caused by increased water loss in the urine.	Document type of IV fluids and amount of total intake.
	Assess and record • HR, RR, and BP every 4 hours and PRN • IV fluids and condition of IV site every hour • laboratory values as indicated. Report any abnormalities to the physician. • signs/symptoms of deficient fluid volume (such as those listed under Assessment) every 4 hours and PRN	Provides information about fluid status of patient. If patient has fluid volume deficit, the HR will increase at first, and eventually decrease. The RR will increase. The BP will eventually decrease. It is necessary to record the amount of IV fluids every hour to make sure the child is not being over or under hydrated. The IV site needs to be assessed every hour for signs of redness or swelling.	Document range of HR, RR, and BP. Document amount of IV fluids and describe condition of IV site along with any interventions needed. Document current laboratory values when indicated. Describe any signs/symptoms of deficient fluid volume noted.
	Check and record urine specific gravity with every void or as indicated.	Urine specific gravity provides information about hydration status.	Document range of urine specific gravity.

(continued)

Primary Nursing Diagnosis: Deficient Fluid Volume *(continued)*

Expected Outcomes	Possible Nursing Interventions	Rationale	Evaluation for Charting
	Assess and record condition of mucous membranes and skin turgor every shift and PRN.	Provides information on hydration status.	Describe status of mucous membranes and skin turgor.
	Weigh child daily on same scale at same time daily. Document results and compare to previous weight.	Decrease in weight may indicate fluid volume deficit due to increased urine output.	Document weight and determine if it was an increase or decrease from the previous weight.
	When indicated, assist with water deprivation testing.	Water deprivation testing can help determine the cause of diabetes insipidus.	Document results of water deprivation testing.
	If indicated, administer desmopressin acetate (DDAVP) on schedule by the prescribed route. Assess and record effectiveness and any side effects noted (e.g., abdominal cramping, tachycardia/bradycardia, or other signs of hypersensitivity).	DDAVP can mimic the effects of antidiuretic hormone and increase water reabsorption.	Document whether DDAVP was administered on schedule. Describe effectiveness and any side effects noted.
TEACHING GOALS Child and/or family will be able to verbalize at least 4 characteristics of deficient fluid volume such as <ul><li>increased number of times child voids</li><li>increased thirst</li><li>weight loss</li><li>rapid heart rate</li><li>cool extremities</li></ul>	Teach child/family about characteristics of deficient fluid volume. Assess and record results.	Increased knowledge will assist the child/family in recognizing and reporting changes in the child's condition.	Document whether teaching was done and describe results.
Child and/or family will be able to verbalize knowledge of care such as <ul><li>medication administration</li><li>monitoring intake and output</li></ul>	Teach child/family about care. Assess and record child's/family's knowledge of and participation in care regarding medication administration, etc.	Education of child/family will allow for accurate care.	Document whether teaching was done and describe results.

Primary Nursing Diagnosis: Deficient Fluid Volume *(continued)*			
Expected Outcomes	**Possible Nursing Interventions**	**Rationale**	**Evaluation for Charting**
• identification of any signs/symptoms of deficient fluid volume (such as those listed under Assessment) • when to contact health care provider			

Nursing Diagnosis Electrolyte Imbalance: Sodium Excess*

Definition Disturbance in the level of the body's sodium

Possibly Related to • Polyuria secondary to lack of ADH

*Non-NANDA diagnosis.

Nursing Diagnosis: Electrolyte imbalance: sodium excess related to polyuria secondary to lack of ADH			
Assessment/Defining Characteristics of Child and/or Family (Subjective & Objective Data): • Increased serum sodium (greater than 145 mEq/L, usually 160 to 200 mEq/L) • Lethargy • Dry mucous membranes • Flushed skin • Intense thirst • Seizures • Coma			
Expected Outcomes	**Possible Nursing Interventions**	**Rationale**	**Evaluation for Charting**
Child will have adequate sodium balance as evidenced by • serum sodium from 138 to 145 mEq/L • appropriate level of consciousness for age • moist mucous membranes • lack of signs/symptoms of sodium excess (such as those listed under Assessment)	Assess and record • signs/symptoms of sodium excess (such as those listed under Assessment) every 4 hours and PRN • appropriate level of consciousness for age • moist mucous membranes • laboratory values, as indicated. Record abnormalities to the physician.	If child experiences sodium excess the child may have a decreased level of consciousness, dry mucous membranes, and high serum sodium levels.	Describe child's neurologic status, mucous membranes status, and any signs/symptoms of sodium excess noted. Document current serum sodium level.

(continued)

Nursing Diagnosis: Electrolyte Imbalance: Sodium Excess *(continued)*

Expected Outcomes	Possible Nursing Interventions	Rationale	Evaluation for Charting
	Administer oral and IV fluids as ordered, including urine output replacement. Intravenous fluids with low sodium (1/16 to 1/8 normal saline) and low glucose (2.5%) concentrations may be used.	Fluids are needed to counteract the increased water loss in the urine.	Document type of IV fluids and amount of total intake.
	Assess and record condition of IV site every hour.	Provides information about the condition of the IV site and allows for interventions if the IV site is red or edematous.	Document condition of IV site and any interventions if needed.
	If indicated, administer desmopressin acetate (DDAVP) on schedule by the prescribed route. Assess and record effectiveness and any side effects noted (e.g., abdominal cramping, tachycardia/bradycardia, or other signs of hypersensitivity).	DDAVP can mimic the effects of antidiuretic hormone and increase water reabsorption, which will help to prevent hypernatremia.	Document whether DDAVP was administered on schedule. Describe effectiveness and any side effects noted.
	Keep accurate record of intake and output.	Increased urinary output may indicate low levels of circulating ADH and increased water loss in the urine.	Document intake and output.
	Provide mouth care every 4 hours and PRN.	Mouth care is necessary to counteract the dry mucous membranes.	Document whether mouth care was done and effectiveness.
TEACHING GOALS Child and/or family will be able to verbalize at least 4 characteristics of electrolyte imbalance: sodium excess such as • lethargy • dry mucous membranes • flushed skin • intense thirst • seizures	Teach child/family about characteristics of electrolyte imbalance: sodium excess. Assess and record results.	Increased knowledge will assist the child/family in recognizing and reporting changes in the child's condition.	Document whether teaching was done and describe results.

	Possible Nursing		**Evaluation for**
Expected Outcomes	**Interventions**	**Rationale**	**Charting**
Child and/or family will be able to verbalize knowledge of care such as • medication administration • monitoring intake and output • identification of any signs/symptoms of electrolyte imbalance: sodium excess (such as those listed under Assessment) • when to contact health care provider	Teach child/family about care. Assess and record child's/family's knowledge of and participation in care regarding medication administration, etc.	Education of child/ family will allow for accurate care.	Document whether teaching was done and describe results.

Nursing Diagnosis: Electrolyte Imbalance: Sodium Excess *(continued)*

Related Nursing Diagnoses

Altered Level of Consciousness*   *related to* hypernatremia

Decreased Cardiac Output   *related to* circulatory compromise secondary to severe fluid volume deficit

Readiness for Enhanced Parenting   *related to*
a. child's hospitalization
b. child's need for chronic medication administration
c. knowledge deficit

Compromised Family Coping   *related to*
a. underlying disease state
b. knowledge deficit
c. child's hospitalization

*Non-NANDA diagnosis.

TWO

DIABETES MELLITUS
MEDICAL DIAGNOSIS

PATHOPHYSIOLOGY The most common endocrine disease of childhood is type 1 diabetes mellitus. In the child with this chronic disease, insulin-producing beta cells in the pancreatic islets of Langerhans have been destroyed or reduced in number, creating a deficiency in insulin. In genetically susceptible children, the beta-cell mass is gradually destroyed by an autoimmune response after exposure to a trigger event (a virus, bacteria, chemical irritant, dietary component). The lack of sufficient insulin adversely affects carbohydrate, protein, and fat metabolism.

Glucose is the primary energy source for most cells. Insulin facilitates the uptake of intravascular glucose by muscle and fat cells, facilitates the storage of glucose (as glycogen) in the liver and muscle cells, and indirectly prevents fat metabolism. Insufficient insulin leads to hyperglycemia because intravascular glucose is unable to enter the cells. The liver responds to lack of intracellular glucose by initiating gluconeogenesis and glycogenolysis, further contributing to the hyperglycemia. Hyperglycemia causes an osmotic diuresis, leading to excessive water loss, electrolyte imbalance, and, eventually, dehydration.

The inability of glucose to enter the cells triggers catabolism. In this process, the body uses fat and protein for energy, and despite increased food intake, weight loss occurs. When fat is used for energy, the liver converts the increased free fatty acids in the blood into ketone bodies. The circulating ketone bodies accumulate in substantial numbers, altering the serum pH, resulting in ketoacidosis. During acidosis, total body potassium can be significantly decreased. Signs of the rise in acetone and ketoacid levels are a fruity breath, Kussmaul breathing, abdominal pains, and vomiting. Once vomiting begins, the excessive fluid loss can no longer be balanced by increased intake, and the child's condition can quickly deteriorate.

The classic presentation of diabetes in children includes a history of polyuria, polydipsia, polyphagia, and weight loss. Many children initially present with ketoacidosis. The child with diabetic ketoacidosis (DKA) exhibits the classic signs and symptoms, but may also have vomiting, dehydration, shortness of breath, abdominal pain, or alteration in the level of consciousness. Hyperglycemia (glucose greater than 300 mg/dL), ketonemia, acidosis (pH less than 7.30, bicarbonate less than 15 mEq/L), glucosuria, and ketonuria are also present in DKA.

Acute treatment of diabetes focuses on returning the child to a balanced metabolic state. Long-term treatment attempts to promote normal growth and development and emphasizes independence and self-management in order to reduce adverse psychosocial effects. Appropriate diabetes management will help prevent the macrovascular and microvascular (i.e., retinopathy, nephropathy, neuropathy) complications of diabetes. Treatment includes child/family education on self-monitoring of blood glucose, insulin administration, diet, exercise, and hyperglycemia/hypoglycemia management. The child with type 1 diabetes is best served by a comprehensive, multidisciplinary approach.

A growing number of children and adolescents are developing type 2 diabetes. Type 2 diabetes mellitus is a combination of both insulin deficiency and insulin resistance. Insulin resistance is the failure of the body to respond to insulin correctly. Children with the highest incidence of having type 2 diabetes are those who are obese and those who have a family history of type 2 diabetes. The high caloric diets and sedentary lifestyle of today's children and adolescents have contributed to the increased incidence of type 2 diabetes mellitus. The presentation of children with type 2 diabetes can vary. They may present with nonketotic hyperglycemia, glucosuria, headaches, acanthosis nigricans, or fatigue. At times they will present with polydipsia and polyuria. The goal of treatment is to achieve near-normal blood glucose levels and A1C values (which reflect the average blood glucose levels for the previous 2 to 3 months), and to prevent long-term diabetes complications. Treatment involves lifestyle changes (diet and exercise) alone or may require oral medications or insulin.

Nursing Care Plan for a Child with Type 1 Diabetes Mellitus

Primary Nursing Diagnosis   Impaired Metabolic Function*

Definition   Imbalance or altered utilization of specific body biochemicals

Possibly Related to   • Insufficient insulin secondary to ineffective beta cells in pancreatic islets
                               • Increased insulin requirements secondary to infection, stress, and/or illness
                               • Unstable serum glucose levels

*Non-NANDA diagnosis.

Primary Nursing Diagnosis: Impaired metabolic function related to insufficient insulin secondary to ineffective beta cells in pancreatic islets; increased insulin requirements secondary to infection, stress, and/or illness; unstable serum glucose levels

Assessment/Defining Characteristics of Child and/or Family (Subjective & Objective Data):

Hyperglycemia, hypoglycemia, or fluctuating blood glucose levels
Signs/symptoms of hyperglycemia (slow onset):

- Polyuria
- Polydipsia
- Polyphagia
- Weight loss
- Enuresis in a previously toilet trained child
- Lethargy or stupor
- Warm, flushed, dry skin
- Weakness

- Nausea/vomiting
- Acetone (fruity) breath
- Abdominal pain
- Kussmaul breathing
- Dehydration
- Glucosuria
- Ketonuria
- Metabolic acidosis

Signs/symptoms of hypoglycemia (rapid onset):

- Excessive sweating
- Faintness
- Dizziness
- Poor coordination
- Pallor
- Cool skin
- Pounding of the heart

- Trembling
- Impaired vision
- Personality changes
- Irritability
- Headache
- Hunger
- Inability to awaken

Expected Outcomes	Possible Nursing Interventions	Rationale	Evaluation for Charting
Child will maintain adequate metabolic function as evidenced by • stable blood glucose level from 70 to 180 mg/dL • lack of signs/symptoms of hyperglycemia (such as those listed under Assessment)	Assess and record • vital signs and neurological status every 1 to 4 hours and PRN • blood glucose levels as ordered and PRN. Fasting, preprandial, peak postprandial, and 3 A.M. blood glucose levels may be needed.	If child experiences altered metabolic function the vital signs will be out of the normal range (can be increased or decreased) and the child can experience decreased level of consciousness as a result of glucose being unable to enter the cells.	Document range of vital signs, blood glucose levels, and any signs/symptoms of hyperglycemia or hypoglycemia. Document amount of IV fluids and describe condition of IV site along with any interventions needed.

(continued)

Primary Nursing Diagnosis: Impaired Metabolic Function *(continued)*

Expected Outcomes	Possible Nursing Interventions	Rationale	Evaluation for Charting
• lack of signs/symptoms of hypoglycemia (such as those listed under Assessment)	Assist child/family with self-monitoring of blood glucose PRN. • signs/symptoms of hyperglycemia or hypoglycemia (such as those listed under Assessment) every 2 to 4 hours and PRN • IV fluids and condition of IV site every hour	Assessing and recording blood glucose levels provides information about hyperglycemia and hypoglycemia and directs needed treatment measures. It is necessary to record the amount of IV fluids every hour to make sure the child is not being over or under hydrated. The IV site needs to be assessed every hour for signs of redness or swelling.	
	Maintain diabetic flow sheet. Include blood glucose levels, insulin dose, injection site, clinical observations, urine test results, and intake and output.	Provides information that helps detects hyperglycemia and hypoglycemia.	Document range of blood glucose levels. Document insulin doses and injections sites used. Document clinical observation results and urine test results. Document intake and output.
	Keep accurate record of intake and output.	Increased urinary output may indicate hyperglycemia, which causes osmotic diuresis and can lead to dehydration.	Document intake and output.
	Weigh child daily on same scale at same time each day. Record weight and compare to previous weight.	Decrease in weight may initially be due to dehydration or may indicate catabolism, which is caused by the inability of glucose to enter the cells.	Document weight and determine if it was an increase or decrease from the previous weight.
	Administer IV maintenance and replacement fluids and supplements (such as potassium bicarbonate) as indicated. Assess and record child's response.	IV fluids are necessary to combat dehydration. Potassium is needed to combat decreased total body potassium.	Document type and amount of IV fluids administered. Describe child's response to therapy.
	When indicated, administer insulin drip following institutional policies for solution and tubing changes and use of a pump. Adjust insulin drip as indicated. Assess and record child's response.	Insulin is administered to facilitate glucose entry into the cells.	Document amount of insulin administered and describe effectiveness and child's response to treatment.

Primary Nursing Diagnosis: Impaired Metabolic Function *(continued)*			
Expected Outcomes	**Possible Nursing Interventions**	**Rationale**	**Evaluation for Charting**
	When indicated, administer subcutaneous insulin on schedule. Assess and record effectiveness.	Insulin is administered to facilitate glucose entry into the cells.	Document amount of insulin administered and describe effectiveness and child's response to treatment.
	If child is hypoglycemic, administer fruit juice (4 oz.), regular soda (4 oz.), or glucose tablets to provide approximately 10 to 15 grams of carbohydrate or 40 calories. Repeat if child does not feel better in 10 to 15 minutes. If severe hypoglycemia occurs and the child is unable to swallow, administer glucagon as indicated. Assess and record child's response.	Carbohydrates are needed to combat hypoglycemia and return child to a balanced metabolic state.	Document any measures used to combat hypoglycemia and the effectiveness of the measures.
TEACHING GOALS Child and/or family will be able to verbalize at least 4 characteristics of impaired metabolic function such as <ul><li>increased number of times child voids</li><li>increased thirst</li><li>weight loss</li><li>lethargy or stupor</li><li>nausea/vomiting</li></ul>	Teach child/family about characteristics of altered metabolic function. Assess and record results.	Increased knowledge will assist the child/family in recognizing and reporting changes in the child's condition.	Document whether teaching was done and describe results.
Child and/or family will be able to verbalize knowledge of care such as <ul><li>glucose monitoring</li><li>insulin dosage adjustment</li><li>insulin administration and site rotation</li><li>food plan (carbohydrate counting) and exercise</li><li>regular eye examination</li><li>foot care</li></ul>	Teach child/family about care. Assess and record child's/family's knowledge of and participation in care regarding glucose monitoring, etc.	Education of child/family will allow for accurate care.	Document whether teaching was done and describe results.

(continued)

	Possible Nursing		Evaluation for
Primary Nursing Diagnosis: Impaired Metabolic Function (continued)			
Expected Outcomes	**Possible Nursing Interventions**	**Rationale**	**Evaluation for Charting**
• nephrotic screening • identification of any signs/symptoms of hyperglycemia and hypoglycemia (such as those listed under Assessment) and the correct action for each • when to contact health care provider			

Nursing Diagnosis   Deficient Fluid Volume

Definition   Decrease in the amount of circulating fluid volume

Possibly Related to   • Osmotic diuresis secondary to hyperglycemia
                          • Vomiting
                          • Decreased oral intake

Nursing Diagnosis: Deficient fluid volume related to osmotic diuresis secondary to hyperglycemia, vomiting, decreased oral intake

Assessment/Defining Characteristics of Child and/or Family (Subjective & Objective Data):
- Polyuria
- Flushed, dry skin
- Dry mucous membranes
- Decreased skin turgor (skin recoil greater than 2 to 3 seconds)
- Weight loss
- Tachycardia
- Tachypnea
- Hypotension
- Lack of tears

Expected Outcomes	**Possible Nursing Interventions**	**Rationale**	**Evaluation for Charting**
Child will have adequate fluid volume as evidenced by • adequate fluid intake, IV and oral (state specific amount of intake needed for each child)	Keep accurate record of intake and output. When indicated, encourage oral fluids.	Increased urinary output may indicate hyperglycemia is present.	Document intake and output.
	Administer IV maintenance and replacement fluids and supplements (such as potassium bicarbonate) as indicated.	Fluids are needed to counteract dehydration from the polyuria that results from hyperglycemia.	Document type of IV fluids and amount of total intake.

Nursing Diagnosis: Deficient Fluid Volume *(continued)*

Expected Outcomes	Possible Nursing Interventions	Rationale	Evaluation for Charting
• adequate urine output (state specific range; 1 to 2 ml/kg/hr) • moist mucous membranes • rapid skin recoil (less than 2 to 3 seconds) • lack of weight loss • heart rate, respiratory rate, and blood pressure within acceptable range (state specific range for each) • urine specific gravity from 1.008 to 1.020 • lack of signs/ symptoms of deficient fluid volume (such as those listed under Assessment)	Assess and record • HR, RR, BP, and urine specific gravity every 4 hours and PRN • IV fluids and condition of IV site every hour • laboratory values as indicated. Report any abnormalities to the physician. • signs/symptoms of deficient fluid volume (such as those listed under Assessment) every 4 hours and PRN	Provides information about fluid status of patient. If patient has fluid volume deficit, the HR will increase at first, and eventually decrease. The RR will increase. The BP will eventually decrease. It is necessary to record the amount of IV fluids every hour to make sure the child is not being over or under hydrated. The IV site needs to be assessed every hour for signs of redness or swelling.	Document range of HR, RR, BP, and urine specific gravity. Document amount of IV fluids and describe condition of IV site along with any interventions needed. Document current laboratory values when indicated. Describe any signs/symptoms of deficient fluid volume noted.
	Provide mouth care every 4 hours and PRN. Record results.	Mouth care is needed because the child is prone to dehydration and dry mucous membranes.	Document whether mouth care was done and describe effectiveness.
	Weigh child daily on same scale at same time of day. Document results and compare to previous weight.	Weight loss is due to dehydration as well as the inability of glucose to enter the cell, which triggers catabolism and results in weight loss.	Document weight and determine if it was an increase or decrease from the previous weight.
TEACHING GOALS Child and/or family will be able to verbalize at least 4 characteristics of deficient fluid volume such as • increased number of times child voids • vomiting • flushed, dry skin • weight loss • rapid heart rate	Teach child/family about characteristics of deficient fluid volume. Assess and record results.	Increased knowledge will assist the child/ family in recognizing and reporting changes in the child's condition.	Document whether teaching was done and describe results.
Child and/or family will be able to verbalize knowledge of care such as • monitoring intake and output	Teach child/family about care. Assess and record child's/family's knowledge of and participation in care regarding monitoring intake and output, etc.	Education of child/ family will allow for accurate care.	Document whether teaching was done and describe results.

(continued)

Nursing Diagnosis: Deficient Fluid Volume *(continued)*			
Expected Outcomes	**Possible Nursing Interventions**	**Rationale**	**Evaluation for Charting**
• identification of any signs/symptoms of deficient fluid volume (such as those listed under Assessment) and the correct action for each • when to contact health care provider			

Nursing Diagnosis

Nursing Diagnosis	Electrolyte Imbalance: Sodium Losses and Potassium Losses*
Definition	Disturbance in the level of the body's sodium and potassium
Possibly Related to	• Sodium losses secondary to vomiting and osmotic diuresis
	• Temporarily increased extracellular potassium (false high) secondary to
	• acidosis
	• insulin deficiency
	• dehydration
	• Potassium losses secondary to
	• polyuria
	• insulin administration
	• dilution resulting from rehydration
	• correction of acidosis (potassium reenters the cell)

*Non-NANDA diagnosis.

Nursing Diagnosis: Electrolyte imbalance: sodium losses and potassium losses related to

- sodium losses secondary to vomiting and osmotic diuresis
- temporarily increased extracellular potassium (false high) secondary to
  1. acidosis
  2. insulin deficiency
  3. dehydration

- potassium losses secondary to
  1. polyuria
  2. insulin administration
  3. dilution resulting from rehydration
  4. correction of acidosis (potassium reenters the cell)

Assessment/Defining Characteristics of Child and/or Family (Subjective & Objective Data):

- Hyponatremia, with the following signs/symptoms
  1. weakness
  2. delirium
- Hyperkalemia, with the following signs/symptoms
  1. EKG changes: spiked T waves, widened QRS complexes, flattened P waves, ectopic beats
  2. weakness
  3. flushed skin

- Hypokalemia, with the following signs/symptoms
  1. EKG changes: flattened T waves, peaked P waves, ectopic beats
  2. hypotension and rapid heart rate
  3. coma

Nursing Diagnosis: Electrolyte Imbalance: Sodium Losses and Potassium Losses *(continued)*

Expected Outcomes	Possible Nursing Interventions	Rationale	Evaluation for Charting
Child will maintain adequate electrolyte balance as evidenced by • serum sodium from 138 to 145 mEq/L • serum potassium from 3.5 to 5.0 mEq/L • normal sinus rhythm and EKG configuration • heart rate within acceptable range (state specific range) • blood pressure within acceptable range (state specific range) • lack of signs/symptoms of electrolyte imbalance (such as those listed under Assessment)	Assess and record • HR and BP every 4 hours • IV fluids and condition of IV site every hour • laboratory values as indicated. Report any abnormalities to the physician. • signs/symptoms of electrolyte imbalance (such as those listed under Assessment) every 4 hours and PRN	Provides information about electrolyte status of patient. If patient has fluid volume deficit, the HR will increase at first, and eventually decrease. The BP will eventually decrease. It is necessary to record the amount of IV fluids every hour to keep make sure the child is not being over or under hydrated. The IV site needs to be assessed every hour for signs of redness or swelling.	Document range of HR and BP. Document amount of IV fluids and describe condition of IV site along with any interventions needed. Document current laboratory values when indicated. Describe any signs/symptoms of electrolyte imbalance noted.
	When indicated, initiate use of a cardiac monitor. Evaluate and record results of EKG strips at least once/shift.	Provides information about serum potassium influence on cardiac rhythm.	Document EKG interpretation.
	Ensure that proper supplements are added to IV fluids.	Supplements are needed to combat the effects of insulin deficiency.	Document amount of supplements needed and any therapeutic measures used to restore electrolyte balance. Describe effectiveness.
TEACHING GOALS Child and/or family will be able to verbalize at least 4 characteristics of electrolyte imbalance: sodium losses and potassium losses such as • weakness • delirium • flushed skin • rapid heart rate • coma	Teach child/family about characteristics of electrolyte imbalance: sodium losses and potassium losses. Assess and record results.	Increased knowledge will assist the child/family in recognizing and reporting changes in the child's condition.	Document whether teaching was done and describe results.

(continued)

Expected Outcomes	Possible Nursing Interventions	Rationale	Evaluation for Charting
Child and/or family will be able to verbalize knowledge of care such as • identification of any signs/symptoms of electrolyte imbalance (such as those listed under Assessment) and the correct action for each • when to contact health care provider	Teach child/family about care. Assess and record child's/family's knowledge of and participation in care regarding identification of any signs/symptoms of electrolyte imbalance, etc.	Education of child/family will allow for accurate care.	Document whether teaching was done and describe results.

Nursing Diagnosis: Electrolyte Imbalance: Sodium Losses and Potassium Losses *(continued)*

Related Nursing Diagnoses

Deficient Knowledge: Child/Parental   *related to*
    a. newly diagnosed illness
    b. child/family request for information
    c. child/family statements of misinformation
    d. noncompliance with child's treatment
    e. mismanagement of child's illness
    f. anxiety regarding care regimen

Imbalanced Nutrition: Less than Body Requirements   *related to* weight loss despite polyphagia secondary to catabolic state

Compromised Family Coping   *related to*
    a. newly diagnosed chronic illness
    b. need for continual monitoring of blood glucose, urine acetone, diet, and exercise on a daily basis
    c. fluctuating blood glucose despite compliance with treatment
    d. frequent hospitalizations
    e. lack of support or financial resources
    f. stress of child's chronic illness on family

THREE

SYNDROME OF INAPPROPRIATE SECRETION OF ANTIDIURETIC HORMONE
MEDICAL DIAGNOSIS

PATHOPHYSIOLOGY The syndrome of inappropriate secretion of antidiuretic hormone (SIADH) occurs when the secretion of antidiuretic hormone (ADH) is inappropriately increased without the presence of a hypovolemic stimuli. Normally ADH is released from the posterior pituitary gland in response to the physiological stimuli of hypovolemia or increased serum osmotic pressure (hyperosmolality), but in SIADH this is not the case. The increased ADH levels in SIADH often involve an abnormal response of the intracranial osmoreceptors of the hypothalamus. Decreased venous return may also stimulate thoracic volume receptors, resulting in water retention and hyponatremia.

The inappropriate or excessive secretion of ADH results in increased reabsorption of water from the renal tubules. This causes intravascular fluid overload, and the fluid then shifts into the intracellular space. Characteristics of SIADH are serum hypoosmolality and hyponatremia associated with urine hyperosmolality and high urine sodium levels. Clinical manifestations, consistent with water intoxication, improve with water restriction.

Syndrome of inappropriate secretion of antidiuretic hormone is associated with a number of clinical conditions, especially those involving the nervous system, such as meningitis, encephalitis, brain tumors and abscesses, Guillain Barré syndrome, and seizures; it can also occur after neurosurgery. Syndrome of inappropriate secretion of antidiuretic hormone may also be a complication of pneumonia, tuberculosis, cystic fibrosis, perinatal asphyxia, repair of mitral valve insufficiency, use of positive pressure ventilators, and use of certain drugs, such as vincristine or vinblastine. Malignant tumors that ectopically produce ADH may cause SIADH as well. In many of these instances, SIADH can be a temporary condition.

Treatment goals for children with SIADH include normalizing the serum sodium and serum osmolality, and decreasing extravascular fluid volume by appropriately restricting fluids. Management of the underlying cause of the SIADH and prevention of neurologic sequelae (due to rapidly falling serum sodium and low serum sodium levels) is essential.

Primary Nursing Diagnosis   Electrolyte Imbalance: Sodium Losses*

Definition   Disturbance in the level of the body's sodium

Possibly Related to   Excessive secretion of ADH resulting in
- increased losses of sodium
- increased intake of water

*Non-NANDA diagnosis.

Primary Nursing Diagnosis: Electrolyte imbalance: sodium losses related to excessive secretion of ADH resulting in increased losses of sodium, increased intake of water

Assessment/Defining Characteristics of Child and/or Family (Subjective & Objective Data):

- Decreased serum sodium (usually less than 130 mEq/L)
- Dilutional hyperkalemia or normal potassium
- Loss of appetite
- Nausea/vomiting
- Headache

- Irritability
- Muscle twitching
- If serum sodium falls below 110 mEq/L: possibly personality changes, including hostility and confusion; possibly neurological abnormalities, such as stupor, seizures, and coma

Expected Outcomes	Possible Nursing Interventions	Rationale	Evaluation for Charting
Child will have adequate sodium balance as evidenced by • serum sodium from 138 to 145 mEq/L • serum potassium from 3.5 to 5.0 mEq/L • adequate urine output (state specific range; 1 to 2 ml/kg/hr) • appropriate level of conciseness for age • lack of nausea/vomiting • lack of signs/symptoms of decreased serum sodium (such as those listed under Assessment)	Assess and record • neurological status every 4 hours and PRN • IV fluids and condition of IV site every hour • laboratory values as indicated. Report any abnormalities to the physician. • signs/symptoms of decreased serum sodium (such as those listed under Assessment) every 4 hours and PRN	Provides information about neurologic, electrolyte, and fluid status of patient. It is necessary to record the amount of IV fluids every hour to make sure the child is not being over or under hydrated. The IV site needs to be assessed every hour for signs of redness or swelling.	Document neurological status. Document amount of IV fluids and describe condition of IV site along with any interventions needed. Document current laboratory values when indicated. Describe any signs/symptoms of electrolyte imbalance noted.
	Keep accurate record of intake and output. Restrict fluids, as indicated, and maintain negative water balance. (Output should exceed intake.)	Fluids may need to be restricted in order to normalize the serum sodium, normalize serum osmolality, and decrease extravascular fluid volume.	Document intake and output.
	If serum sodium is very low, 3% saline with potassium supplements, followed by a loop diuretic (such as furosemide) may be indicated. Assess and record child's response.	This treatment may be necessary in order to normalize the serum sodium, normalize serum osmolality, and decrease extravascular fluid volume.	Describe any therapeutic measures used to restore serum sodium balance. Document their effectiveness.
TEACHING GOALS Child and/or family will be able to verbalize at least 4 characteristics of electrolyte imbalance: sodium excess such as • loss of appetite • nausea/vomiting	Teach child/family about characteristics of electrolyte imbalance: sodium losses. Assess and record results.	Increased knowledge will assist the child/family in recognizing and reporting changes in the child's condition.	Document whether teaching was done and describe results.

Primary Nursing Diagnosis: Electrolyte Imbalance: Sodium Losses *(continued)*

Expected Outcomes	Possible Nursing Interventions	Rationale	Evaluation for Charting
• headache • irritability • lethargy • muscle twitching • personality changes			
Child and/or family will be able to verbalize knowledge of care such as • monitoring intake and output • fluid restriction • medication administration • identification of any signs/symptoms of electrolyte imbalance (such as those listed under Assessment) • when to contact health care provider	Teach child/family about care. Assess and record child's/family's knowledge of and participation in care regarding monitoring intake and output, fluid restriction, etc.	Education of child/family will allow for accurate care.	Document whether teaching was done and describe results.

Nursing Diagnosis   Excess Fluid Volume

Definition   Increase in the amount of circulating fluid volume (which can eventually lead to interstitial or intracellular fluid overload)

Possibly Related to   • Increased water reabsorption from renal tubules secondary to excessive ADH secretion

Nursing Diagnosis: Excess fluid volume related to increased water reabsorption from renal tubules secondary to excessive ADH secretion

Assessment/Defining Characteristics of Child and/or Family (Subjective & Objective Data):

- Decreased urine output
- Decreased serum osmolality (less than 273 mOsm/L)
- Decreased serum sodium (usually less than 130 mEq/L)
- Increased urine osmolality (greater than 900 mOsm/L)
- Urine osmolality inappropriately increased compared to serum osmolality
- Increased urine specific gravity (greater than 1.025)
- Increased urine sodium
- Positive water balance, with intake exceeding output
- Edema
- Sudden weight gain
- Irritability

(continued)

Nursing Diagnosis: Excess Fluid Volume *(continued)*

Expected Outcomes	Possible Nursing Interventions	Rationale	Evaluation for Charting
Child will resume appropriate fluid balance as evidenced by • adequate urine output (state specific range; 1 to 2 ml/kg/hr) • serum sodium from 138 to 145 mEq/L • serum osmolality from 280 to 295 mOsm/L • urine osmolality from 500 to 800 mOsm/L • urine specific gravity from 1.008 to 1.020 • lack of sudden 　1. weight gain 　2. edema 　3. irritability • lack of signs/symptoms of excess fluid volume (such as those listed under Assessment)	Keep accurate record of intake and output. Restrict fluid intake, as indicated, and maintain negative water balance, with output exceeding intake.	Fluids may need to be restricted in order to normalize the serum sodium, normalize serum osmolality, and decrease extravascular fluid volume.	Document intake and output.
	If serum sodium is very low, 3% saline with potassium supplements, followed by a loop diuretic (such as furosemide) may be indicated. Assess and record child's response.	This treatment may be necessary in order to normalize the serum sodium, normalize serum osmolality, and decrease extravascular fluid volume.	Describe any therapeutic measures used to restore serum sodium balance. Document their effectiveness.
	Assess and record • IV fluids and condition of IV site every hour • laboratory values as indicated. Report any abnormalities to the physician. • signs/symptoms of excess fluid volume (such as those listed under Assessment) every 4 hours and PRN	It is necessary to record the amount of IV fluids every hour to make sure the child is not being over or under hydrated. The IV site needs to be assessed every hour for signs of redness or swelling.	Document amount of IV fluids and describe condition of IV site along with any interventions needed. Document current laboratory values when indicated. Describe any signs/symptoms of excess fluid volume noted.
	Check and record urine specific gravity every 4 hours or as indicated.	Urine specific gravity provides information about hydration status.	Document range of urine specific gravity.
	Weigh child daily on same scale at same time of day. Document results and compare to previous weight.	Provides information about the child's fluid status. An increase in the weight can indicate fluid retention. A decrease in the weight can indicate dehydration.	Document weight and determine if it was an increase or decrease from the previous weight.
TEACHING GOALS Child and/or family will be able to verbalize at least 4 characteristics of excess fluid volume such as • decreased urine output • swelling • sudden weight gain • irritability	Teach child/family about characteristics of excess fluid volume. Assess and record results.	Increased knowledge will assist the child/family in recognizing and reporting changes in the child's condition.	Document whether teaching was done and describe results.

	Possible Nursing		Evaluation for
Expected Outcomes	**Interventions**	**Rationale**	**Charting**
Child and/or family will be able to verbalize knowledge of care such as • monitoring intake and output • fluid restriction • medication administration • identification of any signs/symptoms of excess fluid volume (such as those listed under Assessment) • when to contact health care provider	Teach child/family about care. Assess and record child's/family's knowledge of and participation in care regarding monitoring intake and output, fluid restriction, etc.	Education of child/family will allow for accurate care.	Document whether teaching was done and describe results.

Nursing Diagnosis: Excess Fluid Volume *(continued)*

Related Nursing Diagnoses

Altered Level of Consciousness* *related to* cerebral edema secondary to hyponatremia resulting from increased intracellular fluid

Compromised Family Coping *related to* child's underlying disease process

Deficient Knowledge: Child/Parental *related to*
  a. child's underlying disease process
  b. treatments and procedures

Disturbed Body Image *related to* edema and sudden weight gain

*Non-NANDA diagnosis.

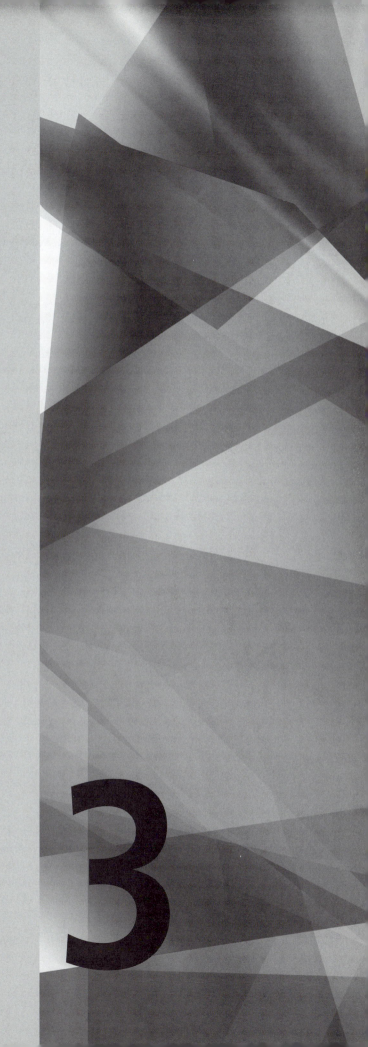

CARE OF CHILDREN WITH FLUID AND ELECTROLYTE IMBALANCE

3

ONE

BURNS
MEDICAL DIAGNOSIS

PATHOPHYSIOLOGY Thermal, electrical, chemical, and radioactive are the four main types of burn injuries. Children ages 4 and younger are at the greatest risk to suffer a burn injury. Their injury rate is twice that of children ages 5 to 14. Scald burns account for two thirds of burn injuries in children younger than 4 years of age. Ten percent of child abuse cases involve burning.

Five interrelated factors are used to determine the severity of a burn: extent of the burn, depth of the burn, age of the child, medical history of the child, and part of the body burned. The extent of the burn injury is determined by estimating the percent of skin area covered by burns, accounting for the changing body proportions and body surface area of the growing child. The degree of involvement of the epidermis, dermis, and underlying structures determines the depth of the burn. In partial-thickness burns, only part of the skin has been damaged; in full-thickness burns, all skin layers are destroyed, including hair follicles, sweat glands, sebaceous glands, and nerves. Subcutaneous tissue, muscle, and bone may also be destroyed.

First- and second-degree burns are partial-thickness burns. In first-degree burns, the epidermis is damaged, resulting in redness, pain, and possibly edema. The wound blanches with pressure, and there is no blistering. Usually, a first-degree burn is able to heal within a week. In a second-degree burn, the injury involves the epidermis and extends into the dermis, resulting in a cherry-red to glassy-white appearance, edema, blister formation, exudate, severe pain, and possible damage to cutaneous nerve endings. A second-degree burn can often heal within 1 to 3 weeks and is commonly caused by a scald injury. With first- and second-degree burns, capillaries, hair follicles, sebaceous glands, and some protective functions usually remain intact. Most partial-thickness burns are able to heal by reepithelialization, especially if protected from further injury and infection.

Third- and fourth-degree burns are full-thickness burns. Third-degree burns vary in appearance from pearly white, tan, or brown to mahogany or black. Blisters are not present, and these burns are rarely painful because nerve endings have been damaged or destroyed. (Often, second-degree burns are also present with full-thickness burns; therefore, the child is not pain free). The tissue of a full-thickness burn is called *eschar*.

Skin grafting is necessary as regeneration is not possible once the dermis and dermal structures are destroyed. Fourth-degree burns have the same characteristics as third-degree, but they extend into structures underlying the dermis, such as muscles, tendons, and bone.

Once the burn injury has occurred, the body responds almost immediately with the complications of burn shock, burn edema, and, if sustained, inhalation injury. Burn injuries result in increased capillary permeability; creating fluid, electrolyte, and protein loss into the interstitium. This leads to edema and possibly hypovolemic shock. Other, noninjured tissues can also swell when the burn exceeds 25% of the child's total body surface area. Various mediators (prostaglandins, histamine, oxygen radicals, etc.) stimulated by the burn injury also impair cardiac contractility and increase vascular resistance, which can contribute to not only hypovolemia and hypoperfusion, but also to tissue ischemia, renal failure, and cardiovascular collapse.

Within a few days of the burn injury the body responds with hypermetabolism, systemic inflammatory response syndrome (SIRS), and becomes at risk for sepsis. A burn injury produces a hypermetabolic state matched by no other disease. Hypermetabolism is characterized by increased use of oxygen, increased heat production, and accelerated protein breakdown, resulting in a negative nitrogen balance and depletion of body protein stores. The short- and long-term consequences of hypermetabolism are numerous, including weight loss, impaired growth, muscle wasting, impaired immunity, delayed wound healing, and increased risk of fractures. The hyperactive immune response to the burn injury causes a generalized inflammation, SIRS, which damages not only the burn wound, but also healthy tissue. Symptoms of SIRS can include tachycardia, tachypnea, leukocytosis, fever, hypotension, shock, or multisystem organ failure. In burn injuries, sepsis remains the leading cause of death, but the infected site is often the lungs and not the burn wound.

Management of children with burns includes fluid resuscitation to prevent shock and replace burn fluid losses, burn wound care, treating the child's pain, preventing infection, nutritional support, and preventing/treating complications. Psychosocial support of the child and family is essential.

Primary Nursing Diagnosis   Deficient Fluid Volume

Definition   Decrease in the amount of circulating fluid volume

Possibly Related to
- Fluid loss from burn wound
- Shift of fluid to interstitium

Primary Nursing Diagnosis: Deficient fluid volume related fluid loss from burn wound, shift of fluid to interstitium

Assessment/Defining Characteristics of Child and/or Family (Subjective & Objective Data):

- Edema
- Decreased urine output
- Tachycardia
- Tachypnea
- Hypotension
- Increased urine specific gravity
- Dry mucous membranes
- Decreased skin turgor (skin recoil greater than 2 to 3 seconds)

Expected Outcomes	Possible Nursing Interventions	Rationale	Evaluation for Charting
Child will have an adequate fluid volume as evidenced by • lack of edema • adequate urine output (state specific range; 1 to 2 ml/kg/hr) • adequate fluid intake, IV and oral (state specific amount of intake needed for each child) • heart rate, respiratory rate, and blood pressure within acceptable range (state specific range for each) • urine specific gravity from 1.008 to 1.020 • moist mucous membranes • rapid skin recoil (less than 2 to 3 seconds) • lack of signs/ symptoms of deficient fluid volume (such as those listed under Assessment)	Keep accurate record of intake and output. When indicated, encourage oral fluids.	Decreased urinary output may indicate burn injury to the vessels causing increased capillary permeability that results in fluid loss into the interstitium. This will cause decreased urine output.	Document intake and output.
	Assess and record • HR, RR, and BP every 4 hours • IV fluids and condition of IV site every hour • signs/symptoms of deficient fluid volume (such as those listed under Assessment) every 4 hours and PRN	Provides information about fluid status of patient. If patient has fluid volume deficit, the HR will increase at first, and eventually decrease. The RR will increase. The BP will eventually decrease. It is necessary to record the amount of IV fluids every hour to make sure the child is not being over or under hydrated. The IV site needs to be assessed every hour for signs of redness or swelling.	Document range of HR, RR, and BP. Document amount of IV fluids and describe condition of IV site along with any interventions needed. Describe any signs/ symptoms of deficient fluid volume noted.
	Check and record urine specific gravity with every void or as indicated.	Urine specific gravity provides information about hydration status.	Document range of urine specific gravity.

(continued)

Primary Nursing Diagnosis: Deficient Fluid Volume *(continued)*

Expected Outcomes	Possible Nursing Interventions	Rationale	Evaluation for Charting
	Assess and record condition of mucous membranes and skin turgor every shift and PRN.	Provides information on hydration status.	Describe status of mucous membranes and skin turgor.
	Weigh child daily on same scale at same time of day. Document results and compare to previous weight.	Changes in weight can indicate hydration status.	Document weight and determine if it was an increase or decrease from the previous weight.
	Provide mouth care every 4 hours and PRN. Record results.	Mouth care is needed because the child is prone to dehydration and dry mucous membranes.	Document whether mouth care was done and describe effectiveness.
TEACHING GOALS Child and/or family will be able to verbalize at least 4 characteristics of deficient fluid volume such as • swelling • decreased number of times child voids • rapid heart rate • dry mucous membranes	Teach child/family about characteristics of deficient fluid volume. Assess and record results.	Increased knowledge will assist the child/family in recognizing and reporting changes in the child's condition.	Document whether teaching was done and describe results.
Child and/or family will be able to verbalize knowledge of care such as • monitoring intake and output • identification of any signs/symptoms of deficient fluid volume (such as those listed under Assessment) • when to contact health care provider	Teach child/family about care. Assess and record child's/family's knowledge of and participation in care regarding monitoring intake and output, etc.	Education of child/family will allow for accurate care.	Document whether teaching was done and describe results.

Nursing Diagnosis   Acute Pain

Definition   Condition in which an individual experiences acute mild to severe pain.

Possibly Related to
- Thermal, electrical, chemical, or radioactive damage to or destruction of the skin and, sometimes, the underlying structures
- Burn dressing changes
- Exposed nerves

Nursing Diagnosis: Acute pain related to thermal, chemical, or radioactive damage to or destruction of the skin and sometimes, the underlying structures; burn dressing changes; exposed nerves

Assessment/Defining Characteristics of Child and/or Family (Subjective & Objective Data):

- Crying or moaning
- Facial grimacing
- Restlessness
- Guarding or protection behavior of burn site
- Physical signs/symptoms (tachycardia, tachypnea, increased blood pressure)
- Altered muscle tone (tenseness or listlessness)
- Verbal expression of pain
- Rating of pain on pain-assessment tool

Expected Outcomes	Possible Nursing Interventions	Rationale	Evaluation for Charting
Child will have decreased pain or be free of severe and/or constant pain as evidenced by • verbal communication of comfort • lack of 1. constant crying or moaning 2. grimacing 3. extreme restlessness 4. guarding or protective behavior of burn area • heart rate within acceptable range (state specific range) • respiratory rate within acceptable range (state specific range) • blood pressure within acceptable range (state specific range) • rating of decreased pain or no pain on pain-assessment tool	Assess and record HR, RR, BP, and any signs/symptoms of pain (such as those listed under Assessment) every 2 to 4 hours and PRN. Use age-appropriate pain-assessment tool.	Provides data regarding the level of pain child is experiencing.	Document range of HR, RR, BP, and degree of pain child was experiencing. Describe any successful measures used to decrease pain.
	Handle child gently.	Helps to minimize pain and promote comfort.	Document if child was handled gently and effectiveness of measure.
	When indicated, administer analgesics on schedule. Assess and record effectiveness.	Analgesics are administered to decrease pain.	Document whether analgesics were administered on schedule. Describe effectiveness and any side effects noted.
	Encourage family members to stay and comfort child when possible.	Helps to comfort and support the child.	Document whether family was able to remain with child and describe effectiveness of their presence.
	Allow family members to participate in care of child when possible.	This may increase the comfort level of the child and thus help child in managing pain.	Document whether family participated in care and if this was successful in helping child with pain management.

(continued)

Nursing Diagnosis: Acute Pain *(continued)*

Expected Outcomes	Possible Nursing Interventions	Rationale	Evaluation for Charting
• lack of signs/ symptoms of pain (such as those listed under Assessment)	Use diversional activities (e.g., music, television, playing games, relaxation) when appropriate.	Diversional activities can distract child and may help to decrease pain.	Document whether diversional activities were successful in helping to manage pain.
	If age appropriate, explain all procedures beforehand.	Allow child some control, which can assist child with pain management.	Describe if this measure was effective in helping child to manage pain.
	If age appropriate, allow the child to participate in planning his or her care. Encourage the child to practice self-care (e.g., bathing, removing dressing).	Allowing child some control can assist child with pain management.	Describe if this measure was effective in helping child to manage pain.
	When indicated, institute additional pain relief measures, such as hypnosis, guided imagery, bed cradle to keep linens off burn area, and special bed mattress. Assess and record effectiveness.	These nonpharmacologic measures may help decrease pain.	Document whether these measures were successful in helping to manage pain.
TEACHING GOALS Child and/or family will be able to verbalize at least 4 characteristics of pain such as • verbal communication of pain or tenderness • crying unrelieved by usual comfort measures • facial grimacing • rapid heart rate	Teach child/family about characteristics of pain. Assess and record results.	Increased knowledge will assist the child/ family in recognizing and reporting changes in the child's condition.	Document whether teaching was done and describe results.
Child and/or family will be able to verbalize knowledge of care such as • medication administration • appropriate diversional activities • identification of any signs/symptoms of pain (such as those listed under Assessment) • when to contact health care provider	Teach child/family about care. Assess and record child's/family's knowledge of and participation in care regarding medication administration, etc.	Education of child/ family will allow for accurate care.	Document whether teaching was done and describe results.

Related Nursing Diagnoses

Risk for Infection	*related to* a. impaired skin integrity b. decreased resistance
Impaired Skin Integrity	*related to* thermal, electrical, chemical, or radioactive injury
Imbalanced Nutrition: Less than Body Requirements	*related to* hypermetabolic state
Impaired Physical Mobility	*related to* a. pain b. dressings and splints
Compromised Family Coping	*related to* a. guilt b. hospitalization of child c. scar formation

TWO

DIARRHEA, DEHYDRATION, AND GASTROENTERITIS
MEDICAL DIAGNOSIS

PATHOPHYSIOLOGY Diarrhea is an increase in the number, frequency, and fluidity of stools. It can be either acute or chronic. The leading cause of illness in children under the age of 5 is acute diarrhea. Chronic diarrhea is defined as lasting longer than 2 weeks. Diarrhea has many different causes. Infection is a common one in children and can be bacterial, viral, or parasitical. The major cause of viral diarrhea is rotavirus. Many organisms are responsible for bacterial diarrhea, including *Campylobacter, Yersinia, Shigella, Salmonella, Staphylococcus aureus*, and *Escherichia coli*. One of the most common parasitic agents to cause diarrhea in children is *Giardia lamblia*. Other causes of diarrhea include food intolerance, such as an allergy to milk; ingestion of toxic substances, such as lead; drug intolerance, such as intolerance of antibiotics; bowel disease, such as Hirschsprung disease; disaccharide deficiencies, such as deficiency of lactase; psychogenic factors, such as emotional stress; malabsorption, such as cystic fibrosis; and localized infections, such as respiratory and urinary tract infections.

Chronic diarrhea is usually caused by chronic conditions such as inflammatory bowel disease, malabsorption syndromes, immune deficiency, food allergy, and lactose intolerance. Proper diagnosis and adequate mangement of the underlying disorder will help alleviate many of the consequences of diarrhea.

Diarrhea results when contents are propelled through the intestines very rapidly, with little time for absorption of digested food, water, and electrolytes. The resultant stool is watery, usually green, and contains undigested fats, undigested carbohydrates, and some undigested protein. Water loss can be up to 10 times the normal rate. Electrolyte imbalance may result with losses of sodium, chloride, bicarbonate, and potassium. Diarrhea resulting in dehydration can eventually lead to hypovolemic shock and can be life threatening in infants and young children.

Age, general health, climate, and environment are factors that can affect an individual's predisposition to diarrhea. Young children and children who are malnourished are more susceptible than others. Warm weather tends to make dehydration worse, and some organisms that cause diarrhea are more prevalent in warmer weather. Diarrhea also occurs more frequently where sanitation and refrigeration are problems and in overcrowded, substandard living conditions. Bowel habits vary considerably among individuals and must be considered when diagnosing diarrhea. Severe diarrhea is most common in infants and usually requires hospitalization.

The categorization of diarrhea can be related to the location in which it occurs along the alimentary tract. Inflammation of the stomach and intestines is called gastroenteritis; inflammation of the small intestines is enteritis; inflammation of the small intestines and colon is enterocolitis; and inflammation of the colon is colitis.

In acute infectious gastroenteritis, there is inflammation of the lining of the stomach and intestines due to an infection by a microorganism: viral, bacterial, or parasitical. Transmission of these organisms can be direct person-to-person contact (as with Shigella; Giardia, which is most common in toddlers; and rotavirus, which is most common in infants), through contaminated food or water (as with Salmonella, Escherichia coli, and Campylobacter), or through contact with family pets (as with Yersinia enterocolitica and Salmonella). Imbalance of the normal flora in the gastrointestinal tract can also cause gastroenteritis (as with C. Difficile). Traveler's diarrhea is most often caused by enterotoxigenic Escherichia coli.

Viral infections damage and destroy the epithelial cells that line the intestinal tract. Bacterial infections can damage the intestinal mucosa in one of three ways: (1) the organism multiplies and adheres to the mucosa, producing an enterotoxin that interacts with the bowel mucosa and causes active water and electrolyte secretion; (2) through an inflammatory process, organisms invade the cells in the epithelium; or (3) organisms multiply intracellularly and penetrate the gut wall. Multiplication of the pathogens may result in production of toxins that lead to fluid and electrolyte shifts. Decreased absorption along with increased secretion into the intestine is secondary to edema of the intestinal mucosa. This leads to diarrhea and dehydration.

Rotavirus is the single most important cause of severe acute gastroenteritis and dehydration in young children throughout the world. In underdeveloped countries where there is poor nutrition, it is a major cause of death of children. Almost all children have been infected by rotavirus by the time they reach 5 years of age, and most children are infected more than once. Severe gastroenteritis is more likely to develop with the initial infection. Rotavirus is primarily transmitted by the fecal-oral route. Rotavirus infection is characterized by vomiting and watery diarrhea. Fever is common. These 3 symptoms, combined with the child's inability to drink, leads to dehydration. Laboratory testing may be necessary to confirm the diagnosis. The key intervention for preventing rotavirus infection is vaccination.

Therapeutic management for rotavirus as well as many other types of diarrhea or gastroenteritis includes hydration, correction of electrolyte imbalance, and as necessary, antipyretics, medications to treat the underlying cause, dietary changes, and prevention of the spread of infection.

Primary Nursing Diagnosis   Deficient Fluid Volume

Definition   Decrease in the amount of circulating fluid volume

Possibly Related to
- An infection:
  - systemic (from a virus, bacteria, or a parasite)
  - local (e.g., respiratory or a urinary tract infection)
- Food intolerance (e.g., mild allergy)
- Drug intolerance (e.g., intolerance of antibiotics)
- Inflammatory bowel disease (e.g., ulcerative colitis)
- Malabsorption (e.g., cystic fibrosis)
- Psychogenic factors (e.g., stress)
- Inflammation of the lining of the stomach and intestine
- Invasion of the stomach and intestine by a microorganism (specify when indicated: viral, bacterial, or protozoal)

Primary Nursing Diagnosis: Deficient fluid volume related to
- an infection:
  1. systemic (from a virus, bacteria, or a parasite)
  2. local (e.g., respiratory or a urinary tract infection)
- food intolerance (e.g., mild allergy)
- drug intolerance (e.g., intolerance of antibiotics)
- inflammatory bowel disease (e.g., ulcerative colitis)
- malabsorption (e.g., cystic fibrosis)
- psychogenic factors (e.g., stress)
- inflammation of the lining of the stomach and intestines
- invasion of the stomach and intestine by a microorganism (specify when indicated: viral, bacterial, or protozoa)

Assessment/Defining Characteristics of Child and/or Family (Subjective & Objective Data):
- Loose, watery stools (can be yellow or green and may contain mucus, pus, blood, and/or sugar)
- Nausea/vomiting
- Abdominal cramping
- Abdominal distention
- Hyperactive bowel sounds
- Weight loss
- Sunken fontanel
- Sunken eyeballs
- Dry mucous membranes
- Decreased skin turgor (skin recoil greater than 2 to 3 seconds)
- Dry mucous membranes
- Decreased urine output
- Increased urine specific gravity
- Fever
- Tachycardia
- Tachypnea
- Hypotension

(continued)

Primary Nursing Diagnosis: Deficient Fluid Volume *(continued)*

Expected Outcomes	Possible Nursing Interventions	Rationale	Evaluation for Charting

Child will have an adequate fluid volume as evidenced by
 	
• adequate fluid intake, IV and oral (state specific amount of intake needed for each child)
• absence of
  1. diarrhea
  2. mucus, pus, blood, and sugar in stool
  3. nausea/vomiting
  4. abdominal cramping and distention
  5. sunken eyeballs
• normal activity of bowel sounds (one every 10 to 30 seconds)
• regaining of weight loss during illness
• flat fontanel
• moist mucous membranes
• rapid skin recoil (less than 2 to 3 seconds)
• adequate urine output (state specific range; 1 to 2 ml/kg/hr)
• Urine specific gravity from 1.008 to 1.020
• Temperature within acceptable range of 36.5°C to 37.2°C
• Heart rate, blood pressure, and respiratory rate within acceptable range (state specific range for each)
• Lack of signs/symptoms of deficient fluid volume (such as those listed under Assessment)
	Keep accurate record of intake and output. Record frequency and characteristics of stools. Measure and record amount and characteristics of any vomitus. If indicated, offer fluids by mouth. Record amount taken and child's tolerance of fluid.	Provides information on child's hydration status. Decreased urine output can indicate dehydration. Characteristics of stools and/or vomitus can help to identify the etiology of the disease.	Document intake and output. Describe characteristics of stools or vomitus.

	Assess and record • HR, RR, BP, and T every 4 hours and PRN • IV fluids and condition of IV site every hour • laboratory values as indicated. Report any abnormalities to the physician. • bowel sounds every shift and PRN • signs/symptoms of deficient fluid volume (such as those listed under Assessment) every 4 hours and PRN	Provides information about fluid status of patient. If patient has deficient fluid volume, the HR will increase at first, and eventually decrease. The RR will increase. The BP will eventually decrease. The T may increase due to the organism causing the disease state. The bowel sounds will be hyperactive in the presence of diarrhea or gastroenteritis. It is necessary to record the amount of IV fluids every hour to make sure the child is not being over or under hydrated. The IV site needs to be assessed every hour for signs of redness or swelling.	Document range of HR, RR, BP, and T. Document amount of IV fluids and describe condition of IV site along with any interventions needed. Document bowel sounds. Document current laboratory values when indicated. Describe any signs/symptoms of deficient fluid volume noted.
	Weigh child daily on same scale at same time of day. Document results and compare to previous weight.	Decrease in weight may be due to increased fluid loss in the stool and indicates the child's hydration status.	Document weight and determine if it was an increase or decrease from the previous weight.
	Check and record urine specific gravity with every void or as indicated.	Urine specific gravity provides information about hydration status.	Document range of urine specific gravity.
	Assess and record condition of mucous membranes and skin turgor every shift and PRN.	Provides information on hydration status.	Describe status of mucous membranes and skin turgor.

Primary Nursing Diagnosis: Deficient Fluid Volume *(continued)*

Expected Outcomes	Possible Nursing Interventions	Rationale	Evaluation for Charting
	Report any of the following to the physician • frequent stooling (more than 3 times in 8 hours) • large amount of vomitus • IV fluids infiltrated and unable to restart	Frequent stooling and large amounts of vomitus can lead to dehydration. IV fluids are critical to sustain adequate hydration.	Describe amount and characteristics of stools and vomitus. Document amount of IV fluids and describe condition of IV site along with any interventions needed.
	Provide mouth care every 4 hours and PRN.	Mouth care is necessary to counteract the dry mucous membranes.	Document whether mouth care was done and describe effectiveness.
TEACHING GOALS Child and/or family will be able to verbalize at least 4 characteristics of deficient fluid volume such as • loose, watery stools • nausea/vomiting • abdominal cramping • abdominal distention • weight loss • decreased urine output • fever	Teach child/family about characteristics of deficient fluid volume. Assess and record results.	Increased knowledge will assist the child/family in recognizing and reporting changes in the child's condition.	Document whether teaching was done and describe results.
Child and/or family will be able to verbalize knowledge of care such as • child's need for appropriate fluids • monitoring intake and output • identification of any signs/symptoms of deficient fluid volume (such as those listed under Assessment) • when to contact health care provider	Teach child/family about care. Assess and record child's/family's knowledge of and participation in care regarding child's need for appropriate fluids, monitoring intake and output, etc.	Education of child/family will allow for accurate care.	Document whether teaching was done and describe results.

Nursing Diagnosis   Risk for Spread of Infection*

Definition   Condition in which the body is invaded by microorganisms that can be transmitted by direct contact

Possibly Related to
- Direct person-to-person contact with infected individual
- Centers that care for children in diapers (e.g., day care, pediatric units)

*Non-NANDA diagnosis.

Nursing Diagnosis: Risk for spread of infection related to direct person-to-person contact with infected individual, centers that care for children in diapers (e.g., day care, pediatric units)

Assessment/Defining Characteristics of Child and/or Family (Subjective & Objective Data)

- Diarrhea
- Vomiting
- Fever
- Tachycardia
- Tachypnea
- Hypotension

Expected Outcomes	Possible Nursing Interventions	Rationale	Evaluation for Charting
Child's infection will not spread to others.	Maintain good hand-washing technique.	Good hand washing is the single most important measure in decreasing spread of infection.	Document whether good hand-washing technique was used.
Child will be free of infection as evidenced by • temperature within acceptable range of 36.5°C to 37.2°C • heart rate within acceptable range (state specific range) • respiratory rate within acceptable range (state specific range) • blood pressure within acceptable range (state specific range)	When indicated, maintain isolation of child according to hospital policy.	Isolating child from others can decrease the spread of infection.	Document whether isolation of child was instituted in accordance with hospital policy.
	Assess and record T, HR, RR, and BP every 4 hours and PRN.	If infection is present, the T, HR, and RR will increase and the BP may decrease.	Document range of T, HR, RR, and BP.
	Maintain infection control protocol of hospital when dealing with body fluids (e.g., vomitus, stools).	Keeping soiled items contained helps to decrease spread of infection.	Document whether disposal of body fluids was done according to hospital protocol.
TEACHING GOALS Child and/or family will be able to verbalize at least 3 characteristics to decrease spread of infection such as • good hand-washing technique • temporary isolation of child from others • sanitary management of body fluids	Teach child/family about characteristics of risk for spread of infection. Assess and record results.	Increased knowledge will assist the child/family in recognizing and reporting changes in the child's condition.	Document whether teaching was done and describe results.

Nursing Diagnosis: Risk for Spread of Infection *(continued)*			
Expected Outcomes	**Possible Nursing Interventions**	**Rationale**	**Evaluation for Charting**
Child and/or family will be able to verbalize knowledge of care such as • good hand-washing technique • proper disposal of soiled items. • identification of any signs/symptoms of spread of infection (such as those listed under Assessment) • when to contact health care provider	Teach child/family about care. Assess and record child's/family's knowledge of and participation in care regarding good hand-washing technique, etc.	Education of child/family will allow for accurate care.	Document whether teaching was done and describe results.

Related Nursing Diagnoses

Electrolyte Imbalance: Sodium Losses and Potassium Losses*	*related to* a. diarrhea b. vomiting
Imbalanced Nutrition: Less than Body Requirements	*related to* a. diarrhea b. vomiting c. increased intestinal mobility
Impaired Skin Integrity	*related to* a. frequent perineal contact with acid stool b. superinfecton of skin related to antibiotic therapy
Acute Pain	*related to* a. abdominal cramping b. abdominal distention c. impaired skin integrity secondary to frequent perineal contact with acid stools
Compromised Family Coping	*related to* hospitalization of child

*Non-NANDA diagnosis.

CARE OF
CHILDREN WITH
GASTROINTESTINAL
DYSFUNCTION

4

ONE

APPENDICITIS
MEDICAL DIAGNOSIS

PATHOPHYSIOLOGY The vermiform appendix is a blind sac located at the end of the cecum and serves no apparent function. Appendicitis, an inflammation of the vermiform appendix, is the most common surgical emergency of childhood, occurring most frequently in older children and adolescents. The walls of the appendix become inflamed when there is a physical obstruction of the lumen. This obstruction can be due to a hard, impacted mass of feces (fecalith), a parasitic infection, stenosis, hyperplasia of lymphoid tissue, tumors, or anatomic defects in the cecum. Obstruction leads to increased intraluminal pressure and distention, which causes compression and ischemia of the mucosal vessels. This compromised blood supply can lead to ulceration and bacterial invasion. Necrosis follows and can result in perforation or rupture, which allows feces and bacteria to escape and contaminate the peritoneal cavity causing peritonitis.

The signs and symptoms of appendicitis are diverse, but the most common findings in children are right lower quadrant pain (McBurney's point), abdominal tenderness, guarding, and vomiting. Other symptoms can include diarrhea, periumbilical pain, fever, and reduced activity. The incidence of rupture in children is higher than in the general adult population (approximately 30–65%), due to the difficulty in evaluating abdominal pain in children. Also, in children, general peritonitis is more common than walled-off abscesses because the omentum is less developed. Ultrasonography and/or computed tomography (CT) with contrast are usually ordered to assist with diagnosis. The earlier appendicitis can be diagnosed, the better the outcome.

Treatment for appendicitis consists of antibiotics, intravenous fluids and electrolytes, and laparotomy for surgical removal of the appendix. Nonperforated acute appendicitis can be treated with laparoscopic surgery. For the child with a ruptured appendix, along with the above treatment, a nasogastric tube may be inserted preoperatively to decompress the gastrointestinal tract. Postoperatively, this child may retain the nasogastric tube until intestinal motility returns and the wound may be left open with a drain. Wound irrigations and wet–to–dry dressings may be ordered to prevent wound infection and abscess formation. Since any sudden, acute illness requiring surgery can be very stressful, psychosocial support for the child and family is imperative.

Postoperative Nursing Care Plan

Primary Nursing Diagnosis   Risk for Further Infection*

Definition Condition in which the body is at risk for being invaded by additional microorganisms

Possibly Related to
- Presence of invading organisms
- Surgical wound
- Compromised postoperative condition
- Spread of organisms to peritoneum

*Non-NANDA diagnosis.

Primary Nursing Diagnosis: Risk for further infection related to presence of invading organism, surgical wound, compromised preoperative condition, spread of organism to peritoneum

Assessment/Defining Characteristics of Child and/or Family (Subjective & Objective Data):

- Fever
- Tachycardia
- Tachypnea
- Hypotension
- Redness
- Swelling
- Purulent wound drainage
- Foul odor
- Lethargy
- Irritability
- Altered white blood cell count (WBC)

Expected Outcomes	Possible Nursing Interventions	Rationale	Evaluation for Charting
Child will be free of infection as evidenced by • temperature within acceptable range of 36.5°C to 37.2°C • heart rate within acceptable range (state specific range) • respiratory rate within acceptable range (state specific range) • blood pressure within acceptable range (state specific range) • wound with minimal clear to serosanguineous drainage • WBC within acceptable range (state specific range) • lack of signs/symptoms of infection (such as those listed under Assessment)	Assess and record T, HR, RR, BP, and any signs/symptoms of infection (such as those listed under Assessment) every 4 hours and PRN.	If infection is present, the T, HR, and RR will increase and the BP may decrease.	Document range of T, HR, RR, and BP. Describe any signs/symptoms of infection noted.
	Maintain good hand-washing technique.	Good hand washing is the single most important measure in decreasing infection.	Document whether good hand-washing technique was used.
	Ensure that wound care is done using aseptic technique.	Aseptic technique is needed to help decrease introduction of pathogens.	Document whether aseptic technique was used during wound care.
	Assess and record amount and characteristics of wound drainage every shift and PRN.	The wound site should have minimal redness and edema. Increase in redness or edema can indicate an infection is present. A change in color of wound drainage (from clear or serosanguineous to yellow, green, etc.) or a change in character of the drainage (from thin minimal amount to copious, thick, foul-smelling drainage) can indicate the presence of an infection.	Describe wound site including amount and characteristics of any drainage.
	If indicated, obtain culture specimens (wound, blood). Check results and notify physician of any abnormalities.	Cultures can indicate if pathogens are present.	Document results of any cultures if available.

(continued)

Primary Nursing Diagnosis: Risk for Further Infection *(continued)*

Expected Outcomes	Possible Nursing Interventions	Rationale	Evaluation for Charting
	Check and record results of WBC. Notify physician if results are out of the acceptable range.	Abnormal WBC results may indicate an infection.	Document WBC results if available.
	Reposition child as indicated. A low Fowler's position will help to localize infection and keep it from spreading upward.	Localizes drainage and helps to decrease spread of infection.	Document how often child was repositioned.
	Administer antibiotics on schedule. Assess and record any side effects (e.g., rash, diarrhea).	Antibiotics are given to combat infection or prophylactically to decrease the chance of getting a further infection.	Document whether antibiotics were administered on schedule. Describe any side effects noted.
	When indicated, administer antipyretics on schedule. Assess and record effectiveness.	Antipyretics are used to reduce fever.	Document whether an antipyretic was needed and describe effectiveness.
	Maintain infection control protocol of hospital when dealing with body fluids (wound drainage).	Keeping soiled items contained helps to decrease spread of infection.	Document whether disposal of body fluids was done according to hospital protocol.
TEACHING GOALS Child and/or family will be able to verbalize at least 4 characteristics of further infection such as • fever • purulent wound drainage • foul odor • lethargy	Teach child/family about characteristics of risk for further infection. Assess and record results.	Increased knowledge will assist the child/family in recognizing and reporting changes in the child's condition.	Document whether teaching was done and describe results.
Child and/or family will be able to verbalize knowledge of care such as • good hand-washing technique • fever control • medication administration • identification of any signs/symptoms of further infection (such as those listed under Assessment) • when to contact health-care provider	Teach child/family about care. Assess and record child's/family's knowledge of and participation in care regarding good hand-washing technique, fever control, medication administration, etc.	Education of child/family will allow for accurate care.	Document whether teaching was done and describe results.

Nursing Diagnosis Deficient Fluid Volume

Definition Decrease in the amount of circulating fluid volume

Possibly Related to
- Nausea/vomiting
- Inability to tolerate oral fluids
- Nasogastric suctioning
- Third spacing of body fluid

Nursing Diagnosis: Deficient fluid volume related to nausea/vomiting, inability to tolerate oral fluids, nasogastric suctioning, third spacing of body fluid

Assessment/Defining Characteristics of Child and/or Family (Subjective & Objective Data):

- Tachycardia
- Tachypnea
- Hypotension
- Abdominal distention
- Prolonged absence of bowel sounds
- Nausea/vomiting
- Dry mucous membranes
- Decreased skin turgor (skin recoil greater than 2 to 3 seconds)
- Decreased urine output
- Increased urine specific gravity

Expected Outcomes	Possible Nursing Interventions	Rationale	Evaluation for Charting
Child will have adequate fluid volume as evidenced by • adequate fluid intake, IV and oral (state specific amount of intake needed for each child) • heart rate, respiratory rate, and blood pressure within acceptable range (state specific range for each) • nondistended abdomen • presence of bowel sounds • absence of nausea/vomiting • moist mucous membranes • adequate urine output (state specific range; 1 to 2 ml/kg/hr) • rapid skin recoil (less than 2 to 3 seconds) • urine specific gravity from 1.008 to 1.020	Keep accurate record of intake and output.	Provides information on child's hydration status.	Document intake and output.
	If indicated, keep NPO or offer oral fluids when bowel sounds are present.	Oral fluids need to be restricted until peristalsis has returned postoperatively in order to prevent abdominal distention.	Describe tolerance of oral fluids.
	Assess and record • IV fluids and condition of IV site every hour • HR, RR, and BP every 4 hours and PRN • bowel sounds every 4 hours and PRN • any signs/symptoms of deficient fluid volume every 4 hours and PRN	Provides information about fluid status of patient. If patient has deficient fluid volume, the HR will increase at first, and eventually decrease. The RR will increase. The BP will eventually decrease. The bowel sounds will be hypoactive in the postoperative period until peristalsis returns. It is necessary to record the amount of IV fluids every hour to make sure the child is not being over or under hydrated. The IV site needs to be assessed every hour for signs of redness or swelling.	Document range of HR, RR, and BP. Document amount of IV fluids and describe condition of IV site along with any interventions needed. Document bowel sounds. Describe any signs/symptoms of deficient fluid volume noted.

(continued)

Nursing Diagnosis: Deficient Fluid Volume (*continued*)

Expected Outcomes	Possible Nursing Interventions	Rationale	Evaluation for Charting
• lack of signs/ symptoms of deficient fluid volume (such as those listed under Assessment)	If indicated, measure and record abdominal girth every shift and PRN.	An increase in abdominal girth indicates abdominal distention, which can be an early sign of infection.	When indicated, document current abdominal girth and determine whether it has increased since the previous measurement.
	If indicated, ensure that nasogastric tube is patent and connected to low intermittent suction. Measure and record drainage. Irrigate as indicated.	A nasogastric tube is used to provide gastric drainage.	Describe amount and characteristics of naso-gastric drainage.
	Check and record urine specific gravity with every void or as indicated.	Urine specific gravity provides information about hydration status.	Document range of urine specific gravity.
	Assess and record condition of mucous membranes and skin turgor every shift and PRN.	Provides information on hydration status.	Describe status of mucous membranes and skin turgor.
TEACHING GOALS Child and/or family will be able to verbalize at least 4 characteristics of deficient fluid volume such as • abdominal distention • nausea/vomiting • dry mucous membranes • decreased urine output	Teach child/family about characteristics of defi-cient fluid volume. Assess and record results.	Increased knowledge will assist the child/ family in recognizing and reporting changes in the child's condition.	Document whether teaching was done and describe results.
Child and/or family will be able to verbalize knowledge of care such as • child's need for appropriate fluids • monitoring intake and output • identification of any signs/symptoms of deficient fluid volume (such as those listed under Assessment) • when to contact health-care provider	Teach child/family about care. Assess and record child's/family's knowl-edge of and participation in care regarding child's need for appropriate fluids, monitoring intake and output, etc.	Education of child/ family will allow for accurate care.	Document whether teaching was done and describe results.

Related Nursing Diagnoses

Acute Pain	*related to* a. surgical incision b. invasive procedures
Compromised Family Coping	*related to* a. surgical procedure b. child's hospitalization c. emergency nature of the illness
Electrolyte Imbalance (Specify)*	*related to* a. fluid volume deficit b. loss of electrolytes from nasogastric suctioning
Altered Nutrition: Less than Body Requirements	*related to* a. nausea/vomiting b. inability to tolerate food or fluids by mouth
Fear: Child	*related to* a. pain b. hospitalization c. unfamiliar surroundings d. forced contact with strangers e. treatments and procedures

*Non-NANDA diagnosis.

TWO

BOWEL OBSTRUCTION
MEDICAL DIAGNOSIS

PATHOPHYSIOLOGY Obstruction of the bowel occurs when either a disturbance in the muscular contractility of the bowel or a decrease/occlusion in the patency of the lumen of the bowel mechanically hinders the passage of intestinal contents. Surgical intervention is often necessary to correct the obstruction. The child's postoperative recovery is directly related to the preoperative state of the bowel, the presence of intraperitoneal infection, and whether or not an anastomosis was performed.

Intussusception

Intussusception is a telescoping of a portion of the intestine into a distal portion of the intestine. It is the most common intestinal obstruction in children ages 3 months to 5 years. It most commonly occurs between 6 and 11 months of age. The ileocecal valve is the most common site for intussusception to occur. In most cases of intussusception, the cause is unknown; other possibilities include Meckel's diverticulum, an ileal polyp, lymphosarcoma, and adenovirus infections. The lumen of the bowel involved in the intussusception is partially obstructed and the vascular flow (venous return) compromised, resulting in inflammation, edema, and bleeding. When complete bowel obstruction occurs, strangulation of the bowel can result with obstruction of arterial flow. If untreated, intussusception causes intestinal gangrene, perforation, peritonitis, and/or death. Prognosis is directly related to the duration of the intussusception prior to treatment.

The onset of intussusception is often sudden. The infant or child has paroxysmal attacks of severe, colicky abdominal pain accompanied by crying or screaming, and vomiting. The knees are drawn up to the chest and the infant/child can be restless, diaphoretic, and/or pale. Between the attacks of abdominal pain, the child may at first show no abnormal signs. As the condition worsens, the child becomes lethargic and weak. The abdomen becomes distended, vomitus may be bile stained, and the presence of blood and mucus gives the stool a currant-jelly-like appearance. Eventually, the child may present in a shock-like state, with a weak, thready pulse, shallow respirations, grunting, and a fever as high as 41°C.

Intussusception reduction is usually an emergency procedure. If the child is not exhibiting signs of shock, peritonitis, or perforation, the intussusception may be reduced by the hydrostatic pressure of air or a barium enema. Ultrasonography can be used to assist with the enema. If surgical intervention is necessary, manual reduction is first attempted. If the intussusception is not reducible by surgical manipulation, the involved bowel must be resected.

Malrotation and Volvulus

Malrotation occurs when the fetal bowel fails to rotate into its normal position. In most cases of malrotation, the cecum fails to move to the right lower quadrant and can eventually cause obstruction. Obstruction occurs if the duodenum becomes trapped behind peritoneal bands, anchoring the abnormally placed cecum, or if the mesentery of the small intestine is not attached properly, allowing twisting of the intestine upon itself. This twisting is called volvulus. It can cause the bowel's blood supply to be compromised, resulting in bowel necrosis.

Children with malrotation of the gut and with volvulus usually present as 1) a neonate with a sudden onset of bilious vomiting and abdominal pain, 2) an infant in the first few months of life with a history of bile-stained emesis after feedings, that now appears like a bowel obstruction, or 3) an older infant or child with failure to thrive and severe feeding intolerance. Abdominal distention may not be present early on, but radiographic films of the abdomen will show multiple distended bowel loops and a large bowel devoid of gas. In some cases of volvulus, vascular collapse occurs so rapidly that the child presents in shock preceded by vomiting but with few other abdominal findings. The sooner the child goes to surgery, the lower the morbidity and mortality of this condition.

After correction of fluid and electrolyte disturbances and/or shock, a laparotomy is performed. Prior to surgery, a nasogastric tube may be placed and antibiotics given to cover gram-positive, gram-negative, and anaerobic flora. During surgery the volvulus is untwisted, the bands between the cecum and the abdominal wall are divided, and the large intestine is straightened. Bowel resection and a jejunostomy or ileostomy may be necessary if a large portion of the bowel has been compromised.

Primary Nursing Diagnosis   Deficient Fluid Volume

Definition   Decrease in the amount of circulating fluid volume

Possibly Related to
- Vomiting
- Third spacing of fluid secondary to infection
- Nasogastric drainage
- Inability to tolerate oral fluids

Primary Nursing Diagnosis: Deficient fluid volume related to vomiting, third spacing of fluid secondary to infection, nasogastric drainage, inability to tolerate oral fluids

Assessment/Defining Characteristics of Child and/or Family (Subjective & Objective Data):

- Vomiting
- Dry mucous membranes
- Decreased skin turgor (skin recoil greater than 2 to 3 seconds)
- Decreased urine output
- Increased urine specific gravity
- Tachycardia
- Tachypnea
- Hypotension
- Sunken fontanel
- Prolonged absence of bowel sounds
- Absence of tears when crying

Expected Outcomes	Possible Nursing Interventions	Rationale	Evaluation for Charting
Child will have adequate fluid volume as evidenced by - adequate fluid intake, IV and oral (state specific amount of intake needed for each child) - heart rate, respiratory rate, and blood pressure within acceptable range (state specific range for each) - moist mucous membranes - rapid skin recoil (less than 2 to 3 seconds) - adequate urine output (state specific range; 1 to 2 ml/kg/hr) - urine specific gravity from 1.008 to 1.020 - absence of vomiting - nondistended abdomen	Keep accurate record of intake and output.	Provides information on child's hydration status.	Document intake and output.
	Assess and record - IV fluids and condition of IV site every hour - HR, RR, and BP every 4 hours and PRN - bowel sounds every 4 hours and PRN - any signs/symptoms of deficient fluid volume (such as those listed under Assessment) every 4 hours and PRN	Provides information about fluid status of patient. If patient has deficient fluid volume, the HR will increase at first, and eventually decrease. The RR will increase. The BP will eventually decrease. The bowel sounds will be hypoactive in the postoperative period until peristalsis returns. It is necessary to record the amount of IV fluids every hour to make sure the child is not being over or under hydrated. The IV site needs to be assessed every hour for signs of redness or swelling.	Document range of HR, RR, and BP. Document amount of IV fluids and describe condition of IV site along with any interventions needed. Describe bowel sounds and any signs/symptoms of deficient fluid volume noted.

(continued)

Primary Nursing Diagnosis: Deficient Fluid Volume *(continued)*

Expected Outcomes	Possible Nursing Interventions	Rationale	Evaluation for Charting
• flat fontanel • presence of bowel sounds • presence of tears when crying • lack of signs/symptoms of deficient fluid volume (such as those listed under Assessment)	When indicated, • keep NPO. • ensure that nasogastric tube is patent and connected to low inter-mittent suction or to gravity drainage. Irrigate to maintain patency. Measure and record drainage. • replace nasogastric tube output with indicated type and amount of IV fluids. • start child on clear liquids (after the return of bowel function) and advance as tolerated.	A nasogastric tube is used to provide gastric drainage.	Document whether child was NPO or record amount and tolerance of any liquids. Describe amount and characteristics of nasogastric drainage.
	If indicated, measure and record abdominal girth every shift and PRN.	An increase in abdominal girth indicates abdominal distention.	When indicated, document current abdominal girth and determine whether it has increased since the previous measurement.
	Check and record urine specific gravity with every void or as indicated.	Urine specific gravity provides information about hydration status.	Document range of urine specific gravity.
	When indicated, administer IV colloids followed by IV diuretics on schedule. Assess and record effectiveness.	Colloids are administered for the purpose of allowing extravascular fluid to return to the vascular system. Diuretics are then given in order to rid the body of fluid overload.	In indicated, describe effectiveness of colloids and diuretics.
TEACHING GOALS Child and/or family will be able to verbalize at least 4 characteristics of deficient fluid volume such as • abdominal distention • nausea/vomiting • dry mucous membranes • decreased urine output	Teach child/family about characteristics of deficient fluid volume. Assess and record results.	Increased knowledge will assist the child/family in recognizing and reporting changes in the child's condition.	Document whether teaching was done and describe results.

Primary Nursing Diagnosis: Deficient Fluid Volume *(continued)*

Expected Outcomes	Possible Nursing Interventions	Rationale	Evaluation for Charting
Child and/or family will be able to verbalize knowledge of care such as • child's need for appropriate fluids • monitoring intake and output • identification of any signs/symptoms of deficient fluid volume (such as those listed under Assessment) • when to contact health-care provider	Teach child/family about care. Assess and record child's/family's knowledge of and participation in care regarding child's need for appropriate fluids, monitoring intake and output, etc.	Education of child/family will allow for accurate care.	Document whether teaching was done and describe results.

Nursing Diagnosis   Risk for Infection

Definition   Condition in which the body is at risk for being invaded by microorganisms

Possibly Related to
- Necrotic bowel and/or the release of intestinal contents into the peritoneal cavity, which may cause peritonitis
- Presence of invading organisms
- Surgical wound
- Compromised preoperative and postoperative condition

Nursing Diagnosis: Risk for infection related to necrotic bowel and/or the release of intestinal contents into the peritoneal cavity, which may cause peritonitis; presence of invading microorganisms; surgical wound; compromised preoperative and postoperative condition

Assessment/Defining Characteristics of Child and/or Family (Subjective & Objective Data):
- Fever
- Tachycardia
- Tachypnea
- Hypotension
- Abdominal pain and/or tenderness
- Abdominal distention
- Lethargy
- Diminished or absent bowel sounds
- Vomiting
- Diaphoresis
- Increased white blood cell count (WBC)
- Pallor

(continued)

Nursing Diagnosis: Risk for Infection *(continued)*

Expected Outcomes	Possible Nursing Interventions	Rationale	Evaluation for Charting

Child will be free of infection as evidenced by
 	
• body temperature within acceptable range of 36.5°C to 37.2°C
• heart rate within acceptable range (state specific range)
• respiratory rate within acceptable range (state specific range)
• blood pressure within acceptable range (state specific range)
• lack of abdominal pain/tenderness
• WBC within acceptable range (state specific range)
• presence of bowel sounds
• lack of
  1. lethargy
  2. diaphoresis
  3. vomiting
  4. pallor
• lack of signs/symptoms of infection (such as those listed under Assessment)
	Assess and record T, HR, RR, BP, and any signs/symptoms of infection (such as those listed under Assessment) every 4 hours and PRN.	If infection is present, the T, HR, and RR will increase and the BP may decrease.	Document range of T, HR, RR, and BP. Describe any signs/symptoms of infection noted.

	Maintain good hand-washing technique.	Good hand washing is the single most important measure in decreasing infection.	Document whether good hand-washing technique was used.
	Check and record results of WBC. Notify physician if results are out of the acceptable range.	Abnormal WBC results may indicate an infection.	Document WBC results if available.
	Administer antibiotics on schedule. Assess and record any side effects (e.g., rash, diarrhea).	Antibiotics are given to combat infection or prophylactically to decrease the chance of getting a further infection.	Document whether antibiotics were administered on schedule. Describe any side effects noted.
	When indicated, administer antipyretics on schedule. Assess and record effectiveness.	Antipyretics are used to reduce fever.	Document whether an antipyretic was needed and describe effectiveness.
	Maintain infection control protocol of hospital when dealing with body fluids.	Keeping soiled items contained helps to decrease spread of infection.	Document whether disposal of body fluids was done according to hospital protocol.
TEACHING GOALS Child and/or family will be able to verbalize at least 4 characteristics of infection such as • fever • purulent wound drainage • foul odor • lethargy	Teach child/family about characteristics of risk for infection. Assess and record results.	Increased knowledge will assist the child/family in recognizing and reporting changes in the child's condition.	Document whether teaching was done and describe results.

Nursing Diagnosis: Risk for Infection *(continued)*

Expected Outcomes	Possible Nursing Interventions	Rationale	Evaluation for Charting
Child and/or family will be able to verbalize knowledge of care such as • good hand-washing technique • fever control • identification of any signs/symptoms of infection (such as those listed under Assessment) • when to contact health-care provider	Teach child/family about care. Assess and record child's/family's knowledge of and participation in care regarding good hand-washing technique, fever control, etc.	Education of child/family will allow for accurate care.	Document whether teaching was done and describe results.

Related Nursing Diagnoses

Electrolyte Imbalance (Specify)* *related to*
    a. vomiting
    b. intestinal obstruction
    c. necrotic bowel

Pain *related to*
    a. intestinal vascular compromise
    b. intestinal obstruction

Ineffective Tissue Perfusion (GI) *related to*
    a. intestinal vascular compromise
    b. intestinal obstruction

Anxiety: Child/Parental *related to*
    a. pain of the child
    b. emergency surgery
    c. outcome of the surgery

Fear: Child *related to*
    a. pain
    b. hospitalization
    c. treatments and procedures
    d. surgery
    e. forced contact with strangers
    f. unfamiliar surroundings

Compromised Family Coping *related to*
    a. situational health crisis of child
    b. surgery
    c. hospitalization

*Non-NANDA diagnosis.

| THREE |

CLEFT LIP AND CLEFT PALATE
MEDICAL DIAGNOSIS

PATHOPHYSIOLOGY Cleft lip and cleft palate occur early in pregnancy when the sides of the lips and roof of the mouth do not fuse together as they should. Cleft lip and cleft palate are the most common of all facial anomalies, occurring in about 1 of 700 births in the United States. They may occur together or separately. Cleft lip, with or without cleft palate, is more common in boys than in girls. Isolated cleft palate occurs more often in girls. The etiology of cleft lip and cleft palate is multifactorial; genetics as well as many environmental factors can be involved. Parents with a family history of a cleft are at higher risk of having an infant with a cleft. Environmental factors putting an infant at higher risk for developing a cleft include exposure in early pregnancy to cigarette smoke, alcohol, illicit drugs, medications, or herbal remedies. Cleft lip and/or cleft palate can be part of a number of syndromes.

Cleft lip results when the nasal and maxillary processes do not fuse during embryonic development. It can be detected prenatally by ultrasound at 13 to 16 weeks gestation. Cleft lip can vary from a slight indentation in the vermilion border to a widely opened cleft extending into the floor of the nose. Along with varying degrees of nasal distortions, dental anomalies such as supernumerary, deformed, or absent teeth may accompany cleft lip. Cleft lip may be unilateral or bilateral and usually involves the maxillary alveolar ridge. Unilateral cleft lip is usually on the left side. Bilateral cleft lip is often associated with cleft palate.

Cleft palate results when the two palatal shelves fail to fuse. The deformity varies in degree from involving only the uvula to extending into the soft and hard palates, or into the nasal cavity. Cleft palate can be unilateral, bilateral, or midline. Occasionally, small submucosal clefts or soft palate clefts may be diagnosed in an older infant or child after they begin exhibiting symptoms.

Infants with cleft lip alone usually do not have feeding difficulties. Speech impairments and problems with tooth development may occur. Infants with cleft palate, with or without cleft lip, usually have feeding difficulties, impaired speech, and are more susceptible to ear infections. Feeding an infant with cleft lip and/or cleft palate prior to surgery can be very challenging. The severity of the deformity will determine the difficulty of sucking for the infant and the types of adjustments necessary to maintain adequate caloric intake.

Cleft lip repair is usually performed prior to 3 months of age if the infant has shown adequate weight gain. The infant should also be free of any infections. Usually during surgery, the lip is sutured together and then a stabilization device is applied to take tension off the suture line. Depending on the severity of the original deformity, revisions or nasal and cosmetic surgery may be needed as the child grows.

The timing of the surgical correction for cleft palate is individualized, depending on the size, shape, and degree of deformity. The goals for corrective surgery include joining the cleft segments, promoting intelligible and pleasant speech, reducing nasal regurgitation, and avoiding injury to the growing maxilla. Traditionally, correction is generally performed between 6 and 18 months of age to protect formation of tooth buds and prevent the formation of faulty speech habits. Again, revisions or additional reconstruction may be necessary as the child grows.

Nasoalveolar molding (NAM) is a nonsurgical method of reshaping the gums, lip, and nostrils before cleft lip and cleft palate surgery. The molding plate is worn by the infant 24 hours a day and it helps lessen the severity of the cleft by gently directing the growth of the gums. Approximately 3 to 6 months after birth, when the molding is complete, surgery is performed. The NAM usually reduces the size of the gap of the cleft, resulting in less tension when the surgeon closes the cleft, producing a better final result of the first surgery. Hopefully, this will mean fewer surgeries later for the child.

For all infants with a cleft, postoperatively, the goals are to maintain a clean incision and to avoid strain on the suture line. Prevention of atelectasis and pneumonia is also important. Maintaining adequate nutritional intake for the infant and helping the family cope with the infant's facial deformity and special care requirements remain priorities. Complications associated with cleft lip and cleft palate include recurrent otitis media, hearing loss, dental decay, displacement of the maxillary arches, malposition of the teeth, and speech defects. Care of an infant with cleft lip and/or palate will require the efforts of a multidisciplinary team to address all the potential issues that may arise. The team may include the pediatrician, pediatric plastic/craniofacial surgeon, dietician, speech therapist, occupational therapist, pediatric dentist, otolaryngologist, audiologist, orthodontist, genetic counselor, social worker, and nurse coordinator.

Preoperative Nursing Care Plan

Primary Nursing Diagnosis   Imbalanced Nutrition: Less than Body Requirements

Definition — Insufficient nutrients to meet body requirements

Possibly Related to
- Sucking difficulties secondary to congenital orofacial defect prohibiting the infant from making an adequate seal around the nipple
- Parental anxiety and frustration secondary to infant's tendency to choke on feedings

Primary Nursing Diagnosis: Imbalanced nutrition: less than body requirements related to sucking difficulties secondary to congenital orofacial defect prohibiting the infant from making an adequate seal around the nipple, parental anxiety and frustration secondary to infant's tendency to choke on feedings

Assessment/Defining Characteristics of Child and/or Family (Subjective & Objective Data):
- Inadequate weight gain
- Episodes of gagging and choking
- Formula returned through the infant's nose

Expected Outcomes	Possible Nursing Interventions	Rationale	Evaluation for Charting
Infant will be adequately nourished as evidenced by • steady weight gain • lack of or decreased episodes of gagging, choking, or formula returned through the nose • sufficient caloric consumption (state range of calories needed for each infant)	Keep accurate record of intake and output.	Provides information on child's hydration status.	Document intake and output.
	Assess and record any signs/symptoms of imbalanced nutrition (such as those listed under Assessment) every 4 hours and PRN.	Provides information on nutritional status of infant.	Describe any signs/symptoms of imbalanced nutrition noted.
	Weigh infant daily on same scale at same time of day. Document results and compare to previous weight.	Decrease in weight may be due to feeding difficulties (such as those described under Assessment).	Document weight and determine if it was an increase or decrease from the previous weight.
	If indicated, maintain and record daily calorie counts.	Provides information on actual caloric intake.	Document calorie count if indicated.
	Place infant in an upright or semi-sitting position during feeding. After feedings, place in an infant seat or on the side with head of bed elevated at a 30° angle.	Upright or semi-erect position during and after feedings helps to decrease the possibility of aspiration. It also makes swallowing easier.	Describe how infant tolerated feedings. Document effectiveness of positioning and feeding technique used.

(continued)

	Primary Nursing Diagnosis: Imbalanced Nutrition: Less than Body Requirements *(continued)*		
Expected Outcomes	**Possible Nursing Interventions**	**Rationale**	**Evaluation for Charting**
	Use an appropriate nipple for each infant (e.g., long and soft, crosscut, preemie, Breck feeder, or lamb's, etc). Place the nipple firmly in the infant's mouth on the side opposite the cleft.	The various nipples are needed in order to help prevent aspiration and to encourage development of the sucking muscles.	Document which type of nipple was used and its effectiveness.
	Burp infant frequently, every 15 to 30 ml (infants have a tendency to swallow large amounts of air). To avoid distressing the infant, remove the nipple from the infant's mouth only for burping or when coughing warrants removal. When indicated, limit feeding times to 30 to 45 minutes.	Frequent burping can help to keep the stomach from becoming overdistended. Shorter feeding times can prevent infant fatigue.	Describe any successful measures used to promote adequate caloric intake.
	When indicated, feed the infant with a rubber-tipped medicine dropper, an Asepto syringe with a rubber tip, or a "gravity flow" nipple attached to a squeezable plastic bottle.	These interventions can assist with feeding the infant when other measures are unsuccessful.	Describe any successful measures used to promote adequate caloric intake.
	Teach family the ESSR method (enlarge nipple, stimulate sucking, swallow and rest). Assess and record results.	These measures can assist giving the infant the appropriate caloric intake.	Describe any successful measures used to provide adequate caloric intake.
	When indicated, assist the mother with techniques to facilitate breast-feeding. Refer the mother to a local La Leche League chapter.	This intervention can assist the mother who wants to breast feed her infant to be successful in getting the infant to take the appropriate amount of calories.	Describe any successful measures used to promote breast feeding and adequate caloric intake.
TEACHING GOALS Family will be able to verbalize at least 4 characteristics of imbalanced nutrition such as • inadequate weight gain • inadequate caloric intake • gagging • choking	Teach family about characteristics of imbalanced nutrition. Assess and record results.	Increased knowledge will assist the family in recognizing and reporting changes in the child's condition.	Document whether teaching was done and describe results.

Primary Nursing Diagnosis: Imbalanced Nutrition: Less than Body Requirements *(continued)*			
Expected Outcomes	**Possible Nursing Interventions**	**Rationale**	**Evaluation for Charting**
Family will be able to verbalize knowledge of care such as • feeding techniques • monitoring intake and output • identification of any signs/symptoms of imbalanced nutrition (such as those listed under Assessment) • when to contact health-care provider	Teach family about care. Assess and record family's knowledge of and participation in care regarding feeding techniques, etc.	Education of family will allow for accurate care.	Document whether teaching was done and describe results.

Related Nursing Diagnoses

Risk for Aspiration   *related to* exposed nasal cavities and a direct pathway created by the cleft to the nasopharynx

Risk for Infection   *related to* insufficient drainage of the middle ear secondary to the cleft defect

Anxiety: Parental   *related to*
a. upcoming surgery
b. unknown outcomes of upcoming surgery

Deficient Knowledge: Parental   *related to*
a. feeding techniques
b. origin of defect
c. surgical procedure

Compromised Family Coping   *related to* difficulty bonding secondary to deformity

Postoperative Nursing Care Plan

Primary Nursing Diagnosis   Risk for Infection

Definition   Condition in which the body is at risk for being invaded by microorganisms

Possibly Related to
• Surgical repair of cleft lip and/or cleft palate
• Strain of sutures on repaired lip or palate
• Trauma to sutures of repaired lip or palate
• Residual of formula on the surgical site providing a medium for the growth of pathogens
• Aspiration of secretions or formula

Primary Nursing Diagnosis: Risk for infection related to surgical repair of cleft lip and/or cleft palate, strain of sutures on repaired lip or palate, trauma to sutures of repaired lip or palate, residual of formula on the surgical site providing a medium for the growth of pathogens, aspiration of secretions or formula

Assessment/Defining Characteristics of Child and/or Family (Subjective & Objective Data):

- Fever
- Tachycardia
- Tachypnea
- Hypotension
- Redness, swelling, or drainage at suture line
- Nonapproximated edges of suture line
- Altered white blood cell count (WBC)
- Abnormal breath sounds
- Lethargy

Expected Outcomes	Possible Nursing Interventions	Rationale	Evaluation for Charting
Infant will be free of infection as evidenced by • body temperature within acceptable range of 36.5°C to 37.2°C • heart rate within acceptable range (state specific range) • respiratory rate within acceptable range (state specific range) • blood pressure within acceptable range (state specific range) • clean and intact incision • WBC within acceptable range (state specific range) • clear and equal breath sounds bilaterally A & P • lack of signs/symptoms of infection (such as those listed under Assessment)	Assess and record T, HR, RR, BP, breath sounds, and any signs/symptoms of infection (such as those listed under Assessment) every 4 hours and PRN.	If infection is present, the T, HR, and RR will increase and the BP may decrease. The breath sounds will be abnormal (crackles, etc.) if infection is present.	Document range of T, HR, RR, and BP. Describe breath sounds and any signs/symptoms of infection noted.
	Maintain good hand-washing technique.	Good hand washing is the single most important measure in decreasing infection.	Document whether good hand-washing technique was used.
	Clean the suture line on schedule and per institutional policy. A solution of 1:2 hydrogen peroxide and saline (or water) applied with a cotton-tipped applicator may be used. If ordered, apply antibiotic ointment to suture line on schedule.	These measures are necessary to help prevent accumulation of bacteria, which can lead to infection of the incision.	Describe incision site. Document if incision site was cleaned and if antibiotic ointment was applied on schedule.
	Apply elbow/arm restraints to prevent infant from traumatizing the suture line by trying to put fingers or objects into the mouth. Remove restraints every 2 hours and PRN.	Trauma to the suture line can lead to contamination and possible infection. Periodic removal of restraints allows for exercising of the infant's arms, and provides opportunities for skin care and play.	Document whether elbow/arm restraints were used. Describe condition of child's skin under restraints.
	When indicated, use a medicine dropper, Asepto syringe or other special appliances to feed the infant. Place the dropper or syringe in the mouth	These feeding measures prevent trauma to the suture line, which can help to decrease the growth of bacteria that can lead to infection.	Describe feeding measures used and their effectiveness.

Primary Nursing Diagnosis: Risk for Infection *(continued)*

Expected Outcomes	Possible Nursing Interventions	Rationale	Evaluation for Charting
	from the side to avoid the suture line. Avoid using straws, pacifier, or spoon. Infants with palate repairs should not be tube, syringe, or fork-fed.		
	After feeding, rinse the infant's mouth with water to remove any milk residue.	Prevents accumulation of milk, which could encourage bacteria to grow.	Document whether the infant's mouth was rinsed after feedings.
	Position infant on the side or back, keeping the head of the bed elevated, or use an infant seat. When indicated, apply a jacket restraint to prevent the infant from rolling onto the abdomen and rubbing the face on the bed.	The head elevated position can prevent aspiration. It also enhances lung expansion and allows drainage of the upper lobes. This along with preventing trauma to the suture line can help to decrease the growth of bacteria.	Document position placement of infant and any successful measures used to prevent trauma to the suture line.
	When indicated, place the infant in a partial-side-lying position to facilitate the drainage of copious serosanguineous secretions. After cleft palate repair, the infant may require gentle oral suctioning PRN.	Allowing drainage of secretions can help to prevent the growth of bacteria. Suctioning may be required to prevent aspiration of secretions.	Document position placement of infant. Describe amount and characteristic of secretions. If suctioning was necessary, document how often it was needed.
	Check and record results of WBC. Notify physician if results are out of the acceptable range.	Abnormal WBC results may indicate an infection.	Document WBC results if available.
	When indicated, administer antibiotics on schedule. Assess and record any side effects (e.g., rash, diarrhea).	Antibiotics are given to combat infection or prophylactically to decrease the chance of getting an infection.	Document whether antibiotics were administered on schedule. Describe any side effects noted.
	When indicated, administer antipyretics on schedule. Assess and record effectiveness.	Antipyretics are used to reduce fever.	Document whether an antipyretic was needed and describe effectiveness.

(continued)

Primary Nursing Diagnosis: Risk for Infection (*continued*)

Expected Outcomes	Possible Nursing Interventions	Rationale	Evaluation for Charting
TEACHING GOALS Family will be able to verbalize at least 4 characteristics of infection such as • fever • rapid respiratory rate • redness, swelling or drainage at suture line • lethargy	Teach family about characteristics of risk for infection. Assess and record results.	Increased knowledge will assist the family in recognizing and reporting changes in the child's condition.	Document whether teaching was done and describe results.
Family will be able to verbalize knowledge of care such as • good hand-washing technique • fever control • cleaning of suture line • medication administration • identification of any signs/symptoms of further infection (such as those listed under Assessment) • when to contact health-care provider	Teach family about care. Assess and record family's knowledge of and participation in care regarding good hand-washing technique, fever control, cleaning of suture line, etc.	Education of family will allow for accurate care.	Document whether teaching was done and describe results.

Related Nursing Diagnoses

Impaired Skin Integrity	*related to* a. surgical closure of cleft lip and/or cleft palate b. strain of sutures on repaired lip or palate c. trauma to sutures of repaired lip or palate
Acute Pain	*related to* surgical correction of the cleft
Anxiety: Infant	*related to* a. restrained arms and/or body b. inability to suck or use pacifier c. inability to get hands to mouth
Anxiety: Parental	*related to* a. outcome of surgery b. potential for future surgery c. home care d. potential for child to have speech defects, hearing loss, or dental decay
Deficient Knowledge: Parental	*related to* home care of infant
Imbalanced Nutrition: Less than Body Requirements	*related to* feeding difficulties

FOUR

ESOPHAGEAL ATRESIA AND TRACHEOESOPHAGEAL FISTULA
MEDICAL DIAGNOSIS

PATHOPHYSIOLOGY In esophageal atresia, the embryonic foregut fails to develop, and the esophagus ends in a blind pouch; a tracheoesophageal fistula (TEF, T-E fistula) is a connection (fistula) between the trachea and the esophagus. Normally the foregut lengthens and separates to form two parallel channels (the esophagus and the trachea) during the fourth and fifth weeks of gestation. If there is defective separation or altered cellular growth during this separation, anomalies involving the esophagus and the trachea, such as TEF, result. The five most frequently seen forms of esophageal atresia and TEF are **Type A**, esophageal atresia only (5% to 8%); **Type B** (rare), esophageal atresia with a proximal TEF; **Type C**, esophageal atresia with a distal TEF (80% to 95% of all cases); **Type D** (rare), esophageal atresia with proximal and distal TEF; and **Type E**, (4%) TEF with no esophageal atresia (also called H type).

Diagnosis is established by gently passing a radiopaque catheter into the esophagus until resistance is met. Attempts to aspirate gastric contents and to auscultate introduced air into the stomach will be unsuccessful when esophageal atresia is present. Radiographic studies and bronchoscopy are necessary to determine the extent of the defect and the location of the fistula(s).

Esophageal atresia and TEF are rare malformations that can occur as separate entities or together. The incidence of these defects is estimated at 1 in every 3,000 to 4,500 live births. There is no sex difference in occurrence, and heredity has not been implicated as a factor. Approximately one-third of affected infants are premature, and more than one-half also have other congenital anomalies, such as vertebral, anorectal, cardiovascular, renal, and limb abnormalities. A history of polyhydramnios prenatally is common due to the inability of the amniotic fluid to reach the gastrointestinal tract of the fetus.

Major clinical manifestations of Type C, esophageal atresia and distal TEF, the most common form of the defect, include excessive pharyngeal secretions, drooling, bubbling from the mouth and nose, coughing, choking, and cyanosis. The infant may also stop breathing. The cyanosis results from laryngospasms, which occur as a compensatory mechanism to try to prevent aspiration of the overflow secretions from the esophageal blind pouch into the trachea. Abdominal distention is present due to air shunting across the fistula. When the gastric contents are regurgitated through the fistula into the trachea, a chemical pneumonitis occurs.

Treatment is aimed at preventing aspiration pneumonia and at maintaining adequate hydration and nutrition of the infant until surgical repair of the defect can be performed. Initially, the infant does not receive anything by mouth and is positioned so that secretions will drain, and to prevent aspiration pneumonia. Antibiotic therapy is often started.

Sometimes the malformation can be corrected in one operation, but at other times it requires two or more procedures. If it can be repaired in one procedure, a thoracotomy is done with TEF ligation and an end-to-end anastomosis of the esophagus. When staged operations are necessary (due to prematurity, multiple anomalies, poor condition of the infant, or insufficient length of the two segments of the esophagus), palliative measures used include ligation of the TEF, a gastrostomy for gastric decompression and feedings, and a cervical esophagostomy to allow for drainage of oral secretions. Complications following reconstructive surgery include strictures or leaks of the esophageal anastomosis site, esophageal motility problems, and respiratory problems. After corrective surgery, a large number of infants have tracheomalacia and gastroesophageal reflux, often requiring further surgical treatment.

Preoperative Nursing Care Plan

Primary Nursing Diagnosis Risk for Aspiration

Definition State in which an individual is at risk for entry of extraneous secretions, foods, fluids, or foreign bodies into the tracheobronchial passages

Possibly Related to
- Overflow of saliva from the proximal esophageal pouch
- Reflux of gastric secretions up the distal esophagus into the trachea via the fistula

Primary Nursing Diagnosis: Risk for aspiration related to overflow of saliva from the proximal esophageal pouch, reflux of gastric secretions up the distal esophagus into the trachea via the fistula

Assessment/Defining Characteristics of Child and/or Family (Subjective & Objective Data):

- Diminished breath sounds
- Excessive pharyngeal secretions
- Drooling
- Bubbling from the mouth and nose
- Coughing

- Choking
- Cyanosis
- Abdominal distention with air
- Intraabdominal pressure (usually resulting from crying)

Expected Outcomes	Possible Nursing Interventions	Rationale	Evaluation for Charting
Infant will be free of signs/symptoms of aspiration as evidenced by • clear and equal breath sounds bilaterally A & P • lack of 1. excessive secretions 2. drooling 3. bubbling from the mouth and nose 4. coughing 5. choking 6. cyanosis 7. abdominal distention	Assess and record breath sounds and any signs/symptoms of aspiration (such as those listed under Assessment) every 4 hours and PRN.	Abnormal breath sounds such as crackles could indicate aspiration.	Describe breath sounds and state any sign/symptoms of aspiration noted.
	Position infant supine with head elevated at least 30°.	This position helps to minimize reflux of gastric secretions into the trachea.	Document if infant was maintained in the supine head elevated position and its effectiveness in reducing reflux.
	Suction (either continuously or intermittently) esophageal blind pouch. Ensure that catheter is changed per hospital protocol. Record the amount and characteristics of secretions.	This intervention is necessary to help prevent aspiration of overflow secretions into the trachea.	Document whether suctioning was continuous or intermittent. Describe amount and characteristics of secretions.
	If a nasogastric tube is in place, connect it to gravity drainage.	This allows air to escape from the abdomen.	Document whether a nasogastric tube was connected to gravity drainage.
	Keep infant NPO. Assess and record IV fluids and condition of IV site every hour.	Infants need to be NPO in order to prevent aspiration. It is necessary to record the amount of IV fluids every hour to make sure the child is not being over or under hydrated. The IV site needs to be assessed every hour for signs of redness or swelling.	Document whether infant was NPO. Document amount of IV fluid intake and condition of IV site along with any interventions needed.

Primary Nursing Diagnosis: Risk for Aspiration *(continued)*			
Expected Outcomes	**Possible Nursing Interventions**	**Rationale**	**Evaluation for Charting**
	If indicated, administer antibiotics on schedule. Assess and record any side effects (e.g., rash, diarrhea).	Antibiotics are given to combat infection or prophylactically to decrease the chance of getting an infection.	Document whether antibiotics were administered on schedule. Describe any side effects noted.
	When indicated, ensure that humidified oxygen is administered in the correct amount and route. Assess and record effectiveness of therapy.	Humidified oxygen will dilate the pulmonary vasculature, which increases surface area available for gas exchange. Extra source oxygen will also allow for better oxygenation to body tissues.	Document amount and route of oxygen delivery. Describe effectiveness.
TEACHING GOALS Family will be able to verbalize at least 4 characteristics of risk for aspiration such as • excessive secretions • drooling • bubbling from nose and mouth • coughing • choking • cyanosis • nasal flaring	Teach family about characteristics of risk for aspiration. Assess and record results.	Increased knowledge will assist the family in recognizing and reporting changes in the child's condition.	Document whether teaching was done and describe results.
Family will be able to verbalize knowledge of care such as • positioning of infant • identification of any signs/symptoms of risk for aspiration (such as those listed under Assessment) • when to contact health-care provider	Teach family about care. Assess and record family's knowledge of and participation in care regarding positioning of infant, etc.	Education of family will allow for accurate care.	Document whether teaching was done and describe results.

Related Nursing Diagnoses

Ineffective Breathing Pattern	*related to* aspiration
Deficient Knowledge: Parental	*related to* a. infant's disease state b. cause of defect c. home care of infant d. sensory overload e. cognitive or cultural-language limitations
Risk for Infection	*related to* a. possibility of aspiration b. invasive procedures
Fear: Parental	*related to* a. impending surgery for infant b. outcome of surgery
Compromised Family Coping	*related to* a. birth of imperfect infant b. need for the infant to have surgery

Postoperative Nursing Care Plan

Primary Nursing Diagnosis   Ineffective Airway Clearance

Definition	Condition in which secretions cannot adequately be cleared from the airways
Possibly Related to	• Excessive secretions • Postoperative complications

Primary Nursing Diagnosis: Ineffective airway clearance related to excessive secretions, postoperative complications

Assessment/Defining Characteristics of Child and/or Family (Subjective & Objective Data):
- Tachypnea
- Diminished breath sounds
- Retractions
- Pallor
- Cyanosis

Expected Outcomes	Possible Nursing Interventions	Rationale	Evaluation for Charting

Infant will have adequate airway clearance as evidenced by
 	
• respiratory rate from 30 to 60 breaths/minute
• clear and equal breath sounds bilaterally A & P
• lack of
  1. retractions
  2. pallor
  3. cyanosis
	Assess and record RR, breath sounds and any signs/symptoms of ineffective airway clearance (such as those listed under Assessment) every 2 to 4 hours and PRN.	If infant experiences ineffective airway clearance the RR will increase and the breath sounds may be abnormal.	Document range of RR. Describe breath sounds and any signs/symptoms of ineffective airway clearance noted.

Primary Nursing Diagnosis: Ineffective Airway Clearance *(continued)*

Expected Outcomes	Possible Nursing Interventions	Rationale	Evaluation for Charting
	Suction infant PRN. Ensure that suction catheters are marked and that catheters are not passed further than a point just above the anastomosis site. Assess and record amount and characteristics of secretions.	Suctioning needs to be done PRN in order to clear secretions. The catheters need to be marked in order to prevent trauma to the anastomosis site.	Describe amount and characteristics of secretions.
	Position infant with the head slightly elevated. Ensure that infant does not hyperextend the neck and pull on the sutured esophagus. Change infant from the back to either side every 2 hours.	The head elevated position allows the lungs to fully expand. Hyperextending the neck can result in stress on the anastomosis site. Changing the infant's position every 2 hours can help to decrease the chance of postoperative pulmonary complications.	Document whether infant was positioned with the head slightly elevated. Document if infant's position was changed every 2 hours.
	When indicated, ensure chest physiotherapy (only vibration over the suture line) is performed on schedule. Assess and record effectiveness of treatments.	Chest percussion loosens secretions and positioning can help to assist the flow of secretions out of the lungs by gravity. This will help to decrease the chance of postoperative pulmonary complications.	Document whether chest physiotherapy was done on schedule. Describe effectiveness and infant's response to treatment.
	Ensure that chest tube system is intact and that negative pressure is maintained. Follow institutional policy for care of chest tubes to maintain patency and assess for air leaks. Record condition of chest tube sites every shift and PRN. Assess and record amount and characteristics of any drainage.	Chest tubes can drain air and/or fluid from the pleural space. They are needed to reexpand the lungs after surgical procedures in which the chest cavity was opened.	Describe condition of chest tube site and indicate whether chest tubes were functioning properly. Describe amount and characteristics of chest tube drainage.

(continued)

	Possible Nursing		Evaluation for
Expected Outcomes	**Interventions**	**Rationale**	**Charting**

Primary Nursing Diagnosis: Ineffective Airway Clearance *(continued)*

Expected Outcomes	Possible Nursing Interventions	Rationale	Evaluation for Charting
TEACHING GOALS Family will be able to verbalize at least 4 characteristics of ineffective airway clearance such as • rapid respiratory rate • retractions • pallor • cyanosis	Teach family about characteristics of ineffective airway clearance. Assess and record results.	Increased knowledge will assist the family in recognizing and reporting changes in the child's condition.	Document whether teaching was done and describe results.
Family will be able to verbalize knowledge of care such as • positioning • chest physiotherapy • suctioning PRN • identification of any signs/symptoms of ineffective airway clearance (such as those listed under Assessment) • when to contact health-care provider	Teach family about care. Assess and record family's knowledge of and participation in care regarding positioning, etc.	Education of family will allow for accurate care.	Document whether teaching was done and describe results.

Related Nursing Diagnoses

Imbalanced Nutrition: Less than Body Requirements	*related to* a. inability to tolerate PO fluids b. healing status of esophageal anastomosis
Acute Pain	*related to* surgical incision
Deficient Fluid Volume	*related to* a. inability to tolerate oral fluids b. high risk for respiratory difficulty
Risk for Infection	*related to* a. surgical procedure b. invasive procedures (e.g., IV, chest tubes)
Compromised FamilyCoping	*related to* a. hospitalization of infant b. home care of infant

FIVE

GASTROESOPHAGEAL REFLUX
MEDICAL DIAGNOSIS

PATHOPHYSIOLOGY Gastroesophageal reflux (GER) is the retrograde passage of gastric contents into the esophagus. GER is a common gastrointestinal disorder in infants and children. Physiologic reflux, which occurs when emesis and regurgitation are infrequent, can often spontaneously resolve by 1 year of age. The most likely primary mechanism of action in GER is the inappropriate, transient relaxations of the lower esophageal sphincter, allowing frequent reflux of gastric contents into the esophagus.

Gastroesophageal reflux disease (GERD) is more serious. The esophageal mucosa is inflamed and becomes hypersensitive from the repeated exposure to gastric acid. The gastric refluxate also stimulates the airway reflexes. Clinical manifestations of GERD for children under the age of 4 can include, along with emesis and regurgitation, poor weight gain, esophagitis, neurobehavioral changes (irritability), and respiratory symptoms (such as wheezing, cough, and pneumonia). Children older than 4 with GERD, have symptoms that mimic reflux in older children and adults, such as heartburn and abdominal pain, with a declining frequency of vomiting. Children at risk for GERD include those with esophageal atresia repair, hiatal hernia, neurologic disorders, asthma, and cystic fibrosis.

Diagnosis is established by taking a health history, which includes the child's feeding pattern, and doing a thorough physical examination. Several diagnostic tests, including barium swallow, upper GI series, pH probe monitoring, endoscopy with esophageal biopsy, gastroesophageal scintigraphy, and esophageal manometry are available to measure the frequency of acid-related injury and/or the severity of GER.

Treatment goals for GER and GERD include alleviating the symptoms, preventing and/or treating complications and promoting mucosal healing. Lifestyle changes that may be recommended include small, frequent feedings, burping frequently, avoiding overfeeding, placing the infant in a head elevated (30°) position, use of hypoallergenic formula, and thickened feedings. Medications are used primarily to reduce gastric acid secretion and its untoward effects. They can include antacids or histamine receptor antagonists (H2 blockers) such as cimetidine, ranitidine, or famotidine, or proton pump inhibitors (PPI) such as omeprazole and lansoprazole. Infants and children who do not respond to medical management may need surgical intervention to prevent complications such as aspiration pneumonia, prolonged esophagitis (which can lead to blood loss and anemia), and weight loss (which may lead to failure to thrive). The Nissen fundoplication is the most commonly performed antireflux surgical procedure. This procedure entails a 360° wrapping of the fundus of the stomach around the base of the esophagus.

Primary Nursing Diagnosis   Imbalanced Nutrition: Less Than Body Requirements

Definition   Insufficient nutrients to meet body requirements

Possibly Related to   • Chronic vomiting or regurgitation

Primary Nursing Diagnosis: Imbalanced nutrition: less than body requirements related to chronic vomiting or regurgitation

Assessment/Defining Characteristics of Child and/or Family (Subjective & Objective Data):
- Excessive vomiting
- Infant readily eating again after vomiting
- Irritability
- Vomitus not containing bile
- Weight loss or failure to gain weight

Expected Outcomes	Possible Nursing Interventions	Rationale	Evaluation for Charting
Infant will be adequately nourished as evidenced by • adequate amount of calories absorbed (state specific amount for each infant) • steady weight gain or lack of weight loss • decreased incidence of vomiting • lack of signs/ symptoms of imbalanced nutrition (such as those listed under Assessment)	Keep accurate record of intake and output. Record emesis: amount, frequency, characteristics, and relationship to feeding.	Provides information on infant's hydration status. Characteristics of emesis can help to identify the etiology of the disease (without bile, etc.)	Document intake and output. Describe characteristics of emesis.
	Assess and record any signs/symptoms of imbalanced nutrition (such as those listed under Assessment) every 4 hours and PRN.	Helps to establish the nutritional status.	Describe any sign/ symptoms of imbalanced nutrition noted.
	Weigh infant daily on same scale at same time each day without clothes. Record results and compare to previous weight.	Weight helps to determine the infant's hydration and nutritional status.	Document weight and determine if it was an increase or decrease from the previous weight.
	Ensure that infant receives small, frequent feedings (every 2 to 3 hours). When indicated, thicken formula with rice cereal. The nipple opening may need to be enlarged for easier sucking. Keep infant in an upright position during feeding, feed slowly, and burp often (after every 30 ml). Position infant with head elevated at a 30° to 45° angle for at least 1 hour after feedings.	These interventions promote retention of feedings and decrease the chance of aspiration.	Document how infant tolerated feedings. Describe any successful measures used.
	Organize nursing care so that medications and baths are given, vital signs assessed, etc. prior to feedings.	This will allow infant to better tolerate feedings.	Describe effectiveness of these measures.

Primary Nursing Diagnosis: Imbalanced Nutrition: Less than Body Requirements (continued)

Expected Outcomes	Possible Nursing Interventions	Rationale	Evaluation for Charting
	Administer medications (cimetidine, ranitidine) on schedule. Assess and record effectiveness and any side effects noted (e.g., agitation, nausea).	These medications allow infant to better tolerate feedings by either promoting gastric emptying or neutralizing gastric acid.	Document whether medications were administered on schedule. Describe effectiveness and any side effects noted.
TEACHING GOALS Family will be able to verbalize at least 4 characteristics of imbalanced nutrition such as • excessive vomiting • infant readily eating again after vomiting • vomitus not containing bile • weight loss or failure to gain weight	Teach family about characteristics of imbalanced nutrition. Assess and record results.	Increased knowledge will assist the family in recognizing and reporting changes in the infant's condition.	Document whether teaching was done and describe results.
Family will be able to verbalize knowledge of care such as • feeding techniques • positioning of infant during and after feedings • medication administration • identification of any signs/symptoms of imbalanced nutrition (such as those listed under Assessment) • when to contact health-care provider	Teach family about care. Assess and record family's knowledge of and participation in care regarding feeding techniques, positioning of infant during and after feedings, medication administration, etc.	Education of family will allow for accurate care.	Document whether teaching was done and describe results.

Nursing Diagnosis Risk for Aspiration

Definition State in which an individual is at risk for entry of extraneous secretions, foods, fluids, or foreign bodies into the tracheobronchial passages

Possibly Related to
• Excessive vomiting
• Reflux of gastric contents into the esophagus

Nursing Diagnosis: Risk for aspiration related to excessive vomiting, reflux of gastric contents into the esophagus

Assessment/Defining Characteristics of Child and/or Family (Subjective & Objective Data):

- Recurrent upper respiratory infections
- Tachypnea
- Wheezing
- Unequal breath sounds
- Apnea
- Dyspnea
- Coughing
- Choking

Expected Outcomes	Possible Nursing Interventions	Rationale	Evaluation for Charting

Infant will be free of signs/symptoms of aspiration as evidenced by
 	
• absence of respiration infection
• respiratory rate within acceptable range (state specific range)
• clear and equal breath sounds bilaterally A & P
• lack of
  1. apnea
  2. dyspnea
  3. coughing
  4. choking
	Assess and record RR, breath sounds, and any signs/symptoms of aspiration (such as those listed under Assessment) every 4 hours and PRN.	If aspiration has occurred the RR will increase, and abnormal breath sounds may be present.	Document range of RR. Describe breath sounds and any signs/symptoms of aspiration noted.

	Ensure that infant receives small, frequent feedings (every 2 to 3 hours). When indicated, thicken formula with rice cereal. The nipple opening may need to be enlarged for easier sucking. Keep infant in an upright position during feeding, feed slowly, and burp often (after every 30 ml). Position infant with head elevated at a 30° to 45° angle for at least 1 hour after feedings.	These interventions promote retention of feedings and decrease the chance of aspiration.	Document how infant tolerated feedings. Describe any successful measures used.
	Organize nursing care so that medications and baths are given, vital signs assessed, etc. prior to feedings.	This will allow infant to better tolerate feedings.	Describe effectiveness of these measures.
	Administer medications (cimetidine, ranitidine) on schedule. Assess and record effectiveness and any side effects noted (e.g., agitation, nausea).	These medications allow infant to better tolerate feedings by either promoting gastric emptying or neutralizing gastric acid.	Document whether medications were administered on schedule. Describe effectiveness and any side effects noted.

	Possible Nursing Interventions	Rationale	Evaluation for Charting
Nursing Diagnosis: Risk for Aspiration *(continued)*			
Expected Outcomes	**Possible Nursing Interventions**	**Rationale**	**Evaluation for Charting**
TEACHING GOALS Family will be able to verbalize at least 4 characteristics of risk for aspiration such as • rapid respirations • wheezing • coughing • choking	Teach family about characteristics of risk for aspiration. Assess and record results.	Increased knowledge will assist the family in recognizing and reporting changes in the infant's condition.	Document whether teaching was done and describe results.
Family will be able to verbalize knowledge of care such as • feeding techniques • positioning of infant during and after feedings • medication administration • identification of any signs/symptoms of risk for aspiration (such as those listed under Assessment) • when to contact health-care provider	Teach family about care. Assess and record family's knowledge of and participation in care regarding feeding techniques, positioning of infant during and after feedings, medication administration, etc.	Education of family will allow for accurate care.	Document whether teaching was done and describe results.

Related Nursing Diagnoses

Risk for Delayed Development: Motor

related to
a. confinement to head-elevated prone position
b. reduced stimulation secondary to prolonged or frequent hospitalization

Risk for Infection

related to inflammation of the esophagus secondary to presence of acid gastric contents in the esophagus

Anxiety: Parental

related to
a. infant's failure to gain weight
b. feeding schedule
c. positioning of infant
d. possibility of aspiration

Deficient Knowledge: Parental

related to
a. disease state
b. care of infant, including feeding schedule, positioning, and appropriate stimulation

SIX

HIRSCHSPRUNG DISEASE
MEDICAL DIAGNOSIS

PATHOPHYSIOLOGY Hirschsprung disease, or aganglionic megacolon, a congenital anomaly, occurs when there is absence or scarcity of autonomic parasympathetic ganglion cells of the submucosal (Meissner's) and myenteric (Auerbach's) plexuses in a segment of the bowel wall. The aganglionic portion results in absence of peristalsis, which causes accumulation of fecal material and mechanical intestinal obstruction. The term megacolon comes from the distention of the bowel proximal to the defect due to the trapped stool in the colon. In addition, the rectal sphincter is unable to relax, preventing evacuation of solids, liquids, or gas and contributing to the obstruction. The length of aganglionic segment of the bowel can vary from a small area (like the internal anal sphincter area) to the entire colon. In the majority of affected children (approximately 80%), the aganglionic segment involves only the rectosigmoid colon.

A major gene has been identified as being involved in Hirschsprung disease. Along with genetic factors, it is thought that the defect is probably caused by a lack of parasympathetic ganglion cell precursor migration during fetal development. Hirschsprung disease occurs in approximately 1 in 5,000 live births, and more commonly in males. It can be an acute or chronic illness.

The severity of bowel involvement determines the clinical manifestations. The chief signs and symptoms in a newborn are failure to pass meconium within 24 to 48 hours after birth, a decreased desire to ingest fluids, abdominal distention, and, possibly, bile stained vomitus. Older infants may present with failure to thrive, constipation, overflow diarrhea, vomiting, and abdominal distention. When the disease goes undiagnosed until childhood, the symptoms include malnutrition, lethargy, muscle wasting, a protuberant abdomen, chronic constipation, and passage of ribbon-like stools. Enterocolitis, inflammation of the small bowel and colon, is a complication of Hirschsprung disease that can occur before or after surgery. With enterocolitis, gastrointestinal bleeding and diarrhea occur due to ischemia and ulceration of the bowel wall.

Hirschsprung disease is diagnosed on the basis of the history, clinical manifestations, including bowel patterns, and various diagnostic studies. Abdominal radiographic studies or barium enema will reveal a distended small bowel and proximal colon with an unexpanded, empty rectum. Anorectal manometry may be done. Rectal biopsy indicating aganglionic bowel segments confirms the diagnosis.

Surgical treatment for infants involves removal of the affected bowel with end-to-end anastomosis to the anal canal. This may be done laparoscopically. Surgical management for severe cases or ill infants usually includes a temporary ostomy or colostomy in a part of the bowel with normal innervation and removal of the aganglionic bowel. Definitive corrective surgery (often a pull-through procedure) is done 3 to 6 months later, and the ostomy is closed. Potential long-term complications after surgery can include anal stricture and incontinence requiring anal dilatations, laxatives, enemas, and dietary changes. For those who have Hirschsprung disease as a chronic illness, lifelong surgical, medical, and psychosocial care may be needed to improve their quality of life.

Nursing Care Plan at Time of Diagnosis

Primary Nursing Diagnosis   Deficient Fluid Volume

Definition   Decrease in the amount of circulating fluid volume

Possibly Related to   • Decreased desire for fluids
                          • Vomiting

Primary Nursing Diagnosis: Deficient fluid volume related to decreased desire for fluids, vomiting

Assessment/Defining Characteristics of Child and/or Family (Subjective & Objective Data):

- Failure to pass meconium within 24 to 48 hours of birth (newborn)
- Feeding problems
- Vomiting (vomitus may include bile or fecal material)
- Hypoproteinemia
- Constipation
- Passage of ribbon like, foul-smelling stools

- Overflow diarrhea
- Dry mucous membranes
- Decreased urine output
- Tachycardia
- Tachypnea
- Hypotension

Expected Outcomes	Possible Nursing Interventions	Rationale	Evaluation for Charting

Child will have an adequate fluid volume as evidenced by
 	
• adequate fluid intake, IV and oral (state specific amount of intake needed for each infant)
• absence of
  1. vomiting
  2. overflow diarrhea
  3. hypoproteinemia
  4. abdominal distention
• moist mucous membranes
• adequate urine output (state specific range; 1 to 2 ml/kg/hr)
• urine specific gravity from 1.008 to 1.020
• heart rate, respiratory rate, and blood pressure within acceptable range (state specific range for each)
• lack of signs/ symptoms of deficient fluid volume (such as those listed under Assessment)
	Keep accurate record of intake and output. Record frequency and characteristics of stools. Measure and record amount and characteristics of any vomitus.	Provides information on child's hydration status. Decreased urine output can indicate dehydration. Characteristics of stools and/or vomitus can help to identify the etiology of the disease.	Document intake and output. Describe characteristics of stools or vomitus.

	Assess and record • IV fluids and condition of IV site every hour • HR, RR, and BP every 4 hours and PRN • signs/symptoms of deficient fluid volume (such as those listed under Assessment) every 4 hours and PRN	Provides information about fluid status of patient. If patient has deficient fluid volume, the HR will increase at first, and eventually decrease. The RR will increase. The BP will eventually decrease. It is necessary to record the amount of IV fluids every hour to make sure the child is not being over or under hydrated. The IV site needs to be assessed every hour for signs of redness or swelling.	Document amount of IV fluids and describe condition of IV site along with any interventions needed. Document range of HR, RR, and BP. Describe any signs/ symptoms of deficient fluid volume noted.
	Check and record urine specific gravity with every void or as indicated.	Urine specific gravity provides information about hydration status.	Document range of urine specific gravity.

(continued)

Primary Nursing Diagnosis: Deficient Fluid Volume *(continued)*			
Expected Outcomes	**Possible Nursing Interventions**	**Rationale**	**Evaluation for Charting**
TEACHING GOALS Child and/or family will be able to verbalize at least 4 characteristics of deficient fluid volume such as • decreased desire for fluids • feeding problems • vomiting • overflow diarrhea • abdominal distention	Teach child/family about characteristics of deficient fluid volume. Assess and record results.	Increased knowledge will assist the child/family in recognizing and reporting changes in the child's condition.	Document whether teaching was done and describe results.
Child and/or family will be able to verbalize knowledge of care such as • child's need for appropriate fluids • monitoring intake and output • identification of any signs/symptoms of deficient fluid volume (such as those listed under Assessment) • when to contact health-care provider	Educate child/family about care. Assess and record child's/family's knowledge of and participation in care regarding child's need for appropriate fluids, monitoring intake and output, etc.	Education of child/family will allow for accurate care.	Document whether teaching was done and describe results.

Related Nursing Diagnoses

Deficient Knowledge: Parental

related to
a. disease state
b. cause of defect
c. home care of child, including colostomy care
d. sensory overload
e. cognitive or cultural-language limitations

Anxiety: Parental

related to
a. hospitalization of child
b. altered home care
c. long-term prognosis

Imbalanced Nutrition: Less than Body Requirements

related to
a. poor feeding
b. vomiting

Acute Pain

related to
a. constipation
b. hunger

Compromised Family Coping *related to*
                      a. impending surgery
                      b. colostomy care
                      c. long-term prognosis

Preoperative Nursing Care Plan for Pull-Through Procedure

Primary Nursing Diagnosis   Anxiety: Parental

Definition   Feeling of apprehension resulting from an unknown cause

Possibly Related to

- Outcome of surgery
- Hospitalization of child
- Treatments and procedures for child

Primary Nursing Diagnosis: Anxiety: parental related to outcome of surgery, hospitalization of child, treatments and procedures for child

Assessment/Defining Characteristics of Child and/or Family (Subjective & Objective Data):

- Verbalization of apprehension or nervousness
- Inability to relax
- Anticipation of misfortune for child during surgery
- Inappropriate or hostile behavior toward health-care team
- Inability to concentrate
- Reports of somatic discomfort

Expected Outcomes	Possible Nursing Interventions	Rationale	Evaluation for Charting
Family will demonstrate decreased anxiety as evidenced by • verbalization of decreased anxiety • ability to relax • lack of statements indicating anticipated misfortune for child during the surgery • lack of inappropriate or hostile behavior toward health care team • ability to concentrate • decreased reports of somatic discomfort	Listen to family's concerns and complaints. Encourage expressions of feelings to health-care team, other family members, or friends regarding the surgery and its implications.	Allows family to express feelings and concerns and provides them with a way to gain knowledge and decrease anxiety about the surgery.	Describe family's behavior, concerns, and complaints. Describe any successful measures used to encourage family to express their feelings and/or decrease their anxiety.
	Remove excess stimulation from the environment.	This will help family to concentrate on information being taught.	Describe successful measures used to decrease stimulation in the environment.
	Record interactions with child/family.	Allows health-care team to tailor the best way to provide care for family and child.	Describe interactions with child and/or family and any successful measures that decreased anxiety.
	Allow family to stay with child as much as possible.	Allowing the family and child to stay together assists child/family in their ability to cope.	Document when family stayed with child. Describe child's/family's behavior.

(continued)

Primary Nursing Diagnosis: Anxiety: Parental *(continued)*			
Expected Outcomes	**Possible Nursing Interventions**	**Rationale**	**Evaluation for Charting**
	Allow child to keep a familiar item with him/her.	A familiar item may comfort the child and ease the family's concern.	Document whether child had a familiar item for comfort and describe effectiveness.
	Dispel any misinformation.	Provides an opportunity for health-care team to correct any misinformation.	Document any misinformation stated by family and measures used to dispel misinformation.
	Explain the surgical procedure. Instruct the family in postoperative and home care. Explain potential changes in the child's behavior after the surgery and upon returning home. Keep explanations simple and concise; use illustrations. Repeat explanations as necessary.	Increased knowledge will help increase understanding and acceptance by the family.	Document whether family was able to verbalize an understanding of explanations regarding the surgery, child's care, and child's condition.
	Answer any questions the family may have regarding the surgery, child's care, or child's condition.	Allowing family to ask questions provides an opportunity to make sure information is correctly understood.	Document whether family had questions and if the questions were sufficiently answered.
TEACHING GOALS Family will be able to verbalize at least 4 characteristics of increased anxiety such as • inability to relax • inappropriate or hostile behavior toward health-care team • inability to concentrate • reports of somatic discomfort • asking the same questions repeatedly	Teach family about characteristics of anxiety. Assess and record results.	Increased knowledge will assist the family in recognizing and reporting changes in their anxiety.	Document whether teaching was done and describe results.

Primary Nursing Diagnosis: Anxiety: Parental *(continued)*			
Expected Outcomes	**Possible Nursing Interventions**	**Rationale**	**Evaluation for Charting**
Family will be able to verbalize knowledge of care regarding • identification of any signs/symptoms of anxiety (such as those listed under Assessment) • when to contact health-care provider	Teach family about care. Assess and record family's knowledge of and participation in care regarding identification of any signs/symptoms of anxiety, etc.	Education of family will allow for accurate care.	Document whether teaching was done and describe results.

Related Nursing Diagnoses

Deficient Knowledge: Parental

related to
a. fear of surgical procedure
b. fear of outcome
c. misconceptions or inaccurate information concerning surgical procedure and outcome

Fear: Child

related to
a. impending surgery
b. hospitalization
c. unfamiliar surroundings
d. forced contact with strangers
e. treatments and procedures

Fear: Family

related to
a. impending surgery
b. outcome of surgery

Compromised Family Coping

related to
a. impending surgery
b. hospitalization of child
c. repeated hospitalization of child

Postoperative Nursing Care Plan

Primary Nursing Diagnosis   Risk for Infection

Definition

Condition in which the body is at risk for being invaded by microorganisms

Possibly Related to

• Surgical wound(s)
• Spread of organisms from bowel

Primary Nursing Diagnosis: Risk for infection related to surgical wound(s), spread of organisms from bowel

Assessment/Defining Characteristics of Child and/or Family (Subjective & Objective Data):

- Fever
- Tachycardia
- Tachypnea
- Hypotension
- Redness
- Swelling
- Purulent wound drainage
- Foul odor
- Lethargy
- Irritability
- Altered white blood cell count (WBC)

Expected Outcomes	Possible Nursing Interventions	Rationale	Evaluation for Charting
Child will be free of infection as evidenced by • axillary temperature within acceptable range of 36.5°C to 37.2°C • heart rate within acceptable range (state specific range) • respiratory rate within acceptable range (state specific range) • blood pressure within acceptable range (state specific range) • a clean wound site with minimal clear to serosanguineous drainage • WBC within acceptable range (state specific range) • lack of signs/ symptoms of infection (such as those listed under Assessment)	Assess and record axillary T (no rectal temperatures), HR, RR, and BP, and any signs/ symptoms of infection (such as those listed under Assessment) every 4 hours and PRN.	If infection is present, the T, HR, and RR will increase and the BP may decrease.	Document range of T, HR, RR, and BP. Describe any signs/symptoms of infection noted.
	Maintain good hand-washing technique.	Good hand-washing is the single most important measure in decreasing infection.	Document whether good hand-washing technique was used.
	Ensure that wound care is done using aseptic technique.	Aseptic technique is needed to help decrease introduction of pathogens.	Document whether aseptic technique was used during wound care.
	Assess and record amount and characteristics of wound drainage every shift and PRN.	The wound site should have minimal redness and edema. Increase in redness or edema can indicate an infection is present. A change in color of wound drainage (from clear or serosanguineous to yellow, green, etc.) or a change in character of the drainage, from thin, minimal amount to copious, thick, foul-smelling drainage) can indicate the presence of an infection.	Describe wound site including amount and characteristics of any drainage.
	If indicated, obtain culture specimens (wound, blood). Check results and notify physician of any abnormalities.	Cultures can indicate if pathogens are present.	Document results of any cultures if available.

Primary Nursing Diagnosis: Risk for Infection *(continued)*

Expected Outcomes	Possible Nursing Interventions	Rationale	Evaluation for Charting
	Check and record results of WBC. Notify physician if results are out of the acceptable range.	Abnormal WBC results may indicate an infection.	Document WBC results if available.
	Reposition child as indicated.	Repositioning helps to decrease the chance of postoperative complications such as pneumonia.	Document how often child was repositioned.
	Administer antibiotics on schedule. Assess and record any side effects (e.g., rash, diarrhea).	Antibiotics are given to combat infection or prophylactically to decrease the chance of getting a further infection.	Document whether antibiotics were administered on schedule. Describe any side effects noted.
	When indicated, administer antipyretics on schedule. Assess and record effectiveness.	Antipyretics are used to reduce fever.	Document whether an antipyretic was needed and describe effectiveness.
	Maintain infection control protocol of hospital when dealing with body fluids (wound drainage).	Keeping soiled items contained helps to decrease spread of infection.	Document whether disposal of body fluids was done according to hospital protocol.
TEACHING GOALS Child and/or family will be able to verbalize at least 4 characteristics of infection such as • fever • purulent wound drainage • foul odor • lethargy	Teach child/family about characteristics of risk for infection. Assess and record results.	Increased knowledge will assist the child/family in recognizing and reporting changes in the child's condition.	Document whether teaching was done and describe results.
Child and/or family will be able to verbalize knowledge of care such as • good hand-washing technique • fever control • identification of any signs/symptoms of infection (such as those listed under Assessment) • when to contact health-care provider	Teach child/family about care. Assess and record child's/family's knowledge of and participation in care regarding good hand-washing technique, fever control, etc.	Education of child/family will allow for accurate care.	Document whether teaching was done and describe results.

Related Nursing Diagnoses

Impaired Skin Integrity	*related to* frequent acidic stools in the perineal area
Acute Pain	*related to* a. surgical incision site(s) b. invasive procedures
Compromised Family Coping	*related to* a. surgical procedure b. child's hospitalization

SEVEN

INFLAMMATORY BOWEL DISEASE
MEDICAL DIAGNOSIS

PATHOPHYSIOLOGY Inflammatory bowel disease (IBD) is used to describe both ulcerative colitis and Crohn's disease, two chronic intestinal disorders. These two diseases have similar epidemiologic, immunologic, and clinical features, but Crohn's disease can be more disabling and severe than ulcerative colitis. Although the causes of IBD are unknown, many infectious, nutritional, immunologic, environmental, and psychogenic factors have been proposed. It is thought that a triggering event, such as a bacterial infection or another immune stimulus, in a genetically predisposed person results in inflammatory bowel disease. Psychological factors, such as stress, may accentuate the symptoms and severity of a relapse but do not contribute to the pathogenesis.

Diagnosis begins with a thorough history and physical, focusing on the nutritional status of the child. Laboratory evaluation may include a complete blood count (to evaluate anemia), erythrocyte sedimentation rate (to assess the body's response to the inflammation), a liver panel, and a variety of other tests. Stool is evaluated for blood, leukocytes, and infectious organisms. A number of radiographic studies, ultrasound, as well as invasive procedures may be ordered. These include an upper gastrointestinal series with small bowel follow-through, computed tomography, and upper endoscopy and colonoscopy with biopsies.

Ulcerative Colitis

Ulcerative colitis is characterized by mucosal ulcerations and diffuse inflammation of the large intestine. The lesion is continuous, spreading to adjacent areas without skipping healthy bowel, but it rarely extends deeper than the submucosa. Thickening of the bowel results from the colonic edema and inflammation. The damaged bowel is ineffective in reabsorbing nutrients, fluid, and electrolytes.

The onset of ulcerative colitis is usually gradual. The child experiences chronic bloody, mucousy diarrhea, fecal urgency, pain, and lower abdominal cramps, especially before defecation. Anorexia with weight loss develops as the diarrhea persists over time. The bowel also takes on a lead pipe appearance, with shortening of the colon, loss of mucosal and haustral folds, and the

development of fibrous tissue and linear strictures. The onset of ulcerative colitis can also be fulminant, with the child experiencing explosive, bloody diarrhea, high fever, and possibly peritonitis and perforation.

Persisting symptoms of ulcerative colitis can delay growth and development. Extraintestinal symptoms, such as skin rash, arthritis, and iritis are rare in children but more common in adolescents and young adults.

Crohn's Disease

Crohn's disease can involve one or more segments of the gut from the mouth to the anus; it most often affects the distal ileum and colon. Diseased bowel is usually separated by healthy bowel (skip lesion), and the lesion is transmural (involving all layers of the bowel). Edema and inflammation contribute to a thickened intestinal wall. Fistulas and fissures can develop between loops of bowel or to other structures, such as the skin or urinary tract, but the inflammation and engorgement on the serosal surface inhibit perforation or spillage of intestinal contents into the peritoneal cavity. Intra-abdominal abscesses, crypt abscesses, and granulomas develop, as does regional lymphatic involvement. Over time, scar tissue and fibrotic strictures form, which can eventually lead to bowel obstruction. The onset of Crohn's disease is subtle. The child will present with crampy abdominal pain, diarrhea, fever, malaise, anorexia, and weight loss. The pain can also be localized periumbilically or in the right lower quadrant. Perianal lesions are also common. Persisting symptoms of Crohn's disease may delay growth and development. Extraintestinal symptoms often accompany Crohn's disease and include arthralgia (common), mouth ulcers, iritis, arthritis (less common), and skin rashes.

TREATMENT The goal of treatment for inflammatory bowel disease is to induce remission of acute symptoms and then to maintain remission over time. Pharmacologic therapy is palliative, not curative, for both ulcerative co litis and Crohn's disease. Medications may include 5-aminosalicylates, corticosteroids, immunomodulators, biologics, and antibiotics. If remission is not attainable with medications, total parenteral nutrition (TPN) and/or an elemental diet may be used in an effort to alleviate symptoms. Surgical intervention to remove affected bowel may be indicated for both diseases. Bowel obstruction, perianal disease, abdominal abscesses, strictures, and toxic megacolon are reasons for surgery. At times, a subtotal colectomy and ileostomy may be done. Ulcerative colitis may be cured with removal of the diseased colon and this can reduce the risk of carcinoma of the colon. Patients with colitis have an increased lifetime risk for the development of colorectal cancer and should be monitored accordingly. Children with Crohn's disease may need to have obstructed, narrowed bowel or fistulous tracks surgically excised; however, there is no cure for Crohn's disease.

Supportive measures are important to the child and family adjusting to IBD. Consultation with psychotherapists and stomal therapists may be beneficial. The National Foundation for Ileitis and Colitis, the United Ostomy Association, and local peer support groups can provide additional support and information.

Primary Nursing Diagnosis   Deficient Fluid Volume

Definition   Decrease in the amount of circulating fluid volume

Possibly Related to   • Diarrhea
                                  • Vomiting

Primary Nursing Diagnosis: Deficient fluid volume related to diarrhea and vomiting			
Assessment/Defining Characteristics of Child and/or Family (Subjective & Objective Data):			
• Severe diarrhea, with frequent, loose, watery stools, which may contain blood, and/or mucus • Vomiting • Weight loss • Anorexia • Abdominal cramping • Abdominal distention • Hyperactive bowel sounds		• Decreased skin turgor (skin recoil greater than 2 to 3 seconds) • Dry mucous membranes • Decreased urine output • Fever (for Crohn's disease) • Tachycardia • Tachypnea • Hypotension	
Expected Outcomes	**Possible Nursing Interventions**	**Rationale**	**Evaluation for Charting**

Child will have an adequate fluid volume as evidenced by
 	
• adequate fluid intake, IV and oral (state specific amount of intake needed for each child)
• absence of
  1. diarrhea
  2. mucus, pus, or blood in stool
  3. vomiting
  4. abdominal cramping and distention
• decreased number and frequency of stools
	Keep accurate record of intake and output. When indicated, encourage oral fluids. Record frequency and characteristics of stools. Measure and record amount and characteristics of any emesis.	Provides information on child's hydration status. Decreased urine output can indicate dehydration. Characteristics of stools and/or vomitus can help to identify the etiology of the disease.	Document intake and output. Describe characteristics of stools or emesis.

	Assess and record • IV fluids and condition of IV site every hour • bowel sounds every shift and PRN • T, HR, RR, and BP every 4 hours and PRN • signs/symptoms of deficient fluid volume (such as those listed under Assessment) every 4 hours and PRN	Provides information about fluid status of patient. If patient has deficient fluid volume, the HR will increase at first, and eventually decrease. The RR will increase. The BP will eventually decrease. It is necessary to record the amount of IV fluids every hour to make sure the child is not	Document amount of IV fluids and describe condition of IV site along with any interventions needed. Describe bowel sounds. Document range of T, HR, RR, and BP. Describe any signs/symptoms of deficient fluid volume noted.

Primary Nursing Diagnosis: Deficient Fluid Volume *(continued)*

Expected Outcomes	Possible Nursing Interventions	Rationale	Evaluation for Charting
• normal activity of bowel sounds (one every 10 to 30 seconds) • regaining of weight lost during exacerbation • adequate urine output (state specific range; 1 to 2 ml/kg/hr) • urine specific gravity from 1.008 to 1.020 • moist mucous membranes • return of appetite • rapid skin recoil (less than 2 to 3 seconds) • temperature within acceptable range of 36.5°C to 37.2°C • heart rate, respiratory rate, and blood pressure within acceptable range (state specific range for each) • lack of signs/symptoms of deficient fluid volume (such as those listed under Assessment)		being over or under hydrated. The IV site needs to be assessed every hour for signs of redness or swelling. Bowel sounds are an indication of peristalsis. Increased T can be a sign of infection.	
	Weigh child on same scale at same time of day. Document results and compare to previous weight.	Weight loss is due to the vomiting and diarrhea and can also indicate the child's hydration status.	Document weight and determine if it was an increase or decrease from the previous weight.
	Check and record urine specific gravity with every void or as indicated.	Urine specific gravity provides information about hydration status.	Document range of urine specific gravity.
	Provide mouth care every 4 hours and PRN.	Mouth care is necessary to counteract the dry mucous membranes.	Document whether mouth care was done and describe effectiveness.
	Administer anti-inflammatory medications (aminosalicylates, corticosteroids) on schedule. Assess and record any side effects (such as nausea, vomiting, bloody diarrhea, leukocytosis, moon faces, acne).	Used to decrease inflammation to the bowel. Aminosalicylates inhibit prostaglandins, which are known to cause diarrhea.	Document whether anti-inflammatory medications were administered on schedule. Describe any side effects noted.
	Administer antibiotics on schedule. Assess and record any side effects (such as nausea, vomiting, overgrowth of candida).	Used to combat any bacteria that may be present.	Document whether antibiotics were administered on schedule. Describe any side effects noted.
TEACHING GOALS Child and/or family will be able to verbalize at least 4 characteristics of deficient fluid volume such as • diarrhea • nausea • weight loss • abdominal cramping • abdominal distention • decreased urine output • fever	Teach child/family about characteristics of deficient fluid volume. Assess and record results.	Increased knowledge will assist the child/family in recognizing and reporting changes in the child's condition.	Document whether teaching was done and describe results.

(continued)

	Primary Nursing Diagnosis: Deficient Fluid Volume (*continued*)		
Expected Outcomes	**Possible Nursing Interventions**	**Rationale**	**Evaluation for Charting**
Child and/or family will be able to verbalize knowledge of care such as • monitoring intake and output • medication administration • identification of any signs/symptoms of deficient fluid volume (such as those listed under Assessment) • when to contact health-care provider	Teach child/family about care. Assess and record child's/family's knowledge of and participation in care regarding monitoring intake and output, medication administration, etc.	Education of child/family will allow for accurate care.	Document whether teaching was done and describe results.

Nursing Diagnosis   Acute Pain

Definition   Condition in which an individual experiences acute mild to severe pain

Possibly Related to   • Abdominal cramping secondary to inflammation and ulceration of the bowel
                          • Perianal fistulas and abscesses

Nursing Diagnosis: Acute pain related to abdominal cramping secondary to inflammation, ulceration of the bowel, and perianal fistulas and abscesses

Assessment/Defining Characteristics of Child and/or Family (Subjective & Objective Data):

• Verbal communication of pain
• Crying or moaning
• Facial grimacing
• For ulcerative colitis: tender abdomen, tenderness upon rectal examination, and lower abdominal pain
• For Crohn's disease: periumbilical pain and/or pain in the right lower quadrant

• Rebound tenderness
• Decreased activity, self-imposed
• Physical signs/symptoms:
  1. tachycardia
  2. tachypnea
  3. increased blood pressure
  4. diaphoresis
• Rating of pain on pain-assessment tool

Expected Outcomes	**Possible Nursing Interventions**	**Rationale**	**Evaluation for Charting**
Child will have decreased pain or be free of severe and/or constant pain as evidenced by • verbal communication of decreased pain or no pain	Assess and record HR, RR, BP, and any signs/symptoms of pain (such as those listed under Assessment) every 2 to 4 hours and PRN. Use age-appropriate pain-assessment tool.	Provides data regarding the level of pain child is experiencing.	Document range of HR, RR, BP, and degree of pain child is experiencing. Describe any successful measures used to decrease pain.

Nursing Diagnosis: Acute Pain *(continued)*

Expected Outcomes	Possible Nursing Interventions	Rationale	Evaluation for Charting
• decrease in or lack of 1. constant crying or moaning 2. facial grimacing 3. extreme restlessness 4. diaphoresis • heart rate within acceptable range (state specific range) • respiratory rate within acceptable range (state specific range) • blood pressure within acceptable range (state specific range) • rating of decreased pain or no pain on pain-assessment tool • increased participation in self-care and in age-appropriate play activities • lack of signs/symptoms of acute pain (such as those listed under Assessment)	Handle child gently.	Helps to minimize pain and promote comfort.	Document if child was handled gently and effectiveness of measure.
	When indicated, administer analgesics on schedule. Assess and record effectiveness.	Analgesics are administered to decrease pain.	Document whether analgesics were administered on schedule. Describe effectiveness and any side effects noted.
	Encourage family members to stay and comfort child when possible.	Helps to comfort and support the child.	Document whether family was able to remain with child and describe effectiveness of their presence.
	Allow family members to participate in care of child when possible.	This may increase the comfort level of the child and thus help child in managing pain.	Document whether family participated in care and if this was successful in helping child with pain management.
	Use diversional activities (e.g., music, television, playing games, relaxation) when appropriate.	Diversional activities can distract child and may help to decrease pain.	Document whether diversional activities were successful in helping to manage pain.
	If age appropriate, explain all procedures beforehand.	Allow child some control, which can assist child with pain management.	Describe if this measure was effective in helping child to manage pain.
	If age appropriate, allow the child to participate in planning his or her care. Encourage the child to practice self-care (e.g., bathing, removing dressing).	Allowing child some control can assist child with pain management.	Describe if this measure was effective in helping child to manage pain.
	When indicated, institute additional pain relief measures, such as hypnosis, guided imagery, and relaxation. Assess and record effectiveness.	These nonpharmacologic measures may help decrease pain.	Document whether these measures were successful in helping to manage pain.
TEACHING GOALS Child and/or family will be able to verbalize at least 4 characteristics of pain such as • verbal communication of pain or tenderness	Teach child/family about characteristics of pain. Assess and record results.	Increased knowledge will assist the child/family in recognizing and reporting changes in the child's condition.	Document whether teaching was done and describe results.

(continued)

Nursing Diagnosis: Acute Pain *(continued)*

Expected Outcomes	Possible Nursing Interventions	Rationale	Evaluation for Charting
• crying unrelieved by usual comfort measures • facial grimacing • rapid heart rate			
Child and/or family will be able to verbalize knowledge of care such as • medication administration • appropriate diversional activities • identification of any signs/symptoms of pain (such as those listed under Assessment) • when to contact health-care provider	Teach child/family about care. Assess and record child's/family's knowledge of and participation in care regarding medication administration, etc.	Education of child/family will allow for accurate care.	Document whether teaching was done and describe results.

Related Nursing Diagnoses

Imbalanced Nutrition: Less than Body Requirements
related to impaired ability to absorb nutrients

Disturbed Body Image
related to
a. disease symptoms
b. medication use, especially steroids
c. colectomy or colostomy
d. altered growth and development

Delayed Growth and Development
related to
a. impaired ability to absorb nutrients
b. large doses of corticosteroids

Compromised Family Coping
related to child's chronic illness

EIGHT

PYLORIC STENOSIS
MEDICAL DIAGNOSIS

PATHOPHYSIOLOGY The pylorus is the opening that allows passage of food from the stomach to the duodenum. Pyloric stenosis, also called hypertrophic pyloric stenosis (HPS), is a thickening of the muscular, circular ring that surrounds the pylorus, leading to eventual obstruction of the gastric outlet. The pylorus not only becomes hypertrophied, but hyperplasia also exists, and there is inflammation and edema of the area, which finally contributes to the complete obstruction of the opening. The thickened muscle can be twice its usual size and may be palpable as an olive-shaped mass in the upper abdomen, just to the right of the umbilicus. Because of the obstruction, food is unable to pass out of the stomach and the infant vomits. The obstruction may also lead to prolonged stasis of gastric fluids, which may cause gastritis. The exact cause of pyloric stenosis is unknown, but immature or lack of innervation of the area may be involved. Other experts theorize that pyloric stenosis may be caused by *Heliobacter pylori*, the same bacteria associated with peptic ulcer disease.

Pyloric stenosis is one of the most common disorders of early infancy, usually presenting during the third to fifth week of life. The condition is thought to occur 2 to 5 times more often in males than in females. Pyloric stenosis occurs in approximately 1 to 4 cases per 1,000 live births, is seen more in white children than in other races, and is most likely to affect full-term infants.

Clinical manifestations of pyloric stenosis vary somewhat, but typically the cardinal sign is vomiting, starting with the regurgitation of small amounts of milk immediately after a feeding and progressing to projectile vomiting (may be 2 to 4 feet) within a week or so. Vomiting can occur during a feeding, immediately after a feeding, or several hours later. The infant will be hungry following the vomiting episode and will eagerly accept a second feeding. Emesis may be blood tinged due to gastritis but will not contain bile. Prolonged vomiting can result in decreased serum levels of both sodium and potassium, a striking decrease in serum chloride levels, and increases in pH and carbon dioxide content (bicarbonate), characterizing hypochloremic alkalosis. Other clinical manifestations include failure to gain weight (or even weight loss), signs and symptoms of dehydration, distended upper abdomen, palpable, olive-shaped mass (distended pylorus), and visible exaggerated gastric peristaltic waves (succession waves) on the surface of the abdomen.

The most common diagnostic test to confirm the diagnosis of pyloric stenosis is an abdominal ultrasound. The size of the pyloric muscle can be accurately measured with this test. Sometimes an upper gastrointestinal radiographic study may be performed and will reveal a narrowed pyloric canal.

Treatment is surgical correction to open the pylorus (pyloromyotomy). An open pyloromyotomy or laparoscopic pyloromyotomy is usually performed. If the infant is dehydrated, or has hypochloremic, hypokalemic metabolic alkalosis, these conditions are corrected prior to surgery. The surgical procedure has a high success rate and a low mortality rate (only 1%). In some countries, treatment of pyloric stenosis with intravenous atropine therapy instead of surgery is being studied.

Preoperative Nursing Care Plan

Primary Nursing Diagnosis   Deficient Fluid Volume

Definition   Decrease in the amount of circulating fluid volume

Possibly Related to   • Vomiting
                              • Dehydration

Primary Nursing Diagnosis: Deficient fluid volume related to vomiting and diarrhea

Assessment/Defining Characteristics of Child and/or Family (Subjective & Objective Data):

- Projectile vomiting
- Abdominal distention
- Tachycardia
- Tachypnea
- Hypotension
- Dry mucosa membranes

- Decreased skin turgor (skin recoil less than 2 to 3 seconds)
- Sunken fontanel
- Sunken eyeballs
- Decreased urine output
- Increased urine specific gravity

Expected Outcomes	Possible Nursing Interventions	Rationale	Evaluation for Charting
Infant will have an adequate fluid volume as evidenced by • adequate fluid intake, IV and oral (state specific amount of intake needed for each infant) • absence of vomiting • nondistended abdomen • heart rate, respiratory rate, and blood pressure within acceptable range (state specific range for each) • moist mucous membranes • rapid skin recoil (less than 2 to 3 seconds) • flat fontanel • lack of sunken eyeballs • adequate urine output (state specific range; 1 to 2 ml/kg/hr) • urine specific gravity from 1.008 to 1.020	Keep accurate record of intake and output. Record emesis: frequency, characteristics, and relationship to feeding.	Provides information on child's hydration status. Decreased urine output can indicate dehydration. Characteristics of emesis can help to identify the etiology of the disease.	Document intake and output. Describe amount, frequency, relationship to feedings, and characteristics of any emesis.
	Assess and record • IV fluids and condition of IV site every hour • HR, RR, and BP every 4 hours and PRN • any signs/symptoms of deficient fluid volume (such as those listed under Assessment) every 4 hours and PRN	Provides information about fluid status of patient. If patient has deficient fluid volume, the HR will increase at first, and eventually decrease. The RR will increase. The BP will eventually decrease. It is necessary to record the amount of IV fluids every hour to make sure the child is not being over or under hydrated. The IV site needs to be assessed every hour for signs of redness or swelling.	Document range of HR, RR, and BP. Document amount of IV fluids and describe condition of IV site along with any interventions needed. Describe any signs/symptoms of deficient fluid volume noted.
	If indicated, maintain NPO status. Provide mouth care every 4 hours and PRN.	Mouth care is necessary to counteract the dry mucous membranes.	If indicated, document whether NPO status was maintained. Document whether mouth care was done and describe effectiveness.
	If oral feedings are ordered, feed slowly with small, frequent feedings. Place in a semierect position. Burp infant at frequent intervals (every 15 to 30 ml) during feedings. After feedings, place on right side in the head-elevated position. Encourage family to participate in feedings.	These interventions help the infant to retain feedings.	Describe any successful measures used to increase retention of feedings.

Primary Nursing Diagnosis: Deficient Fluid Volume *(continued)*

Expected Outcomes	Possible Nursing Interventions	Rationale	Evaluation for Charting
	Organize care to decrease disturbing and handling of infant after feedings.	Enhances infant's retention of feedings.	Describe any successful measures used to assist infant with retention of feedings.
	Check and record urine specific gravity with every void or as indicated.	Urine specific gravity provides information about hydration status.	Document range of urine specific gravity.
	Weigh infant on same scale at same time of day. Document results and compare to previous weight.	Weight helps to determine the infant's hydration and nutritional status.	Document weight and determine if it was an increase or decrease from the previous weight.
	Assess and record condition of mucous membranes and skin turgor every shift and PRN.	Provides information on hydration status.	Describe status of mucous membranes and skin turgor.
TEACHING GOALS Family will be able to verbalize at least 4 characteristics of deficient fluid volume such as • projectile vomiting • abdominal distention • weight loss • dry mucous membranes • decreased urine output	Teach family about characteristics of deficient fluid volume. Assess and record results.	Increased knowledge will assist the family in recognizing and reporting changes in the infant's condition.	Document whether teaching was done and describe results.
Family will be able to verbalize knowledge of care such as • monitoring intake and output • feeding schedule and method of feeding • positioning of infant • identification of any signs/symptoms of deficient fluid volume (such as those listed under Assessment) • when to contact health-care provider	Teach family about care. Assess and record family's knowledge of and participation in care regarding monitoring intake and output, feeding schedule and method of feeding, etc.	Education of family will allow for accurate care.	Document whether teaching was done and describe results.

Related Nursing Diagnoses

Imbalanced Nutrition: Less than Body Requirements	*related to* a. vomiting secondary to thickening of the circular muscle of the pylorus b. vomiting secondary to obstruction of the opening between the stomach and duodenum
Electrolyte Imbalance:	*Sodium Losses and Potassium Losses* related to* a. vomiting b. dehydration
Deficient Knowledge: Parental	*related to* a. disease state b. surgical correction c. postoperative home management
Acute Pain	*related to* a. hunger b. vomiting
Compromised Family Coping	*related to* a. hospitalization of infant b. impending surgery for infant c. knowledge deficit about medical diagnosis

*Non-NANDA diagnosis.

Postoperative Nursing Care Plan

Primary Nursing Diagnosis   Imbalanced Nutrition: Less than Body Requirements

Definition   Insufficient nutrients to meet body requirements

Possibly Related to   • Postoperative vomiting

Primary Nursing Diagnosis: Imbalanced nutrition: less than body requirements related to postoperative vomiting

Assessment/Defining Characteristics of Child and/or Family (Subjective & Objective Data):
- Failure of the bowel sounds to return
- Inability to tolerate oral feedings
- Vomiting
- Weight loss

Expected Outcomes	Possible Nursing Interventions	Rationale	Evaluation for Charting
Infant will be adequately nourished as evidenced by • ability to tolerate oral feedings • lack of vomiting	Keep accurate record of intake and output. Record emesis: frequency, characteristics, and relationship to feeding.	Provides information on child's hydration status. Decreased urine output can indicate dehydration. Characteristics of emesis can help to identify the etiology of the disease.	Document intake and output. Describe amount, frequency, relationship to feedings, and characteristics of any emesis.

Primary Nursing Diagnosis: Imbalanced Nutrition: Less than Body Requirements *(continued)*

Expected Outcomes	Possible Nursing Interventions	Rationale	Evaluation for Charting
• stable weight or lack of weight loss • lack of signs/symptoms of imbalanced nutrition (such as those listed under Assessment)	Assess and record • IV fluids and condition of IV site every hour • any signs/symptoms of imbalanced nutrition (such as those listed under Assessment) every 4 hours and PRN	It is necessary to record the amount of IV fluids every hour to make sure the child is not being over or under hydrated. The IV site needs to be assessed every hour for signs of redness or swelling.	Document amount of IV fluids and describe condition of IV site along with any interventions needed. Describe any signs/symptoms of imbalanced nutrition noted.
	If indicated, maintain NPO status. Provide mouth care every 4 hours and PRN.	Mouth care is necessary to counteract the dry mucous membranes.	If indicated, document whether NPO status was maintained. Document whether mouth care was done and describe effectiveness.
	If oral feedings are ordered, feed slowly with small, frequent feedings. Place in a semierect position. Burp infant at frequent intervals (every 15 to 30 ml) during feedings. After feedings, place on right side in the head-elevated position. Encourage family to participate in feedings.	These interventions help the infant to retain feedings.	Describe any successful measures used to increase retention of feedings.
	Organize care to decrease disturbing and handling of infant after feedings.	Enhances infant's retention of feedings.	Describe any successful measures used to assist infant with retention of feedings.
	Weigh infant on same scale at same time of day. Document results and compare to previous weight.	Weight helps to indicate the infant's hydration and nutritional status.	Document weight and determine if it was an increase or decrease from the previous weight.
TEACHING GOALS Family will be able to verbalize at least 3 characteristics of imbalanced nutrition such as • inability to tolerate oral feedings • vomiting • weight loss	Teach family about characteristics of imbalanced nutrition. Assess and record results.	Increased knowledge will assist the family in recognizing and reporting changes in the infant's condition.	Document whether teaching was done and describe results.

(continued)

	Primary Nursing Diagnosis: Imbalanced Nutrition: Less than Body Requirements *(continued)*		
Expected Outcomes	**Possible Nursing Interventions**	**Rationale**	**Evaluation for Charting**
Family will be able to verbalize knowledge of care such as • monitoring intake and output • feeding schedule and method of feeding • positioning of infant • identification of any signs/symptoms of imbalanced nutrition (such as those listed under Assessment) • when to contact health-care provider	Teach family about care. Assess and record family's knowledge of and participation of care regarding monitoring intake and output, feeding schedule and method of feeding, etc.	Education of family will allow for accurate care.	Document whether teaching was done and describe results.

Related Nursing Diagnoses

Risk for Infection *related to*
a. surgical incision
b. young age of infant
c. invasive procedures (IV)

Deficient Fluid Volume *related to*
a. vomiting
b. dehydration

Acute Pain *related to*
a. surgical incision
b. hunger
c. vomiting and effect on the operative site

Deficient Knowledge: Parental *related to*
a. incision care
b. feeding technique and schedule

Compromised Family Coping *related to*
a. fear of surgery not being successful
b. apprehension and hesitance secondary to prior feeding experience with infant

NINE

SHORT-BOWEL SYNDROME (SHORT-GUT SYNDROME)
MEDICAL DIAGNOSIS

PATHOPHYSIOLOGY Short-bowel syndrome (SBS), also called short-gut syndrome, is the condition in which there is loss of massive amounts of intestine, affecting the ability of the child to digest and absorb a regular diet. Short-bowel syndrome may be congenital or acquired.

The embryologic basis of congenital short-bowel syndrome remains unclear. Congenital SBS is often associated with intestinal malrotation, volvulus, or atresia. Vomiting, diarrhea, and malabsorption can begin at birth if the disease is severe. Congenital SBS, without atresias, is a very rare condition.

In acquired short-bowel syndrome, massive resection of the small intestine during the neonatal period may be required secondary to necrotizing enterocolitis, gastroschisis, malrotation with mid-gut volvulus and infarction, or multiple intestinal atresias. Acquired SBS also occurs when massive amounts of the small intestine are removed because of acute gastrointestinal illnesses. In older infants and children, resection may be necessary because of Crohn's disease or intussusception with gangrenous bowel.

The remaining intestines of most infants with short-bowel syndrome usually adapt to assume the function of the jejunal mucosa. Various problems with malabsorption can result, though, especially if more than 75% of the small bowel has been removed. Malabsorption of vitamin B_{12}, bile salts, iron, calcium, folic acid, or fat-soluble vitamins may occur. The production of lactase, sucrase, and maltase may also decrease. When the ileocecal valve is left in place, it helps regulate transit time and protects against bacterial contamination of the small bowel so that the body can better tolerate the removal of large amounts of bowel. Overgrowth of bacteria can cause increased intestinal gas and diarrhea.

Treatment of infants and children with short-bowel syndrome focuses on promoting adequate nutrition, promoting growth and development, and preventing complications. Continuous enteral feedings via a nasogastric tube or gastrostomy tube should be started as soon as possible after surgery, and advanced as tolerated. Oral feedings may also be offered so that the child learns to suck and swallow, and to prevent future problems with oral hypersensitivity or food aversions. At times long-term use of total parenteral nutrition (TPN) is required. Complications such as fluid and electrolyte imbalance, infection, and perianal skin excoriation due to diarrhea and the excretion of bile acids and enzymes are common. Prolonged TPN therapy along with lack of enteral feedings can lead to cholestasis and liver dysfunction. Complications related to the TPN, such as sepsis, can be life threatening. At the time of the initial bowel resection, an intestinal ostomy may be performed for many of these infants. Further surgery, such as intestinal lengthening procedures, may be indicated for the child to try to delay the intestinal transit time or increase the absorptive surface. Children with short-bowel syndrome may be considered for intestinal transplantation.

Primary Nursing Diagnosis   Imbalanced Nutrition: Less than Body Requirements

Definition   Insufficient nutrients to meet body requirements

Possibly Related to
- Malabsorption
- Diarrhea
- Vomiting

Primary Nursing Diagnosis: Imbalanced nutrition: less than body requirements related to malabsorption, diarrhea, vomiting

Assessment/Defining Characteristics of Child and/or Family (Subjective & Objective Data):
- Diarrhea
- Vomiting
- Malabsorption of vitamins, fat-solution vitamins, calcium, and iron
- Decreased enzymes
- Inadequate weight gain
- Weight loss

Expected Outcomes	Possible Nursing Interventions	Rationale	Evaluation for Charting
Child will be adequately nourished as evidenced by • sufficient caloric consumption— parenteral, oral, or via gastrostomy tube (state specific amount for each child) • steady weight gain or lack of weight loss • lack of 1. vomiting 2. diarrhea 3. vitamin deficiency 4. mineral deficiency • lack of signs/ symptoms of imbalanced nutrition (such as those listed under Assessment)	Keep accurate record of intake and output.	Provides information on child's hydration status. Decreased urine output can indicate dehydration.	Document intake and output.
	Assess and record • IV fluids and condition of IV site every hour • any signs/symptoms of imbalanced nutrition (such as those listed under Assessment) every 4 hours and PRN	It is necessary to record the amount of IV fluids every hour to make sure the child is not being over or under hydrated. The IV site needs to be assessed every hour for signs of redness or swelling.	Document amount of IV fluids and describe condition of IV site along with any interventions needed. Describe any signs/symptoms of imbalanced nutrition noted.
	Weigh child on same scale at same time of day. Document results and compare to previous weight.	Weight helps to indicate the child's hydration and nutritional status.	Document weight and determine if it was an increase or decrease from the previous weight.
	Organize care to conserve energy.	Conserving energy will help to maintain adequate nutrition.	Describe any therapeutic measures used to maintain adequate nutrition. Document their effectiveness.
	Maintain and record caloric count as indicated.	Provides information on amount of calories needed for maintenance of weight.	Document caloric count if indicated.
	Administer gastrostomy tube feedings on schedule. Follow institutional policy for care of the gastrostomy tube and site. Note which elemental formula is being used.	Tube feedings may be necessary due to the inability of the child to tolerate oral feedings. It may also be indicated to bypass a portion of the bowel that cannot absorb nutrients.	Document amount and type of tube feeding administered. Describe child's tolerance of feeding.

Primary Nursing Diagnosis: Imbalanced Nutrition: Less than Body Requirements (*continued*)

Expected Outcomes	Possible Nursing Interventions	Rationale	Evaluation for Charting
	When indicated, administer total parenteral nutrition (TPN) and intralipids. Follow institutional policy for maintenance of TPN and intralipid line and site. Assess and record urine glucose, protein, ketones, and pH every 4 to 8 hours and PRN. Check and record serum glucose and lipid levels as indicated.	TPN and intralipids are indicated when the bowel is unable to absorb sufficient calories by other means (oral or tube feedings). Monitoring urine glucose, protein, and ketones is necessary to assess renal function. Monitoring serum glucose and lipid levels is necessary to assess liver function.	Document care of TPN and intralipid lines. Describe condition of IV site. Document range of urine glucose, protein and ketones values. Document serum glucose and lipid values.
	If indicated, administer vitamins on schedule. Assess and record any side effects (e.g., nausea, unpleasant taste).	Vitamins may be indicated to help make sure the child is adequately nourished.	Document whether vitamins were administered on schedule. Describe any side effects noted.
	If indicated, administer antireflux medications on schedule. Assess and record any side effects (e.g., drowsiness, fatigue).	Antireflux medications may be indicated to help enhance digestion of nutrients.	Document whether antireflux medications were administered on schedule. Describe any side effects noted.
	If indicated, administer antibiotics on schedule. Assess and record any side effects (e.g., rash, diarrhea).	Antibiotics may be indicated to help prevent infection as a result of imbalanced nutrition and invasive procedures.	Document whether antibiotics were administered on schedule. Describe any side effects noted.
	When indicated, initiate consultation with dietitian and visiting nurse.	Provides family support for care of the child.	Document whether any consultations were made.
TEACHING GOALS Child and/or family will be able to verbalize at least 4 characteristics of imbalanced nutrition such as • diarrhea • vomiting • inadequate weight gain • weight loss	Teach child/family about characteristics of imbalanced nutrition. Assess and record results.	Increased knowledge will assist the child/family in recognizing and reporting changes in the child's condition.	Document whether teaching was done and describe results.

(*continued*)

	Primary Nursing Diagnosis: Imbalanced Nutrition: Less than Body Requirements *(continued)*		
Expected Outcomes	**Possible Nursing Interventions**	**Rationale**	**Evaluation for Charting**
Child and/or family will be able to verbalize knowledge of care such as • type and amount of feedings • monitoring child's weight gain and caloric consumption • medication administration • gastrostomy tube and site, as indicated • central line, as indicated • feeding schedule and method of feeding • positioning of infant • identification of any signs/symptoms of imbalanced nutrition (such as those listed under Assessment) • when to contact health-care provider	Teach child/family about care. Assess and record child's/family's knowledge of and participation in care regarding type and amount of feeding, monitoring child's weight gain and caloric consumption, etc.	Education of child/family will allow for accurate care.	Document whether teaching was done and describe results.

Nursing Diagnosis Deficient Fluid Volume

Definition Decrease in the amount of circulating fluid volume

Possibly Related to
• Vomiting
• Diarrhea
• Insufficient free water in feedings

Nursing Diagnosis: Deficient fluid volume related to vomiting, diarrhea, insufficient free water in feedings
Assessment/Defining Characteristics of Child and/or Family (Subjective & Objective Data):

Assessment/Defining Characteristics of Child and/or Family (Subjective & Objective Data):

• Vomiting
• Frequent liquid stools
• Weight loss
• Decreased skin turgor (skin recoil greater than 2 to 3 seconds)
• Dry mucous membranes

• Decreased urine output
• Increase in urine specific gravity
• Absence of tears
• Tachycardia
• Hypotension

Nursing Diagnosis: Deficient Fluid Volume *(continued)*

Expected Outcomes	Possible Nursing Interventions	Rationale	Evaluation for Charting

Child will have adequate fluid volume as evidenced by
 	
• adequate fluid intake: oral, IV, or feeding tube (state specific amount of intake needed for each child)
• absence of
  1. diarrhea
  2. vomiting
• Adequate urine output (state specific range; 1 to 2 ml/kg/hr)
• urine specific gravity from 1.008 to 1.020
• moist mucous membranes
• rapid skin recoil (less than 2 to 3 seconds)
• tears present when crying
• heart rate and blood pressure within acceptable range (state specific range for each)
• lack of signs/symptoms of deficient fluid volume (such as those listed under Assessment)
	Keep accurate record of intake and output. When indicated, encourage oral fluids. Record emesis and diarrhea, including frequency, amount, and characteristics (including consistency, color, pH, and reducing substance).	Provides information on child's hydration status. Decreased urine output can indicate dehydration. Characteristics of stools and/or vomitus can help to clarify its origin.	Document intake and output. Describe characteristics of stools or emesis.

	Assess and record • IV fluids and condition of IV site every hour • HR and BP every 4 hours and PRN • signs/symptoms of deficient fluid volume (such as those listed under Assessment) every 4 hours and PRN	Provides information about fluid status of patient. If patient has deficient fluid volume, the HR will increase at first, and eventually decrease. The BP will eventually decrease. It is necessary to record the amount of IV fluids every hour to make sure the child is not being over or under hydrated. The IV site needs to be assessed every hour for signs of redness or swelling.	Document amount of IV fluids and describe condition of IV site along with any interventions needed. Document range of HR and BP. Describe any signs/symptoms of deficient fluid volume noted.
	Weigh child on same scale at same time of day. Document results and compare to previous weight.	Weight helps to indicate the child's hydration and nutritional status.	Document weight and determine if it was an increase or decrease from the previous weight.
	Check and record urine specific gravity with every void or as indicated.	Urine specific gravity provides information about hydration status.	Document range of urine specific gravity.
	Provide mouth care every 4 hours and PRN.	Mouth care is necessary to counteract the dry mucous membranes.	Document whether mouth care was done and describe effectiveness.
TEACHING GOALS Child and/or family will be able to verbalize at least 4 characteristics of deficient fluid volume such as • vomiting • frequent liquid stools • weight loss • decreased urine output	Teach child/family about characteristics of deficient fluid volume. Assess and record results.	Increased knowledge will assist the child/family in recognizing and reporting changes in the child's condition.	Document whether teaching was done and describe results.

(continued)

Nursing Diagnosis: Deficient Fluid Volume (continued)			
Expected Outcomes	**Possible Nursing Interventions**	**Rationale**	**Evaluation for Charting**
Child and/or family will be able to verbalize knowledge of care such as • child's need for appropriate fluids • monitoring intake and output • identification of any signs/symptoms of deficient fluid volume (such as those listed under Assessment) • when to contact health-care provider	Teach child/family about care. Assess and record child's/family's knowledge of and participation in care regarding child's need for appropriate fluids, monitoring intake and output, etc.	Education of child/family will allow for accurate care.	Document whether teaching was done and describe results.

Related Nursing Diagnoses

Impaired Skin Integrity *related to*
a. irritation of skin by bile salts and enzymes in stools
b. caustic diarrhea

Delayed Growth and Development *related to*
a. malabsorption
b. nonoral feeding methods
c. restricted mobility
d. frequent hospitalizations

Electrolyte Imbalance: (Specify)* *related to*
a. vomiting
b. diarrhea
c. malabsorption

Deficient Knowledge: Parental *related to* home management

*Non-NANDA diagnosis.

CARE OF
CHILDREN WITH
HEMOPOIETIC
DYSFUNCTION
AND NEOPLASMS

5

ONE

HEMOPHILIA
MEDICAL DIAGNOSIS

PATHOPHYSIOLOGY Hemophilia is the term used to describe a group of hereditary bleeding disorders in which one of the factors needed for blood coagulation is deficient. This deficiency leads to repeated bleeding into soft tissues, muscles, and joint capsules. Approximately 85% of affected individuals have hemophilia A, which results from a deficiency of factor VIII. The next most common is hemophilia B, also known as Christmas disease, which results from a factor IX deficiency. Hemophilia is an X-linked recessive disorder and primarily affects males. It is transmitted about 60 to 70% of the time by an unaffected female carrier to male offspring. It can also result from a spontaneous genetic mutation. Approximately one-third of all individuals affected with hemophilia have no family history of the disease.

Individuals with hemophilia can be classified into three groups according to the severity of the factor deficiency. Those who are mildly affected have 5 to 50% of the functioning factor present, moderately affected individuals have 1 to 5% present, and severely affected individuals have less than 1% of the functioning factor present. The severe form can result in spontaneous bleeding without any precipitous trauma. Approximately 60 to 70% of children with hemophilia are diagnosed with the severe form of the disease.

Chorionic villus sampling and amniocentesis are two prenatal tests that can identify affected children before birth. Genetic testing to identify carriers is also increasingly being used. Evaluating the child's history, physical and laboratory data can make the diagnosis. Laboratory findings that are positive for hemophilia include a prolonged partial thromboplastin time (PTT) and low levels of factor VIII or IX coagulant levels. Prothrombin time (PT), thrombin time (TT), fibrinogen, and platelet count are normal.

The classic sign of hemophilia is prolonged bleeding anywhere in the body. Bleeding is likely to occur after minor falls or bumps, loss of deciduous teeth, circumcision, or immunizations. Children with less severe deficiencies may not begin to have bleeding episodes until early childhood when they become active. Hemarthrosis (bleeding into a joint cavity) can occur in joints such as the knee, elbow, or ankle. The bleeding can cause joint swelling, tenderness, and pain; repeated bleeds can result in destruction of the joint. Prophylactic treatment with factor replacement may be needed in children who develop these "target joints" in which they have repeated bleeds. Trauma to the head is dangerous and can lead to bleeding in the central nervous system or death. The other most severe hemorrhages involve the throat, abdomen, and limb compartments.

Therapeutic management consists of prevention, early treatment of bleeding with replacement of the deficient factor, and prevention of complications associated with bleeding. Products used to treat hemophilia are recombinant factor VIII concentrate and for less severe bleeding in mild hemophilia, desmopressin acetate (DDAVP). For those with hemophilia B, recombinant factor IX is used. Cryoprecipitate is no longer used. Elevation, immobilization, pressure, and application of cold can be used as local comfort measures. Analgesics (non-aspirin-containing drugs or nonsteroidal anti-inflammatory drugs) and corticosteroids may also be part of the medical therapy. Special efforts are needed to ensure a safe environment, such as padding the crib and playpen for infants and young children. Older children should be encouraged to participate in noncontact sports such as swimming, hiking, or bicycling. Active hemophiliac children seem to bleed less than those who are sedentary. Strengthening the muscles around the joints may decrease the number of spontaneous bleeding episodes.

Another complication in children receiving frequent factor replacement is the development of immunoglobulin G antibodies directed against either factor VIII or IX. A hematologist should be consulted for treatment of these children. Due to the use of purified plasma-derived or recombinant factor concentrates, viral infections (human immunodeficiency virus, hepatitis) from contaminated factor products are no longer a problem for those who use these products.

Since the development of factor concentrates, home management is now possible. The parent and child are taught to do venipuncture and to administer factor concentrates at home.

Primary Nursing Diagnosis   Impaired Hematologic Function*

Definition   Disturbance in blood cells

Possibly Related to   • Decrease in clotting factor VIII or
                                   IX resulting in hemorrhage

*Non-NANDA diagnosis.

Primary Nursing Diagnosis: Impaired hematologic function related to decrease in clotting factor VIII or IX resulting in hemorrhage

Assessment/Defining Characteristics of Child and/or Family (Subjective & Objective Data):

• Mild/moderate/severe/frequent/spontaneous bleeding episodes of
  1. skin
  2. mucous membranes
  3. joints (causing warmth, redness, swelling, pain, stiffness, tingling, and/or loss of movement)
  4. viscera (causing hematuria and/or black, tarry stools)
  5. central nervous system (causing headache, slurred speech, and/or loss of consciousness)
     • Prolonged partial thromboplastin time (PTT)
     • Low levels of factor VIII or IX coagulant levels
     • Tachycardia
     • Hypotension

Expected Outcomes	Possible Nursing Interventions	Rationale	Evaluation for Charting
Child will have increased hematologic function as evidenced by • lack of new areas of bleeding • elevation of deficient clotting factor to desired level (specify) • heart rate and blood pressure within acceptable range (state specific range for each) • lack of signs/symptoms of impaired hematologic function (such as those listed under Assessment)	Assess and record any new areas bleeding every 4 hours and PRN. If bleeding has occurred, assess and record HR and BP every 1 to 2 hours and PRN.	If bleeding has occurred, the HR will increase and the BP will decrease.	Describe any new areas bleeding noted. If bleeding has occurred, document ranges of HR and BP.
	Handle child gently. Implement bleeding precautions (such as avoidance of IM and subcutaneous injections, rectal temperature, caution with tape, etc.).	Helps to minimize pain, trauma (that can precipitate bleeding) and promote comfort.	Document whether child was handled gently and describe effectiveness of measure.
	Assist child in limiting activity by providing diversional activities (e.g., television, books).	Helps to minimize bleeding episodes.	Describe effectiveness of diversional activities in limiting activity.
	Immobilize and elevate any affected joints. Record effectiveness.	Reduces bleeding, swelling, and pain to affected area, which helps to prevent joint degeneration.	Describe effectiveness of immobilization and elevation to affected area.

(continued)

Primary Nursing Diagnosis: Impaired Hematologic Function (*continued*)

Expected Outcomes	Possible Nursing Interventions	Rationale	Evaluation for Charting
	Check and record results of PTT. Notify physician if results are more prolonged than previous results.	Prolonged PTT results in increased bleeding by decreasing clotting time.	Document results of PTT. Indicate whether it has increased or decreased from previous results.
	When indicated, perform passive range-of-motion exercises after bleeding has stopped. Record results.	Strengthens joints and muscle. Helps to prevent joint degeneration.	Describe effectiveness of range-of-motion exercises.
	Administer antihemophilic factor as indicated. Adhere to institutional policy and current guidelines for administration of products. Assess and record effectiveness and any side effects (e.g., flushing, urticaria, nausea/vomiting).	Provides needed factors for clotting of blood.	Document whether antihemophilic factor was administered according to institutional policy. Describe effectiveness of antihemophilic factor.
	If indicated, administer steroids on schedule. Assess and record effectiveness and any side effects (e.g., gastrointestinal distress, nausea).	Used to reduce inflammation in the joints.	Document whether steroids were administered on schedule. Describe effectiveness and any side effects noted.
	If indicated, administer aminocaproic acid on schedule. Assess and record effectiveness and any side effects noted (e.g., nausea, vomiting).	Applied locally to prevent clot destruction.	Document whether aminocaproic acid was administered on schedule. Describe effectiveness and any side effects noted.
TEACHING GOALS Child and/or family will be able to verbalize characteristics of impaired hematologic function such as • mild/moderate/severe/frequent/spontaneous bleeding episodes	Teach child/family about characteristics of impaired hematologic function (such as those listed under Assessment). Assess and record results.	Increased knowledge will assist the child/family in recognizing and reporting changes in the child's condition.	Document whether teaching was done and describe results.

Primary Nursing Diagnosis: Impaired Hematologic Function (*continued*)

Expected Outcomes	Possible Nursing Interventions	Rationale	Evaluation for Charting
Child and/or family will be able to verbalize knowledge of care such as • protection of child from injury by providing a safe environment (padded sides of crib and playpen, use of car seats in automobiles, etc.) • recognition and management of bleeding episodes by 1. applying pressure to area for 10 to 15 minutes 2. immobilizing and elevating the area above the level of the heart 3. applying cold to promote vasoconstriction • prevention of joint degeneration by 1. elevating and immobilizing the joint 2. performing passive range-of-motion exercises after the bleeding has stopped 3. assisting with physical therapy when indicted • venipuncture technique and medication administration • assessing for medication reaction (e.g., chills, fever, shaking, urticaria, flushing, nausea/vomiting) • fostering of child's independence when child is ready • having child wear Medic Alert identification	Teach child/family about care. Assess and record child's/family's knowledge of and participation in care regarding protection of child from injury by providing a safe environment, recognition and management of bleeding episodes, medication administration, etc.	Education of child/family will allow for accurate care.	Document whether teaching was done and describe results.

(*continued*)

Primary Nursing Diagnosis: Impaired Hematologic Function *(continued)*			
Expected Outcomes	**Possible Nursing Interventions**	**Rationale**	**Evaluation for Charting**
• encouraging child to participate in non-contact sports such as swimming • encourage child to establish good oral hygiene routine including use of a soft-bristle toothbrush • identification of any signs/symptoms of impaired hematologic function (such as those listed under Assessment) • when to contact health-care provider			

Nursing Diagnosis Acute Pain

Definition Condition in which an individual experiences acute mild to severe pain

Possibly Related to • Pressure in a joint or muscle spasms secondary to bleeding into a joint cavity resulting from factor deficiency

Nursing Diagnosis: Acute pain related to pressure in the joint or muscle spasms secondary to bleeding into a joint cavity resulting from factor deficiency			
Assessment/Defining Characteristics of Child and/or Family (Subjective & Objective Data):			

• Inability to move affected joint
• Severe discomfort on movement of involved joint
• Swelling and redness of affected area
• Local increase in skin temperature
• Crying or moaning
• Facial grimacing
• Verbal expression of pain
		• Restlessness
		• Physical signs/symptoms
		  1. tachycardia
		  2. tachypnea
		  3. increased blood pressure
		  4. diaphoresis	

Expected Outcomes	**Possible Nursing Interventions**	**Rationale**	**Evaluation for Charting**
Child will have decreased pain or be free of severe and/or constant pain as evidenced by • decreased swelling and redness of the affected joint	Assess and record HR, RR, BP, and any signs/symptoms of pain (such as those listed under Assessment) every 4 hours and PRN. Use age-appropriate pain-assessment tool.	Provides data regarding the level of pain child is experiencing.	Document range of HR, RR, BP, and degree of pain child is experiencing. Describe any successful measures used to decrease pain.

Nursing Diagnosis: Acute Pain *(continued)*

Expected Outcomes	Possible Nursing Interventions	Rationale	Evaluation for Charting
• decreased skin temperature of the affected joint • lack of constant crying or moaning • verbal communication of decreased pain • lack of facial grimacing and restlessness • heart rate, respiratory rate, and blood pressure with acceptable ranges (state specific range for each) • decreased diaphoresis • lack of signs/symptoms of pain (such as those listed under Assessment)	Handle child gently.	Helps to minimize pain and promote comfort.	Document whether child was handled gently and effectiveness of measure.
	Apply cold packs to help alleviate the pain. Record results.	Helps to decrease swelling which will decrease pain.	Document effectiveness of using cold packs.
	Assist child in limiting activity by providing diversional activities (e.g., television, books).	Diversional activities can distract child and may help to decrease pain.	Document whether diversional activities were successful in helping to manage pain.
	Immobilize and elevate any affected joints.	Reduces bleeding, swelling and pain to affected area, which helps to prevent joint degeneration.	Describe effectiveness of immobilization and elevation to affected area.
	When indicated, perform passive range-of-motion exercises after bleeding has stopped. Record results.	Strengthens joints and muscle. Helps to prevent joint degeneration.	Describe effectiveness of range-of-motion exercises.
	Administer non-aspirin-containing analgesics and/or narcotics on schedule. Assess and record effectiveness.	Analgesics and narcotics reduce pain.	Document whether analgesics and/or narcotics were administered on schedule. Describe effectiveness of pain management.
	Administer antihemophilic factor as indicated. Adhere to institutional policy and current guidelines for administration of products. Assess and record effectiveness and any side effects (e.g., flushing, urticaria, nausea/vomiting).	Provides needed factors for clotting of blood.	Document whether antihemophilic factor was administered and describe effectiveness.
TEACHING GOALS Child and/or family will be able to verbalize at least 4 characteristics of pain such as • inability to move affected joint • severe discomfort on movement of involved joint	Teach child/family about characteristics of pain. Assess and record results.	Increased knowledge will assist the child/family in recognizing and reporting changes in the child's condition.	Document whether teaching was done and describe results.

(continued)

Nursing Diagnosis: Acute Pain *(continued)*			
Expected Outcomes	**Possible Nursing Interventions**	**Rationale**	**Evaluation for Charting**
• swelling and redness of affected area • local increase in skin temperature • facial grimacing • verbal expression of pain			

Child and/or family will be able to verbalize knowledge of care such as
 	
• protection of child from injury by providing a safe environment (padded sides of crib and playpen, use of car seats in automobiles, etc.)
• recognition and management of bleeding episodes by
  1. applying pressure to area for 10 to 15 minutes
  2. immobilizing and elevating the area above the level of the heart
  3. applying cold to promote vasoconstriction
• prevention of joint degeneration by
  1. elevating and immobilizing the joint
  2. performing passive range-of-motion exercises after the bleeding has stopped
  3. assisting with physical therapy when indicated
• medication administration (non-aspirin-containing analgesics)
• venipuncture technique and medication administration
	Teach child/family about care. Assess and record child's/family's knowledge of and participation in care regarding protection of child from injury by providing a safe environment, recognition and management of bleeding episodes, medication administration, etc.	Education of child/family will allow for accurate care.	Document whether teaching was done and describe results.

Nursing Diagnosis: Acute Pain *(continued)*			
Expected Outcomes	**Possible Nursing Interventions**	**Rationale**	**Evaluation for Charting**
• assessing for medication reaction (e.g., chills, fever, shaking, urticaria, flushing, nausea/vomiting) • fostering of child's independence when child is ready • having child wear Medic Alert identification • encouraging child to participate in noncontact sports such as swimming • encourage child to establish good oral hygiene routine including use of a soft-bristle toothbrush • identification of any signs/symptoms of pain (such as those listed under Assessment) • when to contact health-care provider			

Related Nursing Diagnoses

Impaired Physical Mobility	*related to* a. joint pain b. joint swelling c. bleeding episodes
Deficient Knowledge: Child/Family	*related to* a. home management b. disease state
Deficient Fluid Volume	*related to* blood loss out of vascular system
Compromised Family Coping	*related to* a. home management b. child's activity restriction c. genetic nature of disorder

TWO

IDIOPATHIC THROMBOCYTOPENIA PURPURA
MEDICAL DIAGNOSIS

PATHOPHYSIOLOGY Idiopathic thrombocytopenia purpura (ITP), an acquired hemorrhagic disorder characterized by a marked decrease in circulating platelets, is the most common type of childhood thrombocytopenia. Its primary cause is unknown, but it is believed to be due to an autoimmune phenomenon in which platelets become coated with an antiplatelet antibody, which alters the surface of the platelets so they become antigenic and are subsequently destroyed by the reticuloendothelial system in the spleen.

Idiopathic thrombocytopenia purpura can be acute, which is usually self-limiting, or chronic, which is interspersed with periods of remission. The acute form often follows a nonspecific viral infection, such as an upper respiratory infection. The prognosis for acute ITP is excellent, and children usually recover in 6 months. The most common clinical manifestations of either type include a sudden onset of easy bruising, randomly distributed petechiae, and ecchymoses all over the body. Other signs and symptoms include bleeding from mucous membranes (e.g., epistaxis) and internal hemorrhage manifested by hematuria, bloody stools, and menorrhagia.

There is no definitive test used to diagnose ITP. The platelet count is usually reduced to below 20,000 mm³/dL. The tourniquet test (that demonstrates capillary fragility) is positive. Red and white blood cell counts, partial thromboplastin time (PTT), prothrombin time (PT), and hemoglobin concentration are all usually normal. Bone marrow aspiration is useful if aplastic anemia or leukemia is suspected.

Treatment of ITP varies. Activity is usually limited to try to prevent further petechiae and ecchymoses (especially avoidance of contact sports), and aspirin-containing drugs are eliminated. Some physicians do not prescribe any medications and allow the disease to run its course. Others prescribe corticosteroid therapy, although the platelet count will decline as the steroids are tapered. Intravenous immune globulin (IVIG) can be used, as well as anti-D immunoglobulin. Platelet transfusions are not useful because the transfused platelets become coated with the antiplatelet antibody and are destroyed in the spleen.

When the child has ITP for longer than 6 months, they are considered to have chronic ITP. As with the child with acute ITP, they are otherwise well, usually have no underlying disease, and other than contact sports, can participate in all activities of childhood. They receive the same treatment as with acute ITP, but may need steroids, IVIG, or anti-D immunoglobulin before elective surgery, after trauma, or if their platelets remain below 20,000/mm³/dL. Splenectomy is usually reserved as a last resort for children who have recurrent or chronic ITP. After a splenectomy, 60 to 80% of children are free of signs and symptoms of ITP.

Primary Nursing Diagnosis   Impaired Hematologic Function*

Definition   Disturbance in blood cells

Possibly Related to   • Decreased number of circulating platelets

*Non-NANDA diagnosis.

Primary Nursing Diagnosis: Impaired hematologic function related to deceased number of circulating platelets

Assessment/Defining Characteristics of Child and/or Family (Subjective & Objective Data):

- Petechiae
- Ecchymoses
- Tachycardia
- Hypotension
- Bleeding from mucous membranes, including
  1. epistaxis
  2. bleeding gums

  3. hematuria
  4. blood in stools
  5. menorrhagia
- Platelet count below 20,000 mm³/dL

Expected Outcomes	Possible Nursing Interventions	Rationale	Evaluation for Charting

Child will have increased hematologic function as evidenced by
 	
• lack of new areas of petechiae or ecchymoses
• heart rate and blood pressure within acceptable range (state specific range for each)
• lack of bleeding from mucous membranes, including
  1. epistaxis
  2. bleeding gums
  3. hematuria
  4. blood in stools
  5. menorrhagia
• platelet count between 150,000 and 400,000 mm³/dL.
	Assess and record HR, BP, any new areas of petechiae or ecchymoses, and other signs/symptoms of impaired hematologic function every 4 hours and PRN.	Helps to establish hematologic status of child. If bleeding has occurred, the HR will increase and the BP will decrease.	Document range of HR and BP. Describe any new areas of petechiae, ecchymoses, and other signs/symptoms of impaired hematologic function noted.

	Handle child gently. Organize nursing care to avoid trauma to the child's tissues and, when indicated, implement bleeding precautions (e.g., do not use a rectal thermometer, avoid intramuscular injections, provide a soft-bristle toothbrush for child).	Helps to minimize trauma, prevent bleeding, and promote comfort.	Document whether child was handled gently and describe effectiveness of this and other measures.
	Assist child in limiting activity by providing diversional activities (e.g., television, books).	Helps to prevent further petechiae and ecchymoses.	Describe effectiveness of diversional activities in limiting activity.
	Check and record results of platelet count. Notify physician if results are decreased from previous results.	Decreased platelets will result in an increase in petechiae, ecchymoses, and other symptoms.	Document results of platelet count and indicate any change from previous results.
	If indicated, administer steroids and intravenous immune globulin (IVIG) on schedule. Assess and record effectiveness and any side effects (e.g., gastrointestinal distress, nausea, electrolyte imbalance).	Steroids and IVIG help decrease the rate of platelet destruction.	Document whether steroids and IVIG were administered on schedule. Describe effectiveness and any side effects noted.

(continued)

Primary Nursing Diagnosis: Impaired Hematologic Function (*continued*)

Expected Outcomes	Possible Nursing Interventions	Rationale	Evaluation for Charting
	When indicated, administer anti-D immunoglobulin on schedule. Assess and record effectiveness and any side effects (e.g., fever, chills, headache).	Anti-D immunoglobulin helps prolong the survival of the platelets.	Document whether anti-D immunoglobulin was administered on schedule. Describe effectiveness and any side effects noted.
TEACHING GOALS Child and/or family will be able to verbalize at least 4 characteristics of impaired hematologic function such as • petechiae • ecchymoses • epistaxis • bleeding gums	Teach child/family about characteristics of impaired hematologic function. Assess and record results.	Increased knowledge will assist the child/family in recognizing and reporting changes in the child's condition.	Document whether teaching was done and describe results.
Child and/or family will be able to verbalize knowledge of care such as • protection of child from injury by providing a safe environment (padded sides of crib and playpen, use of car seats in automobiles, etc.) • recognition of signs and symptoms of impaired hematologic function (such as those listed under Assessment) • encouraging child to participate in noncontact sports such as swimming • use of non-aspirin-containing medications for pain relief or fever • potential alterations in lifestyle, such as not blowing nose hard, not straining at defecation, using a soft-bristle toothbrush • when indicated, testing of urine (dipstick) and stool (hematest) for blood • when to contact health-care provider	Teach child/family about care. Assess and record child's/family's knowledge of and participation in care regarding protection of child from injury by providing a safe environment, etc.	Education of child/family will allow for accurate care.	Document whether teaching was done and describe results.

Nursing Diagnosis   Fear: Child/Family

Definition   Feeling of apprehension resulting from a known cause

Possibly Related to
- Knowledge deficit concerning disease state
- Unfamiliar surroundings
- Forced contact with strangers
- Treatments and procedures
- Body image disturbance secondary to ecchymoses and petechiae

Nursing Diagnosis: Fear related to knowledge deficit concerning disease state, unfamiliar surroundings, forced contact with strangers, treatments and procedures, body image disturbance secondary to ecchymoses and petechiae

Assessment/Defining Characteristics of Child and/or Family (Subjective & Objective Data):

- Uncooperativeness
- Hostile behavior
- Regressed behavior
- Restlessness
- Inability to recall previously taught information
- Decreased communication
- Decreased attention span
- Verbal expression of fear to the health-care team

Expected Outcomes	Possible Nursing Interventions	Rationale	Evaluation for Charting
Child/family will exhibit only a minimal amount of fear as evidenced by • ability to appropriately relate to family members • lack of hostile behavior • lack of regressed behavior • ability to rest and sleep when indicated • ability to restate information previously taught • ability to participate in care • ability to separate for short periods, when indicated • verbal expression of less fear to members of the health-care team	Assess and record any signs/symptoms of fear demonstrated by child/family (such as those listed under Assessment) every 8 hours and PRN.	Provides information about the level of fear and possibly the source of the fear.	Document level of fear and any identified sources of the fear.
	Decrease child's/family's fear when possible by • encouraging family members to stay with child. • encouraging family members to participate in the child's care. • if possible, having the same nurses and staff care for the child from day to day. • spending extra time with the child when family members are unable to be present. • encouraging family members to bring in familiar articles and toys from home. • explaining to child/family what to expect during procedures.	These measures will help to make the child and family members to be more comfortable and can help to decrease fear.	Document any measures used to help alleviate fear. Document effectiveness of measures.

(continued)

Nursing Diagnosis: Fear: Child/Family *(continued)*

Expected Outcomes	Possible Nursing Interventions	Rationale	Evaluation for Charting
	Initiate age-appropriate play when indicated. Document effectiveness.	Play can help to decrease fears.	Document whether therapeutic play was used and describe its effectiveness.
	Encourage child/family to express fears to the health-care team.	Expression and identification of fears can help the child/family to find ways to manage these fears.	Document any identified fears.
	Reinforce and clarify all information as necessary.	Reinforcing and clarifying information can help decrease fears.	Document whether any information was reinforced and clarified for the family. Describe effectiveness.
	Encourage child/family to meet basic needs, such as eating and resting appropriately. Assist them as needed.	Assist child/family in decreasing stress, which can help to identify and alleviate fears.	Document whether child/family were able to separate for short periods so that family members could meet their own basic needs.
TEACHING GOALS Child and/or family will be able to verbalize at least 4 characteristics of fear such as • uncooperativeness • regressed behavior • hostile behavior • decreased communication • verbal communication of fear	Teach child/family about characteristics of fear. Assess and record results.	Increased knowledge will assist the child/family in recognizing and reporting changes in the child's condition.	Document whether teaching was done and describe results.
Child and/or family will be able to verbalize knowledge of care such as • appropriate diversional activities • identification of any signs/symptoms of fear (such as those listed under Assessment) • when to contact health-care provider	Teach child/family about care. Assess and record child's/family's knowledge of and participation in care regarding appropriate diversional activities, etc.	Education of child/family will allow for accurate care.	Document whether teaching was done and describe results.

Related Nursing Diagnoses

Temporary Impaired Physical Mobility	*related to* decreased circulating platelets
Deficient Knowledge: Child/Family	*related to* a. disease state b. home management
Deficient Fluid Volume	*related to* blood loss
Risk for Infection	*related to* side effects of steroids
Compromised Family Coping	*related to* a. knowledge deficit of disease state b. home management c. child's activity restrictions d. uncertainty of disease course (will child need a splenectomy in the future)

THREE

NEOPLASMS
MEDICAL DIAGNOSIS

PATHOPHYSIOLOGY

Acute Lymphoblastic Leukemia Leukemia is the term used to describe a group of malignancies of the bone marrow and lymphatic system. It is the most common childhood malignancy and its causes are not well understood. Infectious agents, chemical agents, ionizing radiation, and genetic factors may all play a role. The incidence of acute leukemias is increased in certain genetic syndromes, such as Down syndrome or in those children with immune deficiency states, such as Wiskott-Aldrich syndrome.

Leukemias are classified as acute or chronic. Acute leukemias are characterized by the predominance of highly immature white blood cell precursors, or blasts. Chronic leukemias are characterized by proliferation of relatively mature white blood cells. Leukemias are also divided by whether the leukemic cells have characteristics of lymphocyte precursors (lymphoid) or myelocyte precursors (myeloid).

Acute lymphoblastic (lymphocytic) leukemia (ALL) results from malignant changes of the lymphocyte or its precursor and is acute at onset. Of the childhood leukemias, the majorities are ALL and account for 25% of cancers in those younger than 15 years of age, with a marked peak in incidence between 2 and 4 years of age. It is more common in males and whites as compared to blacks. Approximately 90% of all children diagnosed with ALL will be cured.

Classification of leukemia is based on the immune characteristics of the leukemic cells. The condition can be further subdivided according to the morphologic and immunologic features of lymphoblasts (immature white blood cells) and according to the clinical presentation of the child. The subdivisions (determined by cell membrane markers) include T lymphocyte (thymus derived) and B lymphocyte (bone marrow derived).

Leukemias of B-cell lineage account for most of the childhood leukemias. The most common cancer in children is early pre-B cell ALL. These lymphocytes have the common acute lymphocytic leukemia antigen (CALLA) on their surface. This type of ALL is the most responsive to therapy and has the best prognosis. There are several other B-cell subtypes of ALL.

In T cell leukemia, the cell of origin is a lymphocyte that has developed within the thymus. These lymphocytes lack CALLA. Infiltration of the central nervous system, liver, spleen, lymph, and mediastinum is more common in T cell leukemia than in other forms. Adolescents are more likely to get this type of leukemia and the prognosis is not as good.

The leukemic cell possesses qualities that the normal cell does not. The leukemic cells proliferate rapidly by cloning, instead of normal mitosis. This leads to replacement of the bone marrow with abnormal white blood cells (WBCs). In the marrow, these abnormal WBCs also replace the stem cells that produce red blood cells and other blood products (such as platelets), leading to a decrease in the amount of these products. Eventually, the child develops anemia (reduced red blood cells) and thrombocytopenia (reduced amount of platelets). The abnormal WBCs also spill out into the circulation, replacing normally functioning WBCs thereby decreasing the body's ability to fight infection. The leukemic cells also do not differentiate and are resistant to programmed cell death.

The clinical presentation of children with ALL results from the leukemic cells replacing bone marrow components and infiltrating multiple organs. Signs and symptoms can include anorexia, irritability, fatigue, lethargy, headache, fever, pallor, bone pain, bruising, and bleeding. The triad of neutropenia, anemia, and thrombocytopenia is present in the profile of the complete blood cell count (CBC). Bone marrow samples are necessary to delineate the type of leukemia and the appropriate therapy. A lumbar puncture is performed to evaluate any cerebrospinal fluid involvement.

The goals for treatment of ALL include early and continuing remissions. Remission induction, central nervous system prophylaxis, consolidation, and maintenance are the phases of the treatment regimen. Multiple-drug therapy is preferred to the use of a single agent. Bone marrow transplantation is also an option for children with ALL. With such a high cure rate for childhood ALL, many pediatric oncology centers are monitoring and providing follow-up care for the late effects of leukemia therapy.

Hodgkin Disease Hodgkin disease is a malignancy of the lymphoid system. Histology, cell lineage, clinical presentation, and response to treatment differentiate

Hodgkin lymphoma from other lymphomas. Hodgkin lymphoma arises in a single lymph node or anatomic group of nodes and follows a predictable pattern of progression. The pattern begins with painless regional nodal enlargement, followed by extension to adjacent nodes and, without treatment, extranodal involvement of the spleen, liver, lungs, and/or bone marrow. Hodgkin disease is rare before the age of 5, usually occurs between ages 15 and 35, and then again after age 55. It occurs 2 to 3 times more often in males.

Reed-Sternberg cells, giant, multinucleated cells, are diagnostic of Hodgkin disease when associated with certain cellular and architectural-type lesions. There are four subtypes of Hodgkin disease according to Rye classification. The **lymphocytic-predominant** variety, in which almost all cells are mature lymphocytes or a mixture of lymphocytes and benign histocytes, with only an occasional Reed-Sternberg cell, affects 9% of patients. This type has the best prognosis. The most common form, affecting 65% of patients, is the **nodular-sclerosing** variety. In this type, the involved lymph node is divided into nodular cellular areas by broad bands of collagen and a variant of the Reed-Sternberg cell called a lacunar cell. Hodgkin disease of **mixed-cellular** variety is characterized by the accumulation of lymphocytes, plasma cells, eosinophils, histocytes, malignant reticular cells, and Reed-Sternberg cells. This is the second most common form, affecting 22% of patients and found more commonly in those younger than 10 years of age. It often has extranodal involvement. The **lymphocytic-depletion** variety, uncommon in children, and least favorable form of Hodgkin disease, has many bizarre malignant reticular cells and Reed-Sternberg cells, with few lymphocytes. Currently, the World Health Organization (WHO) has replaced the above classification with classical Hodgkin lymphoma (CHL) and the uncommon, nodular lymphocyte-predominant Hodgkin lymphoma (NLPHL).

Staging indicates the extent of disease. The Ann Arbor Staging Classification for Hodgkin Disease is used and is as follows: Stage I disease is limited to a single node, a lymph node region, or a single extra-lymphatic organ or site. Stage II disease involves two or more lymph node regions on the same side of the diaphragm or localized involvement of extralymphatic organ or site and one or more lymph node regions on the same side of the diaphragm. Stage III disease involves lymph node regions on both sides of the di-aphragm and involvement of an extra lymphatic organ or site or involvement of the spleen or both. Stage IV disease has diffuse or disseminated involvement of one or more extralymphatic organs or tissue with or without associated lymph node enlargement. The stages can be further subdivided by the absence (A) or presence (B) of systemic signs and symptoms such as

unexplained fever for at least 3 consecutive days, drenching night sweats, and unintentional weight loss of 10% or greater within 6 months.

Painless, rubbery, mobile, enlarged cervical lymph nodes are the most common presenting feature. Regional inflammation can rarely be found to explain the lymphadenopathy. The patient has few if any systemic symptoms other than anorexia, malaise, and lassitude. Numerous laboratory studies and tests are necessary for diagnosis and staging, starting with a lymph node or tissue biopsy. Computed tomography (CT) and magnetic resonance imaging (MRI), as well as positron emission tomography (PET) may also be used.

Hodgkin disease is treatable, with a good prognosis. Combination chemotherapy, alone or in conjunction with radiation, is highly effective. The intensity of treatment varies with disease presentation, histology, and stage.

Neuroblastoma Neuroblastoma is the most common extracranial solid tumor in children and the most common tumor found in infants during the first year of life. Its cause is unknown. The tumor may arise from any site where neurocrest cells are present along the sympathetic chain, from the posterior cranial fossa to the coccyx. The neurocrest cells form the adrenal medulla, paraganglia, and sympathetic nervous system of the cervical sympathetic chain and the thoracic chain.

Often the primary site is in the abdomen, as the majority of neuroblastomas arise from the adrenal gland or retroperitoneal sympathetic chain. Other sites include the head, neck, chest, or pelvis. If it is located in the abdomen, it usually crosses the midline, which is in contrast to Wilms tumor. Neuroblastoma is usually a firm, gray mass. Most neuroblastomas consist primarily of neuroblastoma cells with little evidence of differentiation. The tumor can invade adjacent tissue, making surgical excision difficult. Neuroblastoma may also extend to the regional lymph nodes via lymphatics. Hematogenous spread usually involves the liver, bones, and bone marrow.

Staging of neuroblastoma indicates the extent of disease. Stage I, a localized primary tumor, with negative lymph nodes, can be completely resected. Stage II disease is a unilateral tumor, with incomplete gross excision, and negative lymph nodes. Stage III disease has the tumor extending across the midline, with or without lymph involvement. Stage IV involves a tumor with distant metastases to the bone, bone marrow, liver, and other organs. Stage IV-S is a special stage in which metastatic disease is limited to the bone marrow, liver, or skin, but not bone.

The clinical manifestations of neuroblastoma vary according to the site of the primary tumor and any metastasis that has occurred. Diagnosis of neuroblastoma can often be made after metastasis has occurred when the child presents with signs of involvement of the nonprimary site. An abdominal mass, fever, irritability, pain from bone metastases, and orbital ecchymoses or proptosis from skull metastases may be present. A history of altered bowel and bladder patterns, anorexia, weight loss, difficulty sleeping, neurological changes, and pain contribute to the diagnosis of neuroblastoma. Numerous diagnostic (CT, MRI, bone scans, etc.) and laboratory evaluations are recommended to make the diagnosis of neuroblastoma and evaluate the degree of metastasis.

Treatment of neuroblastoma involves a variety of combinations of surgery, chemotherapy, and radiation therapy, depending on the stage of disease and the age of the child. The child's prognosis depends on the age of the child at diagnosis and the stage of the disease.

Osteogenic Sarcoma   Osteogenic sarcoma is the most frequently diagnosed malignant primary tumor of the bone. Its onset is most common during the adolescent growth spurt. The cause is unknown. Osteogenic sarcoma, or osteosarcoma, is defined as a primary malignant bone tumor, whose neoplastic cells produce osteoid and osseous tissue. The tumor usually arises in the metaphysis of the long bones, the points of most active growth, but it can also occur in the diaphysis. The tumor arises in the medullary canal of the shaft and breaks through the cortex of the bone to form a soft tissue mass. A single tumor may be the site of diverse differentiating cells, including osteosarcomatous, fibrosarcomatous, and chondrosarcomatous elements. Osteosarcoma can occur in any bone, but the distal femur is the most common site. The proximal tibia and the proximal humerus are other common sites. Metastasis to the lungs frequently occurs.

The most common initial findings of osteogenic sarcoma are pain and, sometimes, swelling at the tumor site. Often these symptoms are attributed to an athletic injury. Later symptoms can include limited movement of the affected extremity, limping or an altered gait, local erythema, and warmth. A number of diagnostic tests (radiographic studies, CT, MRI, bone scan) and laboratory evaluations are done to make the diagnosis.

Treatment for osteogenic sarcoma is aimed toward local control of the primary tumor and prevention of metastasis. A combination of surgery and chemotherapy is often used. Surgery can include amputation or limb salvage procedure. Because osteosarcoma is relatively radio resistant, radiation is reserved for nonresectable tumors of the ribs, pelvis, skull, or for controlling metastatic disease. Prognosis is best when the tumors have low metastatic potential.

Rhabdomyosarcoma   Rhabdomyosarcoma is a malignant tumor of striated muscle cells. It can also originate in tissue that does not contain striated muscle because of its mesenchymal origin. Mesenchyme normally grows into fat, muscle, and bone. Rhabdomyosarcoma accounts for most soft-tissue tumors in childhood. Peak incidence is from 2 to 4 years of age, with a second peak during the adolescent years of 12 to 16. The cause is unknown.

Two major histologic types of rhabdomyosarcoma exist: embryonal and alveolar. The rhabdomyoblasts in the embryonal variety resemble fetal cells at 6 to 8 weeks of development. Approximately 60 to 70% of rhabdomyosarcomas are embryonal and arise from the head, neck, and genitourinary tract. The botryoid type of the embryonal form appears as a cluster of grapes presenting in a body cavity such as the bladder, vagina, nasopharynx, or biliary tract. Spindle cell tumors are another subset of embryonal rhabdomyosarcoma, and occur in the testicular area. The rhabdomyoblasts of alveolar rhabdomyosarcoma resemble fetal cells at 10 to 12 weeks of development and occur most often in the trunk, extremities, and perineum. This variety is seen more commonly in older children and adolescents, and has the poorest prognosis. The pleomorphic rhabdomyosarcoma type is rare in childhood and mixed rhabdomyosarcoma contains more than one of the histologic types.

Staging indicates the extent of the disease. Group I disease is localized, completely removable, with no involvement of regional nodes. Group II involves regional lymph nodes or microscopic residual disease. Group III is indicated by gross residual disease. Group IV has distant metastatic disease at the time of diagnosis.

Rhabdomyosarcoma can present anywhere in the body, causing a variety of symptoms related to the site of the tumor and compression of adjacent organs. Some tumors, such as those close to the eyes, produce symptoms early, whereas other tumors, such as those in the abdomen, may be asymptomatic. Diagnosis of the mass is confirmed by CT, MRI, PET, bone marrow aspiration and biopsy, as well as a number of laboratory evaluations. Treatment can involve a combination of surgery, chemotherapy, and radiation, depending on the location and stage of the tumor.

Wilms Tumor   Wilms tumor, or nephroblastoma, is an embryonal tumor of the kidney that originates from immature renoblast cells. It is the most common abdominal tumor of childhood, and occurs most frequently between 2 and 3 years of age. It occurs in both sexes and in all races with approximately equal frequency. There is an association between Wilms tumor and several congenital anomalies, such as aniridia, hemihypertrophy, and genitourinary anomalies. There is also evidence of a genetic link, as there is increased incidence of Wilms tumor among siblings.

Wilms tumor often extends from the kidney parenchyma into the renal cavity, distorting the renal outline as the residual normal kidney is compressed into a thin rim around the tumor. Wilms tumors are sharply demarcated and variably encapsulated. The tumor is vascular and lends itself to hematogenous spread. The abdomen should not be palpated once Wilms tumor has been diagnosed as the tumor may rupture if manipulated, causing its cells to spread throughout the peritoneal cavity.

Staging of Wilms tumor is performed during surgery. Stage I tumors are limited to the kidney and can be totally resected. Stage II tumors extend beyond the kidney but can still be completely resected. Stage III tumors leave residual nonhematogenous tumors in the abdomen after surgery. Stage IV indicates hematogenous metastases; the most frequent sites of metastasis are the lung, liver, and brain. Stage V tumors have bilateral renal involvement. The histology of the tumor cells is divided into favorable histology or unfavorable histology.

The most common presenting sign in Wilms tumor is an abdominal mass, which is characteristically firm and smooth and is usually asymptomatic. Some children also present with abdominal pain, vomiting, hematuria, dysuria, frequency, anorexia, weight loss, and malaise. Hypertension can also occur, possibly due to pressure on the renal artery, renal ischemia, or increased renin secretion. Numerous laboratory evaluations and diagnostic studies (ultrasound of the abdomen, CT, MRI, and intravenous pyelogram, etc.) are used to make the diagnosis of Wilms tumor.

Treatment protocols are based on the clinical stage and histologic pattern and can include various combinations of surgery, chemotherapy, and radiation. Wilms tumor is one of the most curable childhood tumors. Prognosis is influenced by the specific histology, the stage of the tumor, and the age of the child at the time of diagnosis.

Primary Nursing Diagnosis Risk for Infection

Definition Condition in which the body is at risk for being invaded by microorganisms

Possibly Related to
- Leukopenia
- Neutropenia
- Side effects of chemotherapeutic agents

Primary Nursing Diagnosis: Risk for infection related to leukopenia, neutropenia, side effects of chemotherapeutic agents

Assessment/Defining Characteristics of Child and/or Family (Subjective & Objective Data):

- Fever or drop in temperature
- Weak, rapid pulse
- Tachypnea
- Hypotension
- Altered white blood cell count (WBC)
- Absolute neutrophil count (ANC) < 1,000
- Positive culture results
- Lethargy
- Chills
- Diaphoresis
- Ashen color
- Decreased urine output
- Prolonged capillary refill

- Signs/symptoms from various body systems:
  1. thrush
  2. mouth ulcerations
  3. runny nose
  4. sore throat
  5. dysuria headache
  6. decreased breath sounds
  7. changes in rate and depth of respirations
  8. cloudy or foul-smelling urine
  9. anal fissures
  10. skin breakdown
  11. reddened puncture sites
  12. edematous puncture sites

(continued)

Primary Nursing Diagnosis: Risk for Infection (*continued*)

Expected Outcomes	Possible Nursing Interventions	Rationale	Evaluation for Charting
Child will be free of infection or have decreased symptoms as evidenced by • body temperature within acceptable range of 36.5°C to 37.2°C • heart rate within acceptable range (state specific range) • respiratory within acceptable range (state specific range) • blood pressure within acceptable range (state specific range) • WBC within acceptable range (state specific range) • ANC greater than or equal to 1,000 • clear and equal breath sounds bilaterally A & P • lack of signs/symptoms of infection (such as those listed under Assessment)	Assess and record every 2 to 4 hours and PRN: • T, HR, RR, and BP • breath sounds • any signs/symptoms of infection (such as those listed under Assessment)	If infection is present, the T, HR, and RR will increase and the BP may decrease. The breath sounds will be abnormal if infection is present.	Document range of T, HR, RR, and BP. Describe breath sounds and any signs/symptoms of infection noted.
	Assess and record IV fluids and condition of IV site every hour.	It is necessary to record the amount of IV fluids every hour to make sure the child is not being over or under hydrated. The IV site needs to be assessed every hour for signs of redness or swelling.	Document amount of IV fluids and describe condition of IV site along with any interventions needed.
	Maintain good hand-washing technique.	Good hand washing is the single most important measure in decreasing infection.	Document whether good hand-washing technique was used.
	When indicated obtain cultures (blood, throat, urine).	Cultures are obtained to identify possible sources of infection.	Document whether any cultures were obtained.
	Check and record results of WBC, ANC, chest X-ray, and any cultures. Notify physician of any abnormalities.	Abnormal results may indicate an infection.	Document current results of any testing. Describe any therapeutic measures initiated.
	When indicated, administer antibiotics and antifungals on schedule. Assess and record any side effects (e.g., rash, diarrhea).	Antibiotics and antifungals are given to combat infection.	Document whether antibiotics or antifungals were administered on schedule. Describe any side effects noted.
	When indicated, administer antipyretics on schedule and PRN. Assess and record effectiveness.	Antipyretics are used to reduce fever.	Document whether an antipyretic was needed and describe effectiveness.
	Use aseptic technique for all procedures.	Prevents contamination.	Document if aseptic technique was used for procedures.
	Ensure that child has a private room and that no ill family members, friends, or health-care or institution employees visit the child.	Prevents spread of germs from others to the child.	Document whether anyone coming in contact with the child was ill.

Primary Nursing Diagnosis: Risk for Infection *(continued)*			
Expected Outcomes	**Possible Nursing Interventions**	**Rationale**	**Evaluation for Charting**
	Keep accurate record of intake and output.	Provides information about fluid status of patient.	Document intake and output.
TEACHING GOALS Child and/or family will be able to verbalize at least 4 characteristics of infection such as • fever • chills • ashen color • lethargy	Teach child/family about characteristics of risk for infection. Assess and record results.	Increased knowledge will assist the child/family in recognizing and reporting changes in the child's condition.	Document whether teaching was done and describe results.
Child and/or family will be able to verbalize knowledge of care such as • good hand-washing technique • fever control • medication administration • identification of any signs/symptoms of further infection (such as those listed under Assessment) • when to contact health-care provider	Teach child/family about care. Assess and record child's/family's knowledge of and participation in care regarding good hand-washing technique, fever control, etc.	Education of child/family will allow for accurate care.	Document whether teaching was done and describe results.

Nursing Diagnosis   Grieving: Family

Definition   Feelings of deep sadness and distress

Possibly Related to
• Perceived potential loss of
  • child
  • organ or limb of child
  • various body functions of child
• Disfigurement of child

Nursing Diagnosis: Grieving: family related to perceived potential for
- loss of child
- loss of organ or limb of child
- loss of various body functions of child
- disfigurement of child

Assessment/Defining Characteristics of Child and/or Family (Subjective & Objective Data):
- Verbal expression of grief by the family
- Sadness
- Crying
- Screaming
- Hysteria
- Passivity
- Overprotectiveness or avoidance of child
- Inability to carry on with activities of daily living at optimal level
- Need for repeated explanations or reassurance

Expected Outcomes	Possible Nursing Interventions	Rationale	Evaluation for Charting
Family will grieve appropriately as evidenced by • crying • talking and asking questions about the child • seeking help, support, and advice appropriately • performing activities of daily living • discussing feelings, fears, and concerns about the perceived loss • using available resources • assisting with the child's care	Allow family members to grieve in their own way. Allow time for expression of feelings, fears, and concerns. Give comfort and support.	Provides for the family's emotional needs in a supportive environment and allows for the family to work through the grief process.	Describe any expression of feelings, fears, and concerns by family and any supportive measures provided.
	Encourage the family to spend time with their child. Allow family to participate in care of child when possible (baths, diaper changes, dressing changes, feeding, etc.).	Helps the family feel some control and less powerlessness or helplessness over the situation. Also provides some normality for the child.	Document whether family participated in care.
	Assist family, as needed, in planning for the care of the child.	Decreases stress for the family, which can facilitate their grieving.	Document if assistance was provided to family in planning for the care of the child.
	If possible grant the family's special requests (e.g., to spend time alone with child, to take photographs of child, etc.).	Provides for the emotional needs of the family and helps them work through the grief process.	Document if the family had any special requests and if they were granted.
	If possible, have the same nurses care for the child from day to day.	Consistency and the development of trust for the child and family can help them work through the grief process.	Document if the same nurses were able to consistently care for child.
	Allow family time to meet their own needs and perform activities of daily living.	Allows family to cope with the child's situation, if their needs are met.	Document whether family was able to meet their needs and perform activities of daily living.
	Provide access to resources (e.g., social, spiritual, counseling, financial) and support groups.	Provides resources for the family to assist with their stress and grief.	Document what resources were made available to the family.

Nursing Diagnosis: Grieving: Family *(continued)*			
Expected Outcomes	**Possible Nursing Interventions**	**Rationale**	**Evaluation for Charting**
	Keep family up to date on the condition of the child. Clarify any misperceptions or misinformation for family.	Current and correct information will help increase the family's understanding and acceptance.	Document information shared with the family and describe the family's response.
TEACHING GOALS Child and/or family will be able to verbalize at least 4 characteristics of grieving such as • sadness • crying • inability to do activities of daily living • overprotectiveness or avoidance of child	Teach child/family about characteristics of grieving. Assess and record results.	Increased knowledge will assist the child/family in recognizing and reporting changes in the child's/family's condition.	Document whether teaching was done and describe results.
Child and/or family will be able to verbalize knowledge of grieving such as • stages of grief • potential feelings associated with the grieving process • potential behaviors associated with the grieving process • identification of any signs/symptoms of grief (such as those listed under Assessment) • when to contact health-care provider	Teach child/family about the grieving process. Assess and record child's/family's knowledge of and participation in care regarding stages of grief, etc.	Education of child/family will allow for accurate care. Promotes understanding of the grief process.	Document whether teaching was done and describe results.

Related Nursing Diagnoses

Risk for Injury	*related to* a. decreased number of circulating platelets b. increased fragility of mucous membranes or skin c. side effects of chemotherapeutic agents
Imbalanced Nutrition: Less than Body Requirements	*related to* a. dysphagia secondary to stomatitis b. increased metabolic rate c. insufficient nutrients available for normal cells due to malignant cell utilization of nutrients d. anorexia e. nausea and vomiting
Acute Pain	*related to* a. treatments b. procedures c. side effects of medications
Deficient Knowledge: Child/Parental	*related to* a. disease process b. effects and side effects of chemotherapy c. procedures
Disturbed Body Image	*related to* a. alopecia b. cushingoid features c. weight loss
Activity Intolerance	*related to* decreased oxygenation to tissues secondary to low hemoglobin

FOUR

SICKLE CELL DISEASE
MEDICAL DIAGNOSIS

PATHOPHYSIOLOGY Sickle cell disease is the term applied to a group of inherited (autosomal recessive) hemoglobinopathies. These diseases are characterized by the production of the hemoglobin variant, hemoglobin S (Hb S), in place of the normal adult hemoglobin A (Hb A). The most common forms of sickle cell disease include sickle cell anemia (Hb SS), sickle hemoglobin C disease (Hb SC), and the hemoglobin S beta thalassemia syndromes (Hb S beta thal). Approximately two-thirds of those with sickle cell disease have Hb SS.

The sickle cell disorders can be found in people of African, Mediterranean, Indian, Caribbean, Asian, and Middle Eastern heritage. Newborn screening and follow-up for sickle cell disease and trait exists in most states. Sickle cell disease can be diagnosed by several laboratory tests. These include isoelectric focusing (IEF), hemoglobin electrophoresis (HbEp), high-performance liquid chromography (HPLC), or DNA analysis. Genetic counseling is recommended for individuals and families who have sickle cell disease or trait. The life expectancy has increased significantly for those with sickle cell disease.

Red blood cells contain hemoglobin. The hemoglobin binds to oxygen and then releases the oxygen at a tissue site. Hemoglobin is a complex protein made up of globin molecules and heme (iron-containing) molecules. Oxygenated hemoglobin is bright red in color, giving arterial blood its color. In Hb S, valine replaces glutamic acid in the sixth position of the amino acid beta chain. This substitution reduces the solubility of the deoxygenated Hb S molecule within the red cell. Sickling is the term used to describe the change of the normally round red blood cells into crescent, or half-moon shaped, cells as the Hb S polymerizes and forms tactoids. Sickling can occur in the red blood cells of children with sickle cell anemia when oxygen tension is reduced or as a result of other forms of stress, such as acidosis, infection, dehydration, fever, vigorous exercise, and high altitudes. Usually a red cell can initially resume the round shape upon reoxygenation. After repeated episodes of sickling, however, these normally pliable red cells undergo membrane changes, become stiff and irreversibly sickled, and are eventually destroyed. The stiff, irreversibly sickled cells contribute both to anemia and vaso-occlusion. The red cell life span in individuals with sickle cell disease is reduced from the normal length of 120 days to 10 to 20 days.

Sickle cell disease is a complex condition. Abnormal cellular adhesion, inflammation, coagulation, and vasoconstriction all contribute to the vaso-occlusive condition and induce cumulative damage to tissues and organs. The stressed young blood cells (reticulocytes), unlike mature red blood cells, have adhesion molecules on their surface. The vaso-occlusion that occurs is caused by the adhesion of the sickled cells to the vascular endothelium, and the subsequent inflammatory response. This starts a cycle of adhesion followed by inflammation, followed by increased adhesion. The ongoing process of microvascular occlusion causes ischemic-reperfusion injury, releasing cytokines and free radicals. Many inflammatory mediator levels are also elevated. All these substances contribute to the adhesion-inflammation cycle. Along with red cell membrane abnormalities, the vaso-occlusive process of sickle cell disease is also perpetuated by chronic activation of the coagulation system and nitric oxide depletion (which causes unregulated vasoconstriction). Vaso-occlusion and chronic anemia contribute to tissue hypoxia and organ damage.

Children with sickle cell disease can experience a number of complications, including the following:

- **infections,** especially with *Streptococcus pneumoniae, Staphylococcus aureus, Salmonella* species, *Haemophilus influenza* type b, *Escherichia coli,* and *Klebsiella* species. Infections are a major cause of morbidity and mortality for these children.
- **acute chest syndrome,** characterized by a new pulmonary infiltrate on chest X-ray, chest pain, fever, tachypnea, wheezing, and coughing.
- **acute pain crisis** is the sudden onset of pain probably caused by tissue ischemia and infarction and the resulting inflammatory response. These pain crises are the hallmark of sickle cell disease and are also the most distressing and debilitating symptom for the child. Dactylitis (hand and foot syndrome), characterized by swelling of the soft tissues over the metacarpals or metatarsals and the proximal phalanges of the hands and feet, is the most common cause of pain in infants with sickle cell disease. Those infants who have dactylitis before the age of one are more likely to have severe sickle cell disease.

- **stroke,** which can be thrombotic (or infarctive), hemorrhagic, silent (microvascular), or transient ischemic attacks.
- **acute splenic sequestration crisis** is an enlarged spleen (splenomegaly) with a decrease in the child's baseline hemoglobin and elevated reticulocyte count. The spleen often becomes dysfunctional in young children when the red blood cells pool there. Splenectomy is indicated when the anemia, neutropenia, or thrombocytopenia is severe.
- **aplastic crisis or transient red cell aplasia (TRCA)** is a decrease in hemoglobin associated with reticulocytopenia. Parvovirus B19 is the most common cause of TRCA.
- **hepatic and biliary complications,** including abdominal pain crisis, acute cholecystitis, choledocholithiasis, or sickle hepatopathy.
- **priapism** is a prolonged, unwanted and painful erection of the penis, not relieved by orgasm or ejaculation.
- **avascular necrosis** occurs when blood supply to an area of bone is compromised, which leads to infarction and cellular necrosis.
- **altered growth and development,** especially growth retardation in height and weight.
- **delayed sexual maturation** occurs in both girls and boys. Once puberty does begin, it can progress normally.
- **increased risk of perioperative complications** due to all the potential perioperative stressors to the body.

Comprehensive management of the child with sickle cell disease can greatly improve the prognosis and is best done when the child's primary care physician and a comprehensive sickle cell center share in the child's care. Prevention is key to helping children with sickle cell disease stay well. Treatment involves child/parent education to avoid the triggers of sickling episodes (infection, dehydration, hypoxia, fever, high altitude, vigorous exercise, and emotional stress); management of vaso-occlusive episodes, including hydration and effective analgesia; and treatment with transfusions of red blood cells. Children with sickle cell disease should start on prophylactic penicillin no later than 3 months of age. Pneumococcal, meningococcal, and flu vaccines should be administered along with standard immunizations. Transcranial Doppler ultrasound screening evaluates blood flow velocity to predict risk of stroke and is currently recommended annually for children from 2 to 16 years of age.

The only known cure for sickle cell disease is hematopoietic stem cell transplantation (HSCT). HSCT requires a human leukocyte antigen-matched sibling donor. In the United States, this procedure is only performed in experienced transplant centers and is usually done before end-organ complications occur. The use of red blood cell transfusions for acute manifestations of the disease and stroke prevention, and the use of hydroxyurea (a cytotoxic agent) in severely affected children have greatly reduced morbidity associated with sickle cell disease. Research exploring new treatments and potential cures for sickle cell disease is ongoing.

Primary Nursing Diagnosis   Ineffective Tissue Perfusion

Definition	Inadequate amount of blood and oxygen being delivered to the tissues in the body
Possibly Related to	• Vaso-occlusion
	• Anemia

Primary Nursing Diagnosis: Ineffective tissue perfusion: related to vaso-occlusion, anemia

Assessment/Defining Characteristics of Child and/or Family (Subjective & Objective Data):

- Cool, clammy skin
- Pallor
- Prolonged capillary refill, longer than 2 to 3 seconds
- Fatigue
- Lethargy
- Weakness
- Decrease in activity
- Abdominal distension
- Verbal expression of pain of hands, feet, abdomen, or bone pain
- Splenomegaly
- Stroke
- Decreased hemoglobin
- Dry mucous membranes

Expected Outcomes	Possible Nursing Interventions	Rationale	Evaluation for Charting
Child will have adequate tissue perfusion as evidenced by • skin warm to touch • pink color • brisk capillary refill, within 2 to 3 seconds • increasing activity level • lack of signs/symptoms of ineffective tissue perfusion (such as those listed under Assessment) • hemoglobin at baseline for child • oxygen saturation (via pulse oximeter) 94% to 100% on room air • moist mucous membranes • verbal expression of comfort	Assess and record the following every 4 hours and PRN: • capillary refill • skin temperature and color • condition of mucous membranes • signs/symptoms of ineffective tissue perfusion (such as those listed under Assessment). Notify physician of any abnormalities.	Assessment of capillary refill, skin temperature and color are needed to detect vascular flow problems. Assessment of signs/symptoms of ineffective tissue perfusion is necessary for early detection of problems.	Describe capillary refill, and skin temperature and color. Describe any signs/symptoms of ineffective tissue perfusion noted (such as those listed under Assessment).
	When indicated, ensure that bed rest is maintained or provide rest periods for the child.	Minimal activity helps reduce energy and oxygen expenditure.	Document whether bed rest was indicated and if it was maintained. Describe effectiveness of rest periods.
	When indicated, administer humidified oxygen in the correct amount and route of delivery. Record percent of oxygen and route of delivery. Assess and record effectiveness of therapy.	Oxygen may help prevent further sickling of the cells.	Document amount and route of oxygen delivery. Describe effectiveness.
	Assess and record oxygen saturation every 2 to 4 hours and PRN.	Pulse oximetry detects the oxygen saturation of the blood.	Document range of oxygen saturation.
	Administer fluids, as indicated, both oral and parenteral. Keep accurate record of intake and output.	Provides information on child's hydration status. Adequate hydration helps avoid sickling episodes. Hemodilution helps decrease the effects of the sickled cells.	Document intake and output.

(continued)

Primary Nursing Diagnosis: Ineffective Tissue Perfusion *(continued)*			
Expected Outcomes	**Possible Nursing Interventions**	**Rationale**	**Evaluation for Charting**
	Check and record results of hemoglobin. Notify physician of results.	Adequate hemoglobin for the child will promote effective tissue perfusion.	Document current hemoglobin results and indicate if there has been a change from previous results.
	Administer packed red blood cells or assist with exchange transfusion, as indicated. Adhere to institutional and current guidelines for the administration of blood products. Assess and record effectiveness and any side effects such as transfusion reactions (e.g., chills, fever, shaking, urticaria, flushing, nausea/vomiting) noted.	The administration of packed red blood cells will help increase the child's hemoglobin. An exchange transfusion will decrease the amount of circulating sickled cells.	Document whether packed red blood cells were administered or an exchange transfusion was done. Describe their effectiveness or any side effects noted.
TEACHING GOALS Child and/or family will be able to verbalize at least 4 characteristics of ineffective tissue perfusion such as • cool, clammy skin • pallor • decreased activity • complaints of pain	Teach child/family about characteristics of ineffective tissue perfusion. Assess and record results.	Increased knowledge will assist the child/family in recognizing and reporting changes in the child's condition.	Document whether teaching was done and describe results.
Child and/or family will be able to verbalize knowledge of care such as • promoting child's hydration status • monitoring child's activity • protection against exposure to cold and infection • identification of any signs/symptoms of ineffective tissue perfusion (such as those listed under Assessment) • when to contact health-care provider	Teach child/family about care. Assess and record child's/family's knowledge of and participation in care regarding promoting child's hydration status, etc.	Education of child/family will allow for accurate care.	Document whether teaching was done and describe results.

Nursing Diagnosis   Acute Pain

Definition   Condition in which an individual experiences acute mild to severe pain

Possibly Related to
- Tissue ischemia
- Tissue infarction
- Inflammatory response to tissue injury
  - (All due to vascular occlusion secondary to the sickling of the red blood cells, adhesion of the sickle red cells to the vascular endothelium, and inflammation of the microvasculature)

Nursing Diagnosis: Acute pain related to tissue ischemia, tissue infarction, inflammatory response to tissue injury

Assessment/Defining Characteristics of Child and/or Family (Subjective & Objective Data):

- Verbal communication of pain or tenderness
- Crying or moaning unrelieved by usual comfort measures
- Facial grimacing
- Restlessness
- Irritability
- Physical signs/symptoms (tachycardia, tachypnea/bradypnea, increased blood pressure, diaphoresis)
- Guarding or protective behavior of the painful site
- Altered muscle tone (tense or listless)
- Rating of pain on pain-assessment tool
- Dry mucous membranes
- Pallor

Expected Outcomes	Possible Nursing Interventions	Rationale	Evaluation for Charting
Child will be free of severe and/or constant pain as evidenced by • verbal communication of comfort • lack of constant crying or moaning • lack of extreme restlessness • heart rate within acceptable range (state specific range) • respiratory rate within acceptable range (state specific range) • blood pressure within acceptable range (state specific range) • lack of diaphoresis • lack of signs/symptoms of pain (such as those listed under Assessment) • rating of decreased pain or no pain on pain-assessment tool	Assess and record any signs/symptoms of pain (such as those listed under Assessment) every 2 to 4 hours and PRN. Use age-appropriate pain-assessment tool.	Provides data regarding the level of pain child is experiencing.	Document range of vital signs and degree of pain child is experiencing. Describe any successful measures used to decrease pain.
	Handle child gently. Reposition, immobilize, or elevate the painful area as indicated.	Helps to minimize pain and promote comfort.	Document if child was handled gently and effectiveness of measure.
	When indicated, ensure that bed rest is maintained or provide rest periods for the child. Do not disturb child unless necessary.	Helps to promote comfort, decrease pain, and decrease oxygen expenditure.	Document if bed rest was maintained and effectiveness of rest periods.
	When indicated, administer humidified oxygen in the correct amount and route of delivery. Record percent of oxygen and route of delivery. Assess and record effectiveness of therapy.	Oxygen may help prevent further sickling of the cells.	Document amount and route of oxygen delivery. Describe effectiveness.

(continued)

Nursing Diagnosis: Acute Pain (continued)

Expected Outcomes	Possible Nursing Interventions	Rationale	Evaluation for Charting
• moist mucous membranes • oxygen saturation (via pulse oximeter) 94% to 100% on room air	Assess and record oxygen saturation every 2 to 4 hours and PRN.	Pulse oximetry detects the oxygen saturation of the blood.	Document range of oxygen saturation.
	When indicated, administer analgesics and/or narcotics and adjuvant pain medications on schedule (usually at regular intervals as opposed to PRN). Monitor patient-controlled analgesia (PCA). Assess and record effectiveness.	Analgesics and narcotics are administered to decrease pain. Adjuvant pain medications (such as nonsteroidal anti-inflammatory drugs) provide added pain relief.	Document whether pain medications were administered on schedule. Describe effectiveness and any side effects noted.
	If indicated, consult pain management team.	Provides additional support for pain management.	Document if pain management team was consulted.
	Administer fluids, as indicated, both oral and parenteral. Keep accurate record of intake and output.	Provides information on child's hydration status. Adequate hydration helps avoid sickling episodes. Hemodilution helps decrease the effects of the sickled cells.	Document intake and output.
	Encourage family members to stay and comfort child and participate in care when possible.	Helps to comfort and support the child and can lead to decreased pain.	Document whether family was able to remain with child and describe effectiveness of their presence.
	Use diversional activities (e.g., music, television, playing games, relaxation) when appropriate.	Diversional activities can distract child and may help to decrease pain.	Document whether diversional activities were successful in helping to manage pain.
	If age appropriate, explain all procedures beforehand.	Allows the child some control, which can assist in pain management.	Describe if this measure was effective in helping child manage pain.
	If age appropriate, allow the child to participate in planning his or her care. Encourage the child to practice self-care (e.g., bathing, dressing).	Allowing child some control can assist with pain management.	Describe if this measure was effective in helping child manage pain.

Nursing Diagnosis: Acute Pain *(continued)*

Expected Outcomes	Possible Nursing Interventions	Rationale	Evaluation for Charting
	When indicated, institute additional pain relief measures, such as application of moist heat (warm packs, warm tub baths or whirlpool), massage, guided imagery, or hypnosis. Assess and record effectiveness.	These nonpharmacologic measures may help decrease pain.	Document whether these measures were successful in helping to manage pain.
	When indicated, administer hydroxyurea. Assess and record effectiveness and any side effects (e.g., leukopenia may indicate toxicity).	Hydroxyurea can decrease rate or severity of pain.	Document whether hydroxyurea was administered and describe its effectiveness and any side effects noted.
TEACHING GOALS Child and/or family will be able to verbalize at least 4 characteristics of pain such as • verbal communication of pain or tenderness • crying unrelieved by usual comfort measures • facial grimacing • guarding of painful site	Teach child/family about characteristics of pain. Assess and record results.	Increased knowledge will assist the child/family in recognizing and reporting changes in the child's condition.	Document whether teaching was done and describe results.
Child and/or family will be able to verbalize knowledge of care such as • identification of potential triggers of painful events • medication administration • identification of any signs/symptoms of pain (such as those listed under Assessment) • when to contact health-care provider	Teach child/family about care. Assess and record child's/family's knowledge of and participation in care regarding medication administration, etc.	Education of child/family will allow for accurate care.	Document whether teaching was done and describe results.

Related Nursing Diagnoses

Actual Infection*	*related to* a. bacterial invasion of any organ or body system b. viral invasion of any organ or body system c. granulomatous invasion of any organ or body system d. parasitic invasion of any organ or body system
Activity Intolerance	*related to* a. pain b. fatigue c. shortness of breath d. impaired gas exchange
Deficient Knowledge: Parental	*related to* home management of a child with sickle cell disease
Disturbed Body Image	*related to* a. physical restrictions b. altered growth and development c. sequelae from strokes
Compromised Family Coping	*related to* a. parental guilt b. frequent hospitalization of child with sickle cell disease

*Non-NANDA diagnosis.

CARE OF CHILDREN WITH HEPATIC DYSFUNCTION

6

ONE

CHRONIC LIVER FAILURE
MEDICAL DIAGNOSIS

PATHOPHYSIOLOGY Liver failure results when the liver is unable to maintain its many functions. With this failure, substances normally produced by the liver are absent and those normally removed by the liver accumulate. In children, liver failure most often occurs with chronic liver disease, or with chronic diseases such as cystic fibrosis and hemophilia. Less often, viruses—such as in hepatitis, idiosyncratic reactions to medications, or accidental ingestion of drugs or toxins—cause acute liver failure.

Two common anatomic disorders of the biliary system are biliary atresia and choledochal cysts. Biliary atresia is the complete obstruction of bile flow of the extrahepatic biliary duct system secondary to fibrosis or obliteration, which can progress into the intrahepatic ducts, eventually leading to cirrhosis. Choledochal cysts (congenital cystic dilatation of the common bile duct) may occur at any place along the biliary tree. Cirrhosis is a main complication of these two problems, resulting in portal hypertension, esophageal varices, hepatic coma, and liver failure. Biliary atresia is the most common indication for liver transplantation in pediatric patients.

The liver, one of the most vital organs in the body, performs more than 400 functions. Briefly, these functions include blood storage and filtration; secretion of bile and bilirubin; metabolism of fat, protein, and carbohydrate; synthesis of blood-clotting components; detoxification of hormones, drugs, and other substances; and storage for glycogen, iron, and vitamins A, D, E, and B_{12}. These functions can be affected by inflammatory, obstructive, or degenerative disorders. When the liver is unable to maintain normal body functions, complications arise. Many of the complications are due to cirrhosis.

Cirrhosis occurs as an end stage to many chronic liver diseases and is a result of hepatocyte injury. The hepatocyte injury is followed by necrosis, fibrosis, regeneration, and eventual degeneration. During this degenerative disease process, nodular areas (that replaced injured parenchymal cell mass) and scar tissue (from the hepatocyte response to injury) create a fibrotic and fatty liver. They also impair the intrahepatic blood flow. Cirrhosis can lead to many complications such as ascites, portal hypertension, hepatic encephalopathy, gastrointestinal bleeding, and hepatorenal syndrome.

Liver failure impacts every organ system. The clinical presentation of each child will vary according to the severity of the disease process.

1. The phagocytic activity of Kupffer's cells is decreased; thus, the blood is inadequately filtered as it passes through the liver, making the patient more susceptible to infections.
2. Inadequate amounts of bile salts are manufactured, resulting in decreased emulsification of fats when insufficient quantities of bile salts reach the small intestine. The deposit of excessive bile salts in the skin causes pruritis when these salts are inadequately extracted from the portal venous blood by the liver cells in hepatic disorders such as hepatitis, cholestasis, or extrahepatic biliary obstruction. This process can also cause skin breakdown. Fats too large to enter the circulation are lost in the feces (steatorrhea), a source of high calorie loss. Decreased fat intake can contribute to malnutrition. Reduced absorption of fat-soluble vitamins A, D, E, and K can also occur further adding to malnutrition. Deficiency of vitamin D can cause rickets.
3. Albumin synthesis is decreased and serum albumin levels fall in proportion to the degree of hepatocellular failure. This state of hypoproteinemia can contribute to the formation of ascites (the accumulation of fluid within the peritoneal cavity), peripheral edema, and malnutrition.
4. The liver's production of blood-clotting factors is decreased. Since fat-soluble vitamin K has limited absorption, the production of vitamin K-dependent clotting factors (factors II, VII, IX, and X) is decreased, resulting in a prolonged prothrombin time, easy bruising, and overt bleeding.
5. The liver is unable to remove activated clotting factors from the serum, contributing to the formation of microthrombi and the consumption of platelets, fibrinogen, and other clotting factors.
6. When hepatic circulatory bypasses exist, blood is shunted around the liver directly into the systemic circulation, and ammonia is not converted to urea. Hyperammonemia contributes to hepatic encephalopathy. (Ammonia is formed in the gastrointestinal tract from amino acids following bacterial and enzymatic breakdown of proteins.)

7. The liver is unable to effectively detoxify certain hormones, harmful compounds, and drugs.

8. Serum glucose levels can drop because gluconeogenesis is not completed by the liver. This can compromise cerebral function since glucose is the brain's major energy source.

9. The release of vasoactive substances into the blood contributes to a hyperkinetic circulation.

10. Jaundice occurs due to high levels of bilirubin that the liver is unable to remove (the staining of elastic tissue by conjugated or unconjugated bilirubin).

11. Sodium and water are retained. Significant intravascular fluid loss secondary to ascites or splanchnic sequestration because of portal hypotension causes the heart, adrenal cortex, and kidneys to perceive a decrease in circulating blood volume, stimulating aldosterone secretion, and resulting in renal sodium and water retention.

12. Other common electrolyte imbalances include hypokalemia, due to vomiting, diarrhea, anorexia, hyperaldosteronism, or use of diuretics; hypocalcemia, due to decreased absorption of vitamin D, steatorrhea, and inadequate dietary intake; and hypomagnesemia, due to decreased storage by the liver.

13. The spleen becomes congested and enlarged as increased venous pressures delay blood flow through the splanchnic bed. This hypersplenism can produce thrombocytopenia, anemia, and leukopenia, which in turn can contribute to hypoxemia, increased susceptibility to infection, and increased bleeding tendencies.

14. Ascites elevates the diaphragm and interferes with lung expansion. Intrapulmonary right-to-left shunting can also occur as can hypoxemia.

15. The hepatic enzymes: serum-glutamic oxaloacetic transaminase (SGOT) (aspartate aminotransferase—AST), serum glutamic-pyruvic, transaminase (SGPT) (alanine aminotransferase—ALT), lactate dehydrogenase (LDH), and creatine phosphokinase (CPK) are elevated due to their release into the blood with the destruction of liver cells.

16. Varices develop in the esophagus and rectum due to the intrahepatic fibrosis, which obstructs blood flow. These varices provide collateral circulation, but are thin-walled and prone to bleeding (causing gastrointestinal bleeding).

The child's medical history and liver involvement will determine what laboratory evaluations and other diagnostic studies will be needed. Comprehensive blood chemistries, liver function tests, and hematology and coagulation studies are usually ordered. Ultrasound, computed tomography (CT), endoscopy, and a liver biopsy are also helpful in establishing the diagnosis and degree of liver involvement.

Management of chronic liver failure focuses on treatment of the child's symptoms and complications. Children with end-stage liver disease are assessed for liver transplantation.

Primary Nursing Diagnosis   Impaired Metabolic Function*

Definition   Imbalance or altered utilization of specific body biochemicals

Possibly Related to   • Hepatic damage

*Non-NANDA diagnosis.

Primary Nursing Diagnosis: Impaired metabolic function related to hepatic damage

Assessment/Defining Characteristics of Child and/or Family (Subjective & Objective Data):

- Hypoalbuminemia
- Hyperammonemia
- Prolonged prothrombin time
- Increased hepatic enzymes (SGOT, SGPT, LDH, CPK)
- Hypoglycemia
- Increased total, direct, and indirect bilirubin
- Jaundice
- Easy bruising, nosebleeds, gingival bleeding, bleeding from puncture sights, blood in urine, and/or petechiae
- Dark and foamy urine
- Hyper-Aldosteronism
- Leukopenia

Expected Outcomes	Possible Nursing Interventions	Rationale	Evaluation for Charting
Child will have improved metabolic function as evidenced by • ammonia within acceptable range for child (normal is 15 to 45 mcg/dL) • prothrombin time within acceptable range for child (normal is 12 to 14 seconds) • SGOT (AST) within acceptable range for child (normal is 0 to 40 U/L) • SGPT (ALT) within acceptable range for child (normal is 5 to 35 U/L) • LDH within acceptable range for child (normal is 80 to 120 U/L) • CPK within acceptable range for child (normal is 0 to 70 IU/L) • glucose within acceptable range for child (normal is 60 to 120 mg/dL) • direct bilirubin within acceptable range for child (normal is up to 0.3 mg/dL) • indirect bilirubin within acceptable range for child (normal is 0.1 to 1.0 mg/dL)	Assess and record • IV fluids and condition of IV site every hour • laboratory values as indicated. Report abnormalities to the physician. • signs/symptoms of impaired metabolic function (such as those listed under Assessment) every 4 hours and PRN	If child experiences impaired metabolic function the lab values will be out of the normal range. It is necessary to record the amount of IV fluids every hour to make sure the child is not being over or under hydrated. The IV site needs to be assessed every hour for signs of redness or swelling.	Document current ranges of laboratory values and any signs/symptoms of metabolic dysfunction noted. Document amount of IV fluids and describe condition of IV site along with any interventions needed.
	If indicated, administer lactulose on schedule. Assess and record effectiveness and any side effects (e.g., abdominal cramping, anorexia, diarrhea).	Inhibits ammonia production and lowers ammonia levels.	Document if lactulose was administered on schedule. Describe effectiveness and any side effects noted.
	If indicated, administer antibiotics (neomycin, kanamycin, tetracycline) on schedule. Assess and record any side effects (e.g., nausea, vomiting, loss of appetite).	Antibiotics are used to combat any pathogens that are present and/or because the child has an increased susceptibility to infection as a result of impaired phagocytic function.	Document if antibiotics were administered on schedule. Describe any side effects noted.
	Administer plasma or colloids as indicated. Follow institutional protocol for administration and care of child while receiving medication. Assess and record effectiveness.	Plasma or colloids are administered to correct hypovolemia and coagulopathy.	Document if plasma or colloids were administered on schedule and if hospital protocol was followed. Describe effectiveness.

Primary Nursing Diagnosis: Impaired Metabolic Function (*continued*)

Expected Outcomes	Possible Nursing Interventions	Rationale	Evaluation for Charting
• total bilirubin within acceptable range for child (normal is 0.2 to 0.8 mg/dL) • serum albumin within acceptable range for child (normal is 4.0 to 5.8 g/dL) • WBC within acceptable range for child (state normal range for each child) • lack of signs/symptoms of impaired metabolic function (such as those listed under Assessment)	If indicated, administer diuretics on schedule. Assess and record effectiveness and any side effects (e.g., hypokalemia, vomiting).	Diuretics are used to help decrease fluid overload.	Document if diuretics were administered on schedule. Describe effectiveness and any side effects noted.
	Keep accurate record of intake and output. Record characteristics of all output.	Provides information about fluid status of patient. Decreased output may indicate a shift of the intravascular fluid into the interstitial space. Characteristics of output can help to determine if treatment measures are effective and if additional treatment is indicated.	Document intake and output. Describe characteristics of all output.
TEACHING GOALS			
Child and/or family will be able to verbalize at least 4 characteristics of impaired metabolic function such as • jaundice • easy bruising • nosebleeds • gingival bleeding • dark and foamy urine	Teach child/family about characteristics of impaired metabolic function. Assess and record results.	Increased knowledge will assist the child/family in recognizing and reporting changes in the child's condition.	Document whether teaching was done and describe results.
Child and/or family will be able to verbalize knowledge of care such as • monitoring of intake and output • medication administration • identification of any signs/symptoms of impaired metabolic function (such as those listed under Assessment) and the correct action for each • when to contact health-care provider	Teach child/family about care. Assess and record child's/family's knowledge of and participation in care regarding monitoring intake and output, etc.	Education of child/family will allow for accurate care.	Document whether teaching was done and describe results.

Nursing Diagnosis

Deficient Fluid Volume: Intravascular and/or Excess Fluid Volume: Extravascular or Intravascular

Definition

Decrease in the amount of circulating fluid volume *and/or* interstitial fluid overload *or* increased intravascular volume (which can eventually lead to interstitial or intracellular fluid overload)

Possibly Related to

- Hypoalbuminemia
- Peripheral edema
- Ascites
- Increased serum aldosterone
- Increased antidiuretic hormone
- Hemorrhage

Nursing Diagnosis: Deficient fluid volume: intravascular and/or excess fluid volume: extravascular or intravascular related to

- Hypoalbuminemia
- Peripheral edema
- Ascites
- Increased serum aldosterone
- Increased antidiuretic hormone
- Hemorrhage

Assessment/Defining Characteristics of Child and/or Family (Subjective & Objective Data):

- Tachycardia
- Tachypnea
- Dry mucous membranes
- Hypotension
- Absence of tears
- Decreased skin turgor (skin recoil greater than 2 to 3 seconds)
- Sunken fontanel
- Peripheral edema
- Ascites
- Decreased urine output
- Increased urine specific gravity
- Increased weight
- Vomiting
- Diarrhea
- Increased urine osmolality
- Increased serum osmolality

Expected Outcomes	Possible Nursing Interventions	Rationale	Evaluation for Charting
Child will have improved fluid balance as evidenced by - adequate fluid intake, IV and oral (state specific amount of intake needed for each child) - adequate urine output (state specific range; 1 to 2 ml/kg/hr) - moist mucous membranes - rapid skin recoil (less than 2 to 3 seconds)	Keep accurate record of intake and output. If indicated, maintain fluid and sodium restriction.	Fluids may need to be restricted in order to normalize the serum sodium, normalize serum osmolality, and decrease extravascular fluid volume.	Document intake and output.
	Assess and record - HR, RR, and BP every 4 hours and PRN - IV fluids and condition of IV site every hour	Provides information about fluid status of patient. If patient has fluid imbalance, the HR, RR, B/P, and laboratory values will change. It is necessary to record the	Document range of HR, RR, and BP. Document amount of IV fluids and describe condition of IV site along with any interventions needed. Document current

Nursing Diagnosis: Deficient Fluid Volume: Intravascular and/or Excess Fluid Volume: Extravascular or Intravascular *(continued)*

Expected Outcomes	Possible Nursing Interventions	Rationale	Evaluation for Charting

• urine specific gravity from 1.008 to 1.020
• urine osmolality within acceptable range for child (normal is from 500 to 800 mOsm/L)
• serum osmolality within acceptable range for child (normal is from 280 to 295 mOsm/L)
• heart rate, respiratory rate, and blood pressure within acceptable range (state specific range for each)
• lack of
  1. ascites
  2. peripheral edema
  3. vomiting
  4. diarrhea
• lack of signs/symptoms of fluid imbalance (such as those listed under Assessment)
	• laboratory values as indicated. Report any abnormalities to the physician.
	• signs/symptoms of fluid imbalance (such as those listed under Assessment) every 4 hours and PRN
		amount of IV fluids every hour to make sure the child is not being over or under hydrated. The IV site needs to be assessed every hour for signs of redness or swelling.	laboratory values when indicated. Describe any signs/symptoms of fluid imbalance noted.

	Check and record urine specific gravity with every void or as indicated.	Urine specific gravity provides information about hydration status.	Document range of urine specific gravity.
	Assess and record condition of mucous membranes and skin turgor every shift and PRN.	Provides information on hydration status.	Describe status of mucous membranes and skin turgor.
	Measure and record abdominal girth every shift and PRN.	Increase in abdominal girth can indicate ascites and or hepatosplenomegaly.	Document current abdominal girth and determine whether it has increased or decreased since the previous measurement.
	Weigh child daily on same scale at same time of day. Document results and compare to previous weight.	To assess overall hydration status.	Document weight and determine if it was an increase or decrease from the previous weight.
	Administer plasma or colloids as indicated. Follow institutional protocol for administration and care of child while receiving medication. Assess and record effectiveness.	Plasma or colloids are administered to correct hypovolemia or coagulopathy.	Document if plasma or colloids were administered on schedule and if hospital protocol was followed. Describe effectiveness.
	If indicated, administer diuretics on schedule. Assess and record effectiveness and any side effects (e.g., hypokalemia, vomiting).	Diuretics are used to help decrease fluid overload.	Document if diuretics were administered on schedule. Describe effectiveness and any side effects noted.

(continued)

Nursing Diagnosis: Deficient Fluid Volume: Intravascular and/or Excess Fluid Volume: Extravascular or Intravascular *(continued)*

Expected Outcomes	Possible Nursing Interventions	Rationale	Evaluation for Charting
TEACHING GOALS Child and/or family will be able to verbalize at least 4 characteristics of fluid imbalance such as • dry mucous membranes • absence of tears • decreased urine output • increased weight • vomiting • diarrhea	Teach child/family about characteristics of fluid imbalance. Assess and record results.	Increased knowledge will assist the child/family in recognizing and reporting changes in the child's condition.	Document whether teaching was done and describe results.
Child and/or family will be able to verbalize knowledge of care such as • monitoring of intake and output • medication administration • identification of any signs/symptoms of fluid imbalance (such as those listed under Assessment) and the correct action for each • when to contact health-care provider	Teach child/family about care. Assess and record child's/family's knowledge of and participation in care regarding monitoring intake and output, etc.	Education of child/family will allow for accurate care.	Document whether teaching was done and describe results.

Related Nursing Diagnoses

Impaired Level of Consciousness*

related to
a. increased serum ammonia levels secondary to decreased ammonia excretion and/or reduced conversion to urea
b. increased circulating nitrogenous wastes secondary to decreased liver detoxification of these wastes
c. hypoglycemia
d. decreased storage of vitamins, such as niacin and B vitamins
e. electrolyte imbalances, such as hypocalcemia
f. hypoxemia

Imbalanced Nutrition: Less than Body Requirements	*related to* a. altered metabolism of fats, proteins, and carbohydrates b. decreased absorption of fats c. decreased storage of vitamins and minerals d. anorexia e. hypoalbuminemia
Risk for Infection	*related to* a. decreased activity of Kupffer cells b. malnutrition
Grieving: Family	*related to* a. severity of illness b. change in child's physical appearance c. uncertain prognosis d. potential of not finding a donor (if needed)

*Non-NANDA diagnosis.

7

CARE OF
CHILDREN WITH
INFECTIONS

ACQUIRED IMMUNODEFICIENCY SYNDROME (AIDS)
MEDICAL DIAGNOSIS

PATHOPHYSIOLOGY A child with acquired immunodeficiency syndrome (AIDS) has been infected with the human immunodeficiency virus (HIV), a retrovirus that causes an immune deficiency and eventually destroys the immune system. There are 2 types of HIV that cause AIDS. HIV-1 is more common in the United States and in various other countries; it also has a number of subtypes. HIV-2 is more common in Africa and appears to have a slower progression. The CDC has developed a system to classify pediatric HIV based on clinical and immunological categories. Diagnosis of HIV in children over the age of 18 months is usually made using a combination of clinical signs and symptoms and laboratory tests. Enzyme-linked immunosorbent assay (ELISA) is the test used to diagnose HIV infection, along with one other confirmatory test, such as Western blot or polymerase chain reaction (PCR) tests. To receive a diagnosis of AIDS, a child must have either a CD4+ count below 15% for his or her age group or one of the clinical illnesses that define AIDS. Once a child has been classified in a certain category, he or she may not be reclassified in a less severe category even with improvement in his or her clinical or immunological status. The World Health Organization (WHO) has also developed several systems for diagnosing HIV infection in children based on clinical disease.

The majority of pediatric AIDS patients (90%) acquire the infection during the perinatal period. If the mother receives treatment during pregnancy, the incidence is significantly reduced. The other 10% of children acquire HIV from sexual abuse, prior blood product exposure, or unknown causes. Adolescents have one of the fastest growing rates of HIV infection, due especially to high-risk behaviors (drugs, unprotected sex, etc.).

HIV selectively infects and destroys certain T cells, which are involved in the mediation of cellular immunity and in the regulation of B cell function (the humoral immune system). HIV does this by utilizing the DNA of CD4+ cells to replicate itself. The child infected with HIV experiences the destruction and depletion of CD4+ helper/inducer T cells and a reversal of the helper-to-suppressor T cell ratio, resulting in depression of cellular immunity. The loss of T cell regulation of B cell function leaves the child with AIDS unable to properly respond to new antigens and particularly vulnerable to common bacterial infections. The child also experiences monocyte/macrophage abnormalities, contributing to an increased susceptibility to parasitic and other intracellular infections.

There are 6 phases to the HIV life cycle. Soon after HIV enters the child's bloodstream, it becomes attached to CD4+ T cells. The external surface antigen of the virus binds to the CD4+ receptor of the cell, and then the virus enters the cell and is uncoated (binding and entry). With the help of the reverse transcriptase enzyme, the retroviral RNA is transcribed into DNA (reverse transcription). This newly formed DNA then integrates itself into the CD4+ cell nucleus (integration) or remains unintegrated in the cellular cytoplasm. This integration not only affects cellular gene function, but as the infected cells proliferate, a proviral sequence remains in all progeny cells. An infected cell can continue to actively produce HIV (replication) or can remain latent until stimulated. Cofactors, stimuli that activate the production of HIV, include cytokines and can include certain other viruses as well. The new HIV viruses push through the cell wall (budding) and contain all the components necessary to infect other cells. The host cell is usually destroyed once active replication of the virus occurs. After cellular death, viral particles from the cell are released. The viral particles undergo a process (maturation) and are now ready to infect other cells, leading to the spread of the HIV infection.

Infection by HIV can have a wide spectrum of clinical manifestations varying from no symptoms to severe opportunistic infections, neurological deterioration, pulmonary failure, and/or death. Children with AIDS can present with failure to thrive, recurrent bacterial infections, chronic diarrhea, lymphadenopathy, hepatosplenomegaly, developmental delay, oral candidiasis, and/or lymphoid interstitial pneumonitis (LIP). Since their bodies lack the appropriate cellular response, many children present with two or more opportunistic infections, most commonly *Pneumocystis carinii* pneumonia (PCP). Because children with AIDS are unable to respond to new antigens, they can have many bacterial infections, presenting as pneumonia, meningitis, and sepsis, which can be recurrent and life threatening. Causative organisms include *Haemophilus influenzae, Staphylococcus aureus, Staphylococcus epidermidis, Streptococcus pneumoniae, Streptococcus pyogenes*, and some gram-negative enteric bacteria. A child with AIDS is also susceptible to rare neoplasms.

Generally, antiretroviral therapy is indicated for all infants, children, and adolescents with HIV. The three main groups of antiretroviral drugs are: nucleoside reverse transcriptase inhibitors (NRTIs), non–nucleoside reverse transcriptase inhibitors (NNRTIs), and protease inhibitors (PIs). Each group of drugs interrupts HIV replication at a different point in the life cycle. Most children are given combinations of the antiretroviral drugs. Adjunctive immune therapies can include hyperimmune globulins and cytokines. Prevention of opportunistic infections is also essential. When the CD4+ cell levels fall below a certain level (according to the CDC categories), prophylaxis against PCP, invasive cytomegalovirus infections, and *Mycobacterium avium-intracellulare* should be started. A narrow and accelerated immunization schedule is recommended for children who have HIV infection, always taking into consideration the child's CD4+ cell count. Maintaining adequate nutrition is also essential for HIV-infected children.

A multitude of issues exists for children with HIV infection and their families: physical, psychosocial, societal, ethical, and legal. This illness has many implications for the child and the entire family, requiring compassionate, consistent, and comprehensive care from the health-care system and community.

Primary Nursing Diagnosis   Actual Infection and Risk for Further Infection*

Definition   Condition in which microorganisms have invaded and threaten to further invade the body

Possibly Related to
- Humoral immunosuppression
- Depression of cellular immunity
- Opportunistic agents
- Common bacterial agents
- Malnutrition

*Non-NANDA diagnosis.

Primary Nursing Diagnosis: Actual infection and risk for further infection related to humoral immunosuppression, depression of cellular immunity, opportunistic agents, common bacterial agents, malnutrition

Assessment/Defining Characteristics of Child and/or Family (Subjective & Objective Data):
- Fever
- Tachycardia
- Tachypnea
- Hypotension
- Lymphadenopathy
- Diarrhea (often profuse)
- Nausea/vomiting
- Painful swallowing
- Skin rashes and mucous membrane lesions
- Cough
- Chest pain
- Dyspnea
- Malaise
- Fatigue
- Night sweats
- Change in the level of consciousness/meningeal signs
- Altered complete blood count (CBC) with differential
- Decreased appetite
- Weight loss

(continued)

Primary Nursing Diagnosis: Actual Infection and Risk for Further Infection *(continued)*

Expected Outcomes	Possible Nursing Interventions	Rationale	Evaluation for Charting
Child will be free of secondary infection as evidenced by • body temperature within acceptable range of 36.5°C to 37.2°C • heart rate within acceptable range (state specific range) • respiratory rate within acceptable range (state specific range) • blood pressure within acceptable range (state specific range) • clear and intact skin and mucous membranes • alertness when awake • if age appropriate, orientation to person, place, and time (oriented X3) • CBC within acceptable range (state specific range) • lack of signs/ symptoms of infection (such as those listed under Assessment)	Assess and record T, HR, RR, BP, and any signs/symptoms of infection (such as those listed under Assessment) every 4 hours and PRN.	Provides data on the status of the child's infection. If infection is present, the T, HR, and RR will increase and the BP may decrease.	Document range of T, HR, RR, and BP. Describe any signs/symptoms of infection noted.
	Maintain good hand-washing technique.	Good hand washing is the single most important measure in decreasing infection.	Document whether good hand-washing technique was used.
	Adhere to Centers for Disease Control (CDC) guidelines and/or institutional policy for current precautions/ isolation techniques.	Provides the latest information on the standard of care.	Document maintenance of isolation/precaution techniques.
	When indicated, obtain culture specimens (blood, stool, wound, urine, sputum). Check results and notify physician of any abnormalities.	Identifies infectious agents and guides treatment.	Document current results of any cultures.
	Use tepid baths and cooling blankets as indicated.	Assists in temperature reduction.	Describe any therapeutic measures used to treat the infection.
	Administer antibiotics on schedule. Assess and record any side effects (e.g., rash, diarrhea).	Antibiotics are given to combat infection or prophylactically to decrease the chance of getting a further infection.	Document whether antibiotics were administered on schedule. Describe any side effects noted.
	When indicated, administer antipyretics on schedule. Assess and record effectiveness.	Antipyretics are used to reduce fever.	Document whether an antipyretic was needed and describe effectiveness.
	Administer antiretroviral agents on schedule. Assess and record any side effects (e.g., abdominal pain, anemia).	Inhibits retrovirus life cycle.	Document whether antiretroviral agents were administered on schedule. Describe any side effects noted.
	Administer antiviral agents on schedule. Assess and record any side effects (e.g., nausea, vomiting).	Antiviral agents are given to combat viral infections.	Document whether antiviral agents were administered on schedule. Describe any side effects noted.

Primary Nursing Diagnosis: Actual Infection and Risk for Further Infection *(continued)*

Expected Outcomes	Possible Nursing Interventions	Rationale	Evaluation for Charting
	Administer antifungal agents on schedule. Assess and record any side effects (e.g., fever, hypotension).	Antifungal agents are used to kill fungi and yeast that cause infections.	Document whether antifungal agents were administered on schedule. Describe any side effects noted.
	If indicated, administer IV hyperimmune globulins on schedule (for example VZIG for varicella exposure). Assess and record any side effects (e.g., rash, hives). Administer according to institutional protocol.	Used to help prevent infections or shorten the course of the disease.	Document whether IV hyperimmune globulin was administered on schedule. Describe any side effects noted.
	Check and record results of CBC with differential. Notify physician of any abnormalities.	Abnormal results may indicate an infection.	Document current results of any testing. Describe any therapeutic measures initiated.
TEACHING GOALS Child and/or family will be able to verbalize at least 4 characteristics of infection such as • fever • cough • diarrhea • chest pain • decreased appetite • weight loss	Teach child/family about characteristics of infection. Assess and record results.	Increased knowledge will assist the child/family in recognizing and reporting changes in the child's condition.	Document whether teaching was done and describe results.
Child and/or family will be able to verbalize knowledge of care such as • medication administration • maintenance of modified immunization practices • identification of any signs/symptoms of infection (such as those listed under Assessment) • when to contact health-care provider	Teach child/family about care. Assess and record child's/family's knowledge of and participation in care regarding medication administration, etc.	Education of child/family will allow for accurate care.	Document whether teaching was done and describe results.

Nursing Diagnosis

Nursing Diagnosis Imbalanced Nutrition: Less than Body Requirements

Definition Nutrients insufficient to meet body requirements

Possibly Related to
- Increased metabolic demands secondary to fever, increased respiratory rate, and sepsis
- Nausea/vomiting secondary to infection or side effects of medications
- Diarrhea secondary to gram-negative enteric microorganisms
- Decreased oral intake secondary to painful oral lesions and inflamed esophagus
- Lack of interest in food
- Altered taste sensation

Nursing Diagnosis: Imbalanced nutrition: less than body requirements related to increased metabolic demands secondary to fever, increased respiratory rate, and sepsis; nausea/vomiting secondary to infection or side effects or medications; diarrhea secondary to gram-negative enteric microorganisms; decreased oral intake secondary to painful oral lesions and inflamed esophagus; lack of interest in food; altered taste sensation

Assessment/Defining Characteristics of Child and/or Family (Subjective & Objective Data):
- Anorexia
- Weight loss or failure to gain weight
- Vomiting
- Diarrhea
- Abdominal cramping
- Muscle wasting
- Dysphagia
- Oral lesions

Expected Outcomes	Possible Nursing Interventions	Rationale	Evaluation for Charting

Child will be adequately nourished as evidenced by
 	
• sufficient caloric consumption, parenterally and orally (state specific amount for each child)
• steady weight gain
• lack of
  1. vomiting
  2. diarrhea
  3. abdominal cramping
  4. muscle wasting
  5. dysphagia
• lack of signs/symptoms of imbalanced nutrition (such as those listed under Assessment)
	Keep accurate record of intake and output.	Provides information on child's hydration status.	Document intake and output.

	Assess and record any signs/symptoms of imbalanced nutrition (such as those listed under Assessment) every 4 hours and PRN.	Provides information on nutritional status of child.	Describe any signs/symptoms of imbalanced nutrition noted.
	Weigh child daily on same scale at same time of day. Document results and compare to previous weight.	Decrease in weight may be due to feeding difficulties such as those described under Assessment.	Document weight and determine if it was an increase or decrease from the previous weight.
	If indicated, maintain and record daily calorie counts.	Provides information on actual caloric intake.	Document calorie count if indicated.
	Encourage child to eat by assessing likes/dislikes and, when possible, providing foods that the child likes to eat.	Provides encouragement for child to eat.	Describe any therapeutic measures used to maintain adequate nutrition. Document their effectiveness.

Nursing Diagnosis: Imbalanced Nutrition: Less than Body Requirements *(continued)*

Expected Outcomes	Possible Nursing Interventions	Rationale	Evaluation for Charting
	Offer small, frequent feedings (six small meals per day).	Provides opportunity for increased caloric intake.	Describe any therapeutic measures used to maintain adequate nutrition. Document their effectiveness.
	Provide high-caloric meals, snacks, and supplements.	Provides opportunity for child to meet nutritional requirements.	Describe any therapeutic measures used to maintain adequate nutrition. Document their effectiveness.
	Initiate a nutritional consultation with a pediatric dietitian who will take into account cultural and social factors.	Provides nutritional support and can encourage the child to eat.	Describe any therapeutic measures used to maintain adequate nutrition. Document their effectiveness.
	When indicated, administer tube feedings on schedule. Follow institutional policy for changing and care of the feeding tube.	Provides supplemental nutrition.	When indicated, document whether tube feedings were administered on schedule. Document if institutional policy for changing and care of the feeding tube was followed.
	When indicated, administer total parenteral nutrition (TPN) and intralipids. Follow institutional policy for maintenance of TPN, intralipids line, and dressing. Assess and record serum glucose and lipid levels. Notify physician if levels are out of the normal range.	Provides supplemental nutrition.	When indicated, document whether TPN and intralipids were administered on schedule. Document if institutional policy for maintenance of TPN, intralipids line, and dressing change was followed. Document range of serum glucose and lipid levels.
	Provide oral hygiene. If indicated, provide analgesics prior to meals and snacks.	Helps to improve the integrity of the oral mucous membranes and increases comfort.	Document if oral hygiene was maintained and whether analgesics were administered. Describe effectiveness.
	Administer antiemetics on schedule. Assess and record effectiveness and any side effects (e.g., drowsiness, constipation).	If nausea is decreased, child will be more likely to eat.	Document whether antiemetics were administer on schedule. Describe effectiveness and any side effects noted.

(continued)

Nursing Diagnosis: Imbalanced Nutrition: Less than Body Requirements (*continued*)

Expected Outcomes	Possible Nursing Interventions	Rationale	Evaluation for Charting
	Administer antidiarrheals on schedule. Assess and record effectiveness and any side effects (e.g., constipation, bloating).	Administered to combat diarrhea that can compromise nutritional status.	Document whether antidiarrheal medications were administered on schedule. Describe effectiveness and any side effects noted.
	When indicated, initiate a social services consultation to facilitate obtainment of groceries or food supplements.	Provides support for child and family in meeting the child's nutritional needs.	Describe any therapeutic measures used to maintain adequate nutrition. Document their effectiveness.
TEACHING GOALS Child and/or family will be able to verbalize at least 4 characteristics of imbalanced nutrition such as • anorexia • weight loss or failure to gain weight • vomiting • diarrhea • abdominal cramping	Teach child/family about characteristics of imbalanced nutrition. Assess and record results.	Increased knowledge will assist the child/family in recognizing and reporting changes in the child's condition.	Document whether teaching was done and describe results.
Child and/or family will be able to verbalize knowledge of care such as • medication administration • monitoring intake and output • maintenance of good oral hygiene including regular dental visits • identification of any signs/symptoms of imbalanced nutrition (such as those listed under Assessment) • when to contact health-care provider	Teach child/family about care. Assess and record child's/family's knowledge of and participation in care regarding medication administration, monitoring intake and output, etc.	Education of child/family will allow for accurate care.	Document whether teaching was done and describe results.

Related Nursing Diagnoses

Compromised Family Coping

related to
a. child's terminal illness
b. financial considerations
c. guilt
d. lack of material resources
e. social isolation
f. grieving
g. depression
h. fear
i. parental drug use

Impaired Gas Exchange

related to chronic lung infections

Acute Pain

related to
a. treatments
b. painful swallowing
c. lymphadenopathy
d. dyspnea

Deficient Knowledge:
Child/Family

related to
a. guilt
b. fear
c. sensory overload
d. misconceptions or inaccurate information
e. cognitive or cultural-language limitations
f. home care

Fear: Child/Parental

related to
a. terminal illness
b. death
c. social ramifications of illness

TWO

CELLULITIS
MEDICAL DIAGNOSIS

PATHOPHYSIOLOGY Cellulitis is an inflammation of the skin (dermis) and underlying connective tissue caused by an infection. It usually occurs on the face or extremities as a result of a break in the skin or as a result of trauma. Often, the child has a history of impetigo, folliculitis, recent otitis media, or sinusitis. The infection can occur at or near an open wound, animal bite, intravenous infusion site or even at an area with a vague history of recent trauma. Cellulitis may also result from an abscess.

Cellulitis occurs when bacterial organisms destroy hyaluronic acid, a binding and protective agent known as the cement substance of tissue. In this condition, bacterial organisms produce hyaluronidase (an enzyme that hydrolyzes hyaluronic acid), increasing the permeability of connective tissue and destroying tissue barriers, thus allowing the invasion by and spread of bacteria. The most common bacterial organisms responsible for cellulitis are *Staphylococcus aureus*, beta-hemolytic Group A streptococci, other beta-hemolytic streptococci, *Haemophilus influenzae*, and *Pasteurella multocida*.

Clinical manifestations include redness, edema, tenderness, warmth, and pain in the affected area. Often the regional lymph nodes are enlarged and lymphangitis "streaking" can be seen. The child may also have a fever, chills, and malaise.

Treatment consists of administration of intravenous antibiotics (mild cases can sometimes be treated with oral antibiotics at home), immobilization and elevation of the infected area, and application of warm, moist soaks. Cellulitis is a common occurrence in the pediatric population because of the social nature of young children and their close proximity to other children. Hospitalization is usually indicated for children with systemic symptoms, joint involvement, or cellulitis of the face.

Primary Nursing Diagnosis   Actual Infection*

Definition   Condition in which microorganisms have invaded the body

Possibly Related to   • Bacterial invasion of cellular or connective tissue

*Non-NANDA diagnosis.

Primary Nursing Diagnosis: Actual infection related to bacterial invasion of cellular or connective tissue
Assessment/Defining Characteristics of Child and/or Family (Subjective & Objective Data):
• Redness   • Fever   • Edema   • Tachycardia   • Warm to touch   • Tachypnea   • Red streaks radiating from infected area   • Hypotension   • Tenderness   • Altered white blood cell count (WBC)   • Pain

Primary Nursing Diagnosis: Actual Infection *(continued)*

Expected Outcomes	Possible Nursing Interventions	Rationale	Evaluation for Charting

Child will be free of infection as evidenced by
• body temperature within acceptable range of 36.5°C to 37.2°C
• heart rate within acceptable range (state specific range)
• respiratory rate within acceptable range (state specific range)
• blood pressure within acceptable range (state specific range)
• natural color of skin tissue
• WBC within acceptable range (state specific range)
• lack of the following to the infected area
  1. redness
  2. edema
  3. warm to touch
  4. red streak
  5. tenderness
  6. pain
• lack of signs/symptoms of infection (such as those listed under Assessment)
	Assess and record T, HR, RR, BP, and any signs/symptoms of infection (such as those listed under Assessment) every 4 hours and PRN.	If infection is present, the T, HR, and RR will increase and the BP may decrease.	Document range of T, HR, RR, and BP. Describe any signs/symptoms of infection noted.

	Assess and record IV fluids and condition of IV site every hour.	It is necessary to record the amount of IV fluids every hour to make sure the child is not being over or under hydrated. The IV site needs to be assessed every hour for signs of redness or swelling.	Document amount of IV fluids and describe condition of IV site along with any interventions needed.
	Keep accurate record of intake and output.	Provides information on child's hydration status.	Document intake and output.
	Maintain good hand-washing technique.	Good hand washing is the single most important measure in decreasing infection.	Document whether good hand-washing technique was used.
	Administer antibiotics on schedule. Assess and record any side effects (e.g., rash, diarrhea).	Antibiotics are given to combat infection.	Document whether antibiotics were administered on schedule. Describe any side effects noted.
	Administer antipyretics on schedule. Assess and record effectiveness.	Antipyretics are used to reduce fever.	Document whether an antipyretic was needed and describe effectiveness.
	When indicated, immobilize and elevate infected area and apply warm, moist packs as directed. Assess and record effectiveness. Assess circulation in affected area every 2 to 4 hours. Record every 4 hours and PRN.	Immobilization can be used to reduce tenderness and pain to the infected area. Warm, moist packs result in vasodilatation to the infected area, which increases circulation and promotes healing.	Describe any therapeutic measures used to treat the infection. Document their effectiveness in increasing child's comfort level. Describe circulation in affected area.
	Check and record results of WBC. Notify physician if results are out of the normal range.	Abnormal WBC results may indicate an infection.	Document WBC results if available.

(continued)

| | Possible Nursing | | Evaluation for |
Expected Outcomes	Interventions	Rationale	Charting
TEACHING GOALS Child and/or family will be able to verbalize at least 4 characteristics of infection such as • fever • redness • swelling • warm to touch • red streaks radiating from infected area • tenderness • pain	Teach child/family about characteristics of infection. Assess and record results.	Increased knowledge will assist the child/family in recognizing and reporting changes in the child's condition.	Document whether teaching was done and describe results.
Child and/or family will be able to verbalize knowledge of care such as • good hand-washing technique • fever control • medication administration • identification of any signs/symptoms of infection (such as those listed under Assessment) • when to contact health-care provider	Teach child/family about care. Assess and record child's/family's knowledge of and participation in care regarding good hand-washing technique, medication administration, etc.	Education of child/family will allow for accurate care.	Document whether teaching was done and describe results.

Primary Nursing Diagnosis: Actual Infection *(continued)*

Nursing Diagnosis   Impaired Tissue Integrity

Definition   Interruption of the integrity of or damage to the mucous membrane, integumentary, or subcutaneous tissue

Possibly Related to   • Increased permeability of connective tissue and destruction of the tissue barriers secondary to bacterial invasion

Nursing Diagnosis: Impaired tissue integrity related to increased permeability of connective tissue and destruction of the tissue barriers secondary to bacterial invasion

Assessment/Defining Characteristics of Child and/or Family (Subjective & Objective Data):
- Redness
- Edema
- Warm to touch
- Red streaks radiating from the infected area
- Tenderness
- Pain

Expected Outcomes	Possible Nursing Interventions	Rationale	Evaluation for Charting

Child will be free of signs/symptoms of impaired tissue integrity as evidenced by
 	
• natural color of the skin tissue
• lack of the following to the infected area
  1. redness
  2. edema
  3. warm to touch
  4. red streaks
  5. tenderness
  6. pain
	Assess and record
	
	• condition of tissue surrounding the infected site every 4 hours and PRN
	• IV fluids and condition of IV site every hour
	• signs/symptoms of impaired tissue integrity (such as those listed under Assessment) every 4 hours and PRN
		Condition of tissue surrounding the infected site needs to be clearly documented in order to detect changes. It is necessary to record the amount of IV fluids every hour to make sure the child is not being over or under hydrated. The IV site needs to be assessed every hour for signs of redness or swelling.	Describe condition of tissue surrounding the infected site. Determine if this is a change from the previous assessment findings. Document amount of IV fluids and describe condition of IV site along with any interventions needed. Describe any signs/symptoms of impaired tissue integrity noted.

	Keep accurate record of intake and output.	Provides information on child's hydration status.	Document intake and output.
	Maintain good hand-washing technique.	Good hand washing is the single most important measure in decreasing infection.	Document whether good hand-washing technique was used.
	Administer antibiotics on schedule. Assess and record any side effects (e.g., rash, diarrhea).	Antibiotics are given to combat infection.	Document whether antibiotics were administered on schedule. Describe any side effects noted.
	Administer antipyretics on schedule. Assess and record effectiveness.	Antipyretics are used to reduce fever.	Document whether an antipyretic was needed and describe effectiveness.
	When indicated, immobilize and elevate infected area and apply warm, moist packs as directed. Assess and record effectiveness. Assess circulation in affected area every 2 to 4 hours. Record every 4 hours and PRN.	Immobilization can be used to reduce tenderness and pain to the infected area. Warm, moist packs result in vasodilatation to the infected area, which increases circulation and promotes healing.	Describe any therapeutic measures used to treat the infection. Document their effectiveness in increasing child's comfort level. Describe circulation in affected area.

(continued)

Nursing Diagnosis: Impaired Tissue Integrity (*continued*)			
Expected Outcomes	**Possible Nursing Interventions**	**Rationale**	**Evaluation for Charting**
TEACHING GOALS Child and/or family will be able to verbalize at least 4 characteristics of impaired tissue integrity such as • redness • swelling • warm to touch • red streaks radiating from infected area • pain, tenderness	Teach child/family about characteristics of impaired tissue integrity. Assess and record results.	Increased knowledge will assist the child/family in recognizing and reporting changes in the child's condition.	Document whether teaching was done and describe results.
Child and/or family will be able to verbalize knowledge of care such as • immobilization and elevation of infected area • application of warm, moist packs to the infected area • good hand-washing technique • medication administration • identification of any signs/symptoms of impaired tissue integrity (such as those listed under Assessment) • when to contact health-care provider	Teach child/family about care. Assess and record child's/family's knowledge of and participation in care regarding immobilization and elevation of infected area, etc.	Education of child/family will allow for accurate care.	Document whether teaching was done and describe results.

Related Nursing Diagnoses

Acute Pain   *related to*
                               a. joint involvement
                               b. bacterial invasion

Activity Intolerance   *related to*
                               a. immobilization of infected area
                               b. IV fluids
                               c. warm soaks
                               d. fever

Fear: Child   *related to*
                               a. hospitalization
                               b. treatment and procedures
                               c. altered comfort

Compromised Family Coping   *related to* hospitalization of the child

THREE

KAWASAKI DISEASE
MEDICAL DIAGNOSIS

PATHOPHYSIOLOGY Kawasaki disease (KD) is an acute multisystem vasculitis that usually affects young children (< 5 years of age). The child presents with a high fever, rash, and other symptoms of systemic inflammation (such as inflammation of the meninges, joints, liver, and mucous membranes). The child with KD is at risk for developing coronary artery abnormalities, such as aneurysms and cardiac dysfunction, both of which can be life threatening. KD is one of two leading causes of acquired heart disease in children in the United States. The etiology of KD is unknown, but clinical and epidemiological features suggest an infectious cause that evokes an abnormal immunological response in genetically susceptible children. Peak incidence of KD is between 18 and 24 months of age, with 80% of all cases occurring in children younger than 5 years of age. It rarely occurs in children older than 8 years of age. The male-female ratio is approximately 1.5:1, and boys have a greater risk for aneurysms. Siblings and children of those who have had KD are at increased risk. Although KD can occur in any racial group, the incidence is highest in Asians. There is no evidence for spread by person-to-person contact, and most cases in the United States are reported during the late winter and early spring.

Although the pathogenesis of the vascular changes in KD is not completely understood, it is known that mainly the medium-sized arteries, especially the coronary arteries, are involved. Initially, a progressive inflammatory infiltration of the vessel walls occurs, as the endothelial and smooth muscle cells have become edematous. As the vasculitis progresses, the vessels then lose their structural integrity. Dilation of the arteries and aneurysm formation occurs as the vessels continue to weaken. Diffuse inflammation of the heart (pancarditis), as well as pericardial effusion and valvular insufficiency may develop, causing the child to have congestive heart failure and myocardial dysfunction. As the vessels heal, the inflammation in the pericardium, myocardium, and endocardium begins to decrease steadily. After 6 to 8 weeks, there is no further sign of inflammation and the lesions begin to heal, but scarring, calcification, and stenosis may be present in the affected vessels. The altered condition of the vessels and resultant low blood flow contribute to thrombi formation.

There are three distinct clinical phases in Kawasaki disease. During the acute phase, which lasts 1 to 2 weeks, the child will present with fever and other signs and symptoms of acute inflammation. At 2 to 4 weeks after the onset of symptoms, during the subacute phase, the child's fever resolves, but other symptoms persist. The child continues to be irrritable, has a loss of appetite, conjunctivitis, desquamation around the nails, and thrombocytosis. It is during the subacute phase that coronary artery aneurysms develop. During the convalescent phase, 6 to 8 weeks after the onset of symptoms, all signs and symptoms resolve and laboratory values, which had reflected acute inflammation, return to normal.

The child with KD presents with a high fever that persists for at least 5 days and is unresponsive to antibiotics and antipyretics. Other characteristics appear within several days of the fever, including (1) discrete conjunctival injection without exudate; (2) erythematous mouth and pharynx, strawberry tongue, and red cracked lips; (3) a polymorphous, generalized erythematous rash; (4) changes in the hands and feet consisting of indurative peripheral edema and diffuse erythema of the palms and soles; and (5) a unilateral cervical lymph node enlarged to at least 1.5 cm in diameter. Associated common features include irritability, abdominal pain, vomiting, and diarrhea. Other findings may include urethritis, liver dysfunction, arthritis or arthralgia, aseptic meningitis, gallbladder hydrops, coronary artery abnormalities, and cardiac function abnormalities.

The diagnosis of KD is based on the clinical features, with the exclusion of other possible illnesses, and supported by certain laboratory tests. The classic criteria include fever (104°F or higher) for 5 days, and a minimum of 4 of the 5 characteristic clinical features. It is often difficult to diagnose KD, as many children do not meet the classic diagnostic criteria. These cases are given a diagnosis of "incomplete" or "atypical" KD. The American Heart Association (AHA) has published guidelines to help diagnose and treat KD. These guidelines are supported by the American Academy of Pediatrics (AAP) and recommend using laboratory evaluation and echocardiography to assist with the diagnosis and treatment. The laboratory evaluations are divided into primary and supplementary criteria. C-reactive protein (> 3mg/dL) and erythrocyte sedimentation rate (> 40mm/hr) are the primary laboratory criteria. The supplementary laboratory criteria are: albumin (< or = 3g/d), anemia for age, elevated alanine aminotransferase level, platelet count $> 450 \times 10^3$/uL after 7 days of fever, white blood cell count $> 15 \times 10^3$/uL, and urine > 10 white blood cells/high powered field.

Treatment goals focus on minimizing damage to the myocardium and re-establishing patency and flow of the arteries. The current treatment of KD involves the administration of high-dose intravenous immune globulin (IVIG) therapy along with high-dose aspirin therapy (for its anti-inflammatory and antiplatelet effects). Most children have a rapid response to this therapy, with 90% being afebrile by 48 hours. After 10 days of illness, IVIG is only used for those children with persistent fever, accompanied by evidence of continued systemic inflammation and/or coronary aneurysm. In children with coronary aneurysms and giant aneurysms, additional anticoagulant therapy may be needed. Long-term aspirin therapy may be required for the children who have coronary abnormalities. Children with KD may need to have their immunization schedule adjusted to avoid the administration of the live-virus vaccines for 11 months after receiving IVIG. The American Heart Association recommends that all children who have had KD be monitored for myocardial ischemia, valvular insufficiency, dyslipidemia, and hypertension.

Primary Nursing Diagnosis   Decreased Cardiac Output

Definition   Decrease in the amount of blood that leaves the left ventricle

Possibly Related to
- Multisystem vasculitis
- Possibility of thrombus formation
- Inflammation of the heart
- Possibility of dilatation of the coronary arteries
- Scarring, calcification, and stenosis of vessels
- Myocardial dysfunction

Primary Nursing Diagnosis: Decreased cardiac output related to multisystem vasculitis; possibility of thrombus formation; inflammation of the heart; possibility of dilatation of the coronary vessels; scarring, calcification, and stenosis of vessels; myocardial dysfunction

Assessment/Defining Characteristics of Child and/or Family (Subjective & Objective Data):

- Tachycardia out of proportion to the degree of fever
- Gallop rhythm
- Electrocardiogram (EKG) changes
- Fever
- Tachypnea
- Hypotension
- Arrhythmias
- Peripheral edema
- Elevated erythrocyte sedimentation rate (ESR)
- Elevated C-reactive protein
- Myocarditis
- Anemia
- Thrombocytosis
- Leukocytosis

Expected Outcomes	Possible Nursing Interventions	Rationale	Evaluation for Charting
Child will have adequate cardiac output as evidenced by - heart rate with acceptable range (state specific range) - normal sinus rhythm - temperature within acceptable range of 36.5°C to 37.2°C - respiratory rate within acceptable range (state specific range)	Assess and record the following every 4 hours and PRN - T, HR, RR, and BP - laboratory values - any signs/symptoms of decreased cardiac output (listed under Assessment) every 4 hours and PRN	If child experiences decreased cardiac output (CO) the HR and RR will increase and BP will decrease. If T increases it will increase HR.	Document range of T, HR, RR, and BP. Document current laboratory values. Describe any signs/symptoms of decreased cardiac output noted.

Primary Nursing Diagnosis: Decreased Cardiac Output *(continued)*

Expected Outcomes	Possible Nursing Interventions	Rationale	Evaluation for Charting
• blood pressure within acceptable range (state specific range for each) • ESR within acceptable range (state specific range) • C-reactive protein within acceptable range (state specific range) • WBC within acceptable range (state specific range) • Hbg/Hct within acceptable range (state specific range) • platelet count within acceptable range (state specific range) • lack of 1. arrhythmias 2. peripheral edema 3. myocarditis 4. signs/symptoms of decreased cardiac output (such as those listed under Assessment)	Check and record results of chest X-ray, when indicated.	Changes in chest X-ray results may indicate increased heart size.	Document results of chest X-ray when indicated.
	Administer aspirin on schedule. Assess and record effectiveness and any side effects (e.g., nausea and vomiting).	Administered for its anti-inflammatory and anti-coagulant effect.	Document whether aspirin was administered on schedule. Describe effectiveness and any side effects noted.
	Administer IVIG on schedule. Assess and record any side effects (e.g., as tightness in the chest, vomiting, or hypotension). Assess and record blood pressure every 15 to 30 minutes during infusion (or according to institutional protocol).	Administered for its anti-inflammatory effect.	Document whether IVIG was administered on schedule. Describe any side effects noted.
	Evaluate and record results of EKG strips.	Changes in EKG may indicate decreased cardiac output and/or changes in the myocardium or coronary arteries.	Describe results of EKG when indicated.
	Organize nursing care to allow child uninterrupted rest.	Proper rest will help to decrease workload on the heart.	Document whether child was able to have uninterrupted rest periods.
TEACHING GOALS Child and/or family will be able to verbalize at least 3 characteristics of decreased cardiac output such as • rapid heart rate • fever • peripheral edema	Teach child/family about characteristics of decreased cardiac output. Assess and record results.	Increased knowledge will assist the child/family in recognizing and reporting changes in the child's condition.	Document whether teaching was done and describe results.
Child and/or family will be able to verbalize knowledge of care such as • fever control • medication administration	Teach child/family about care. Assess and record child's/family's knowledge of and participation in care regarding fever control, medication administration, etc.	Education of child/family will allow for accurate care.	Document whether teaching was done and describe results.

(continued)

Primary Nursing Diagnosis: Decreased Cardiac Output *(continued)*			
Expected Outcomes	**Possible Nursing Interventions**	**Rationale**	**Evaluation for Charting**
• sufficient rest periods • identification of any signs/symptoms of decreased cardiac output (such as those listed under Assessment) • when to contact health-care provider			

Nursing Diagnosis Deficient Fluid Volume

Definition Decrease in the amount of circulating fluid volume

Possibly Related to
- High fever
- Decreased oral intake
- Painful dry, red, cracked lips
- Oropharyngeal redness
- Strawberry tongue
- Mouth fissures
- Crusts in the mouth

Nursing Diagnosis: Deficient fluid volume related to high fever; decreased oral intake; painful, dry, red, cracked lips; oropharyngeal redness; strawberry tongue; mouth fissures; crusts in the mouth
Assessment/Defining Characteristics of Child and/or Family (Subjective & Objective Data):

- Fever
- Tachycardia
- Tachypnea
- Hypotension
- Sunken fontanel
- Sunken eyes
- Decreased oral intake
- Painful dry, red, cracked lips
- Oropharyngeal redness
- Strawberry tongue
- Mouth fissures
- Crusts in the mouth
- Decreased skin turgor (skin recoil greater than 2 to 3 seconds)
- Decreased urine output
- Increased urine specific gravity
- Weight loss
- Erythema of palms and soles

Nursing Diagnosis: Deficient Fluid Volume *(continued)*

Expected Outcomes	Possible Nursing Interventions	Rationale	Evaluation for Charting
Child will have an adequate fluid volume as evidenced by • adequate fluid intake, IV and oral (state specific amount of intake needed for each child) • adequate urine output (state specific range; 1 to 2 ml/kg/hr) • flat fontanel • absence of sunken eyes • urine specific gravity from 1.008 to 1.020 • temperature within acceptable range of 36.5°C to 37.2°C • heart rate, respiratory rate, and blood pressure within acceptable range (state specific range for each) • moist mucous membranes • lack of signs/symptoms of deficient fluid volume (such as those listed under Assessment)	Keep accurate record of intake and output. When indicated, encourage oral fluids.	Provides information on child's hydration status. Decreased urine output can indicate dehydration.	Document intake and output.
	Assess and record • HR, RR, and T every 4 hours and PRN • IV fluids and condition of IV site every hour • signs/symptoms of deficient fluid volume (such as those listed under Assessment) every 4 hours and PRN	Provides information about fluid status of patient. If patient has deficient fluid volume, the HR will increase at first, and eventually decrease. The RR will increase. The BP will eventually decrease. The T may increase due to the organism causing the disease state. It is necessary to record the amount of IV fluids every hour to make sure the child is not being over or under hydrated. The IV site needs to be assessed every hour for signs of redness or swelling.	Document range of HR and T. Document amount of IV fluids and describe condition of IV site along with any interventions needed. Describe any signs/symptoms of deficient fluid volume noted.
	Weigh child daily on same scale at same time of day. Document results and compare to previous weight.	Decrease in weight may be due to increased fluid loss from high fever and increased metabolic rate. It indicates the child's hydration status.	Document weight and determine if it was an increase or decrease from the previous weight.
	Check and record urine specific gravity with every void or as indicated.	Urine specific gravity provides information about hydration status.	Document range of urine specific gravity.
	Offer frozen popsicles or ice. If indicated, administer analgesics prior to meals or snacks.	Helps to increase comfort.	Describe any therapeutic measures used to improve fluid volume deficit. Describe effectiveness.
	When indicated, use lubricating ointment to the lips.	Moisturizing lips can help to decrease dryness.	Describe any therapeutic measures used to improve fluid volume deficit. Describe effectiveness.
	Assess and record condition of fontanel, eyes, mucous membranes and skin turgor every shift and PRN.	Provides information on hydration status.	Describe status of fontanel, mucous membranes, eyes, and skin turgor.

(continued)

Nursing Diagnosis: Deficient Fluid Volume *(continued)*			
Expected Outcomes	**Possible Nursing Interventions**	**Rationale**	**Evaluation for Charting**
TEACHING GOALS Child and/or family will be able to verbalize at least 4 characteristics of deficient fluid volume such as • high fever • decreased oral intake • painful dry, red, cracked lips • mouth fissures • weight loss • decreased urine output	Teach child/family about characteristics of deficient fluid volume. Assess and record results.	Increased knowledge will assist the child/family in recognizing and reporting changes in the child's condition.	Document whether teaching was done and describe results.
Child and/or family will be able to verbalize knowledge of care such as • child's need for appropriate fluids • monitoring intake and output • identification of any signs/symptoms of deficient fluid volume (such as those listed under Assessment) • when to contact health-care provider	Teach child/family about care. Assess and record child's/family's knowledge of and participation in care regarding child's need for appropriate fluids, monitoring intake and output, etc.	Education of child/family will allow for accurate care.	Document whether teaching was done and describe results.

Related Nursing Diagnoses

Acute Pain	*related to* a. multisystem vasculitis b. erythematous mouth and pharynx, strawberry tongue, red cracked lips, fissures, and crusts in the mouth c. generalized erythematous rash d. conjunctivitis e. peripheral edema and erythema of the palms and soles f. cervical lymphadenopathy g. joint inflammation
Impaired Skin Integrity	*related to* inflammatory skin changes
Ineffective Tissue Perfusion	*related to* a. vasculitis b. possible thrombus formation

CARE OF
CHILDREN WITH
MUSCULOSKELETAL
DYSFUNCTION

8

ONE

DUCHENNE MUSCULAR DYSTROPHY
MEDICAL DIAGNOSIS

PATHOPHYSIOLOGY Muscular dystrophy is the name of a group of genetically acquired diseases that cause gradual progressive muscle wasting. Duchenne muscular dystrophy (DMD), also called pseudohypertrophic muscular dystrophy, is the most common and most severe form of muscular dystrophy in children. Duchenne muscular dystrophy is an X-linked recessive disorder primarily affecting boys. The incidence is 1 in 3,300 males. New mutations can account for up to one-third of the children with DMD.

Duchenne muscular dystrophy results from mutations of the gene that encodes dystrophin. Dystrophin, a protein product in skeletal muscle, is needed as a muscle membrane stabilizer. Dystrophin is absent in children with DMD. Skeletal and cardiac muscle are primarily affected. Initial muscle weakness and atrophy begin in the proximal muscles, especially of the hips, shoulders, and spine, and present between the ages of 3 and 5. Affected boys exhibit inability to get up from a supine position, difficulty running and jumping, waddling gait, difficulty climbing stairs, and frequent falls. The child has difficulty rising from a sitting or squatting position on the floor and develops Gowers sign (a way of walking the hands up the legs to gradually straighten into a standing position). Between ages 8 and 12, the boys begin to use wheelchairs full time. Although the function of dystrophin in the brain is unknown, many affected boys will require extra help with academics. Curvature of the spine requiring surgical stabilization usually occurs 3 to 4 years after losing ambulation. Joint contractures of the lower extremities develop and the feet assume the typical equinovarus position. The ability for self-care declines in the midteens as the boys lose function of their upper extremities. They often will require nocturnal assisted ventilation. Their schools will need to accommodate for both the physical and learning needs of the child. Eventually, all muscles of the body are affected, including those of the respiratory (oropharyngeal muscles, diaphragm and respiratory musculature) and cardiovascular (myocardium) systems. Death usually results from pulmonary or cardiac complications.

The muscles of children with DMD undergo several histologic changes: nerve fibers degenerate, fat and connective tissue replace muscle fibers, and there is a variation in fiber size and central nuclei. As a compensatory mechanism, adjacent fibers hypertrophy. All of these processes contribute to the pseudo-hypertrophy of the calves, thighs, and upper arms. Pseudohypertrophic muscles are enlarged and feel firmer than normal muscles as a result of the infiltration with fatty tissue and inflammatory cells. The diagnosis of DMD is based primarily on clinical symptoms and confirmed by muscle biopsy, electromyography (EMG), and serum enzyme measurements.

There is no definitive cure for DMD. The goal of treatment is to promote optimal functioning. A regular exercise program of stretching and range of motion, aggressive management of respiratory and cardiac problems, the use of adaptive devices to facilitate activities of daily living, and modifications in the home help to assist ambulation and independence as long as possible. The child should be encouraged to avoid excessively strenuous activities and fatigue. Nutritional management is also a priority to offset the increased risk of obesity for boys with DMD. Currently, corticosteroids are used to delay the progression of muscle weakness and preserve muscle function.

A comprehensive health-care team can best meet the needs of a child with DMD. The family should also be recommended for genetic counseling. The Muscular Dystrophy Association offers support services to these children and their families.

Primary Nursing Diagnosis   Impaired Physical Mobility

Definition   Limited ability of movement

Possibly Related to
- Muscle weakness
- Contractures
- Joint deformities

Primary Nursing Diagnosis: Impaired physical mobility related to muscle weakness, contractures, joint deformities

Assessment/Defining Characteristics of Child and/or Family (Subjective & Objective Data):

- Decreased range of motion
- Contractures
- Muscle weakness
- Fatigue
- Joint deformities
- Muscle atrophy
- Clumsiness
- Falling
- Waddling gait
- Difficulty arising from a sitting position
- Lordosis
- Difficulty climbing stairs

Expected Outcomes	Possible Nursing Interventions	Rationale	Evaluation for Charting
Child will maximize ability of movement as evidenced by (state specific examples for each child)	Assess and record child's activity level at least once/shift and PRN.	Provides a mobility baseline, which can be used to describe increased or decreased activity.	Describe child's level of mobility.
	Assess and record any signs/symptom of impaired physical mobility (such as those listed under Assessment) once/shift and PRN.	Provides information that can assist when planning nursing care for the child.	Describe any signs/ symptoms of impaired physical mobility noted.
	Ensure that child keeps scheduled appointments with occupational therapy and physical therapy as indicated.	Therapy will help maximize ability of movement.	Describe any therapeutic measures used to improve physical mobility. Document their effectiveness.
	Encourage child to participate as much as possible in self-care.	Promotes autonomy.	Document child's ability to participate in self-care.
	Make available activities within child's limitations (state specific examples for each child).	Decreases anxiety and frustration while allowing child to accomplish activities.	Describe any activities in which the child was able to participate.
	Allow adequate rest periods (state specific amount of rest needed for each child).	Maintains ability to participate in usual activities.	Document effectiveness of rest periods.
	Perform scheduled active and passive range-of-motion exercises every 4 hours and PRN.	Helps preserve muscle and joint function.	Document whether range-of-motion exercises were done and their effectiveness.
	Reposition child every 1 to 2 hours.	Helps to prevent skin breakdown.	Document whether child was repositioned on schedule.
	Ensure that child's body stays in proper alignment, whether in bed, chair, or wheelchair.	Maintains position and helps to prevent deformities.	Document whether child was kept in proper alignment.

(continued)

Primary Nursing Diagnosis: Impaired Physical Mobility *(continued)*

Expected Outcomes	Possible Nursing Interventions	Rationale	Evaluation for Charting
	Encourage use of devices such as handrails, foot-boards, and rubber-soled shoes.	Assist in facilitating activities of daily living.	Document whether devices were used and their effectiveness in facilitating activities of daily living.
	Assist child as necessary with use of braces.	Assist with mobility and promote independence.	Document whether braces were used and their effectiveness in increasing mobility.
TEACHING GOALS Child and/or family will be able to verbalize at least 4 characteristics of impaired mobility such as • decreased range of motion • clumsiness • falling • waddling gait • difficulty arising from a sitting position • difficulty climbing stairs	Teach child/family about characteristics of impaired mobility. Assess and record results.	Increased knowledge will assist the child/family in recognizing and reporting changes in the child's condition.	Document whether teaching was done and describe results.
Child and/or family will be able to verbalize knowledge of care such as • correct use of adaptive devices and home modifications • correct handling and positioning technique • appropriate use of resources • identification of any signs/symptoms of impaired mobility (such as those listed under Assessment) • when to contact health-care provider	Teach child/family about care. Assess and record child's/family's knowledge of and participation in care regarding correct use of adaptive devices and home modifications, etc.	Education of child/family will allow for accurate care.	Document whether teaching was done and describe results.

Nursing Diagnosis   Ineffective Breathing Pattern

Definition   Breathing pattern that results in inadequate oxygen consumption (failure to meet the cellular requirements of the body)

Possibly Related to
- Weakness of pulmonary musculature
- Scoliosis
- Lordosis

Nursing Diagnosis: Ineffective breathing pattern related to weakness of pulmonary musculature, scoliosis, lordosis

Assessment/Defining Characteristics of Child and/or Family (Subjective & Objective Data):

- Shallow respirations
- Pooled secretions and/or mucus
- Tachypnea
- Tachycardia
- Diaphoresis
- Pallor or cyanosis
- Crackles and/or rhonchi
- Decreased breath sounds
- Infiltrates revealed on chest X-ray

Expected Outcomes	Possible Nursing Interventions	Rationale	Evaluation for Charting

Child will have effective breathing pattern as evidenced by
 	
• respiratory rate within acceptable range (state specific range)
• clear and equal breath sounds bilaterally A & P
• heart rate within acceptable range (state specific range)
• pink/tan color
• absence of
  1. pallor or cyanosis
  2. crackles and/or rhonchi
  3. diaphoresis
  4. pooled secretions and/or mucus
• oxygen saturation (via pulse oximeter) from 94 to 100% on room air
• clear chest X-ray
	Assess and record RR, HR, breath sounds, and any signs/symptoms of ineffective breathing pattern (such as those listed under Assessment) every 2 to 4 hours and PRN.	If child experiences ineffective breathing pattern the RR and HR will increase and the child will work harder to breathe, exhibiting some of the characteristics of ineffective breathing pattern.	Document range of RR and HR. Describe breath sounds and any signs/symptoms of ineffective breathing pattern noted.

	If indicated, administer humidified oxygen in correct amount and route of delivery. Record percent of oxygen and route of delivery. Assess and record effectiveness of therapy.	Humidified oxygen will dilate the pulmonary vasculature, which increases surface area available for gas exchange. Extra source oxygen will also allow for better oxygenation to body tissues and thus help combat ineffective breathing pattern.	Document amount and route of oxygen delivery. Describe effectiveness.
	Keep head of bed elevated at a 30° angle.	Elevating the head of the bed to a 30° angle causes a shift of the abdominal contents downward and this in turn will allow for increased lung expansion in order to help improve breathing pattern.	Document whether head of bed was kept elevated and describe effectiveness of measure.

(continued)

Nursing Diagnosis: Ineffective Breathing Pattern *(continued)*

Expected Outcomes	Possible Nursing Interventions	Rationale	Evaluation for Charting
	Ensure that chest physio-therapy is done on schedule (including deep breathing, coughing, and use of incentive spirome-try). Record effectiveness and child's response to treatment.	Chest percussion loosens secretions and position-ing can help to assist the flow of secretions out of the lungs by gravity. This will aid in effective breathing pattern.	Document whether chest physiotherapy was done on schedule. Describe effectiveness and child's response to treatment.
	When using a pulse oximeter, record reading every 2 to 4 hours and PRN.	Pulse oximetry detects the oxygen saturation in the blood stream. It is important to detect small changes in oxygen satu-ration before the child starts displaying overt characteristics of ineffec-tive breathing pattern.	Document range of oxygen saturation.
	Check and record results of chest X-ray when indicated.	Changes in chest X-ray results may indicate need for a change in therapy.	Document results of chest X-ray when indicated.
	When indicated, admin-ister antibiotics on sched-ule. Assess and record any side effects (e.g., rash, diarrhea).	Antibiotics combat any invading organisms.	Document whether antibiotics were adminis-tered on schedule. Describe any side effects noted.
TEACHING GOALS Child and/or family will be able to verbalize at least 3 characteristics of ineffective breathing pattern such as • color change from pink/tan to gray or blue • rapid respirations • intolerance of normal activities	Teach child/family about characteristics of ineffec-tive breathing pattern. Assess and record results.	Increased knowledge will assist the child/ family in recognizing and reporting changes in the child's condition.	Document whether teaching was done and describe results.
Child and/or family will be able to verbalize knowledge of care such as • treatments such as chest physiotherapy • head elevated positioning	Teach child/family about care. Assess and record child's/family's knowl-edge of and participation in care regarding chest physiotherapy treatments, etc.	Education of child/ family will allow for accurate care.	Document whether teaching was done and describe results.

Nursing Diagnosis: Ineffective Breathing Pattern (continued)			
Expected Outcomes	**Possible Nursing Interventions**	**Rationale**	**Evaluation for Charting**
• identification of any signs/symptoms of ineffective breathing pattern (such as those listed under Assessment) • when to contact health-care provider			

Related Nursing Diagnoses

Disturbed Body Image   *related to*
a. chronic illness
b. disabling features of the illness
c. limited physical activity
d. weight gain

Self-Care Deficit: (Specify)   *related to*
a. joint contractures and/or deformities
b. muscle weakness

Grieving: Family   *related to* child's debilitating chronic illness

TWO

FRACTURES
MEDICAL DIAGNOSIS

DESCRIPTION A fracture is a break in the continuity of the tissue of the bone. Fractures can be complete, with fragments separated, or incomplete, with fragments remaining attached. They can also be classified as simple (closed) or compound, with one or both ends of the broken bone protruding through an open wound. Fractures account for approximately 10 to 15% of all serious childhood injuries.

Since a child's skeletal structure is not the same as that of an adult, the management and treatment of fractures in children is different than in adults. Children's bones are more easily injured, and fractures can result from minor falls or twists. In children, bones are more flexible, have decreased density, and have a thicker periosteum. The increased flexibility allows the bone to bend 45° or more before breaking. A break in a young child's bone is more often incomplete due to the decreased density of the bone. The thick periosteum can sometimes serve as a hinge and facilitate closed reduction of a fracture. The epiphyseal growth plate, which serves to absorb shock and protect joint surfaces in children, is the weakest point of long bones and consequently a frequent site of damage during trauma. The growth plate is located between the epiphysis and metaphysis of all long bones. If the fracture occurs in this portion of the bone and destroys the germinal layer, it can cause shortening and a progressive angular deformity of the affected limb. If the injury stimulates blood supply to the epiphysis, it can lead to overgrowth of the affected bone. Growth plate injuries account for 15 to 30% of all pediatric fractures. They occur most commonly in boys, during periods of rapid growth, peaking between the ages of 10 and 16. Fractures usually heal faster in children than in adults because of the rich blood supply and high osteogenic activity in children. Children's bones are also continuously being reshaped and reconstructed; this process is called remodeling. Remodeling occurs faster in children than in adults, which promotes rapid healing and therefore the child may not need anatomic alignment. Remodeling depends on the age of the child, the site and type of fracture, and amount of fragmentation.

Most often fractures occur while the child is at play. Young children fall forward onto outstretched arms; older children are injured by bicycle falls, sports-related trauma, and motor vehicle accidents. One of the most common fractures in children younger than 4 years of age is the "toddler's fracture." This occurs when a rotational injury induces a nondisplaced spiral fracture of the tibia. Overall, upper extremity fractures usually happen more frequently. Common fractures in children include a complete fracture; buckle fracture, greenstick fracture, and spiral fracture. A buckle fracture, also called a torus fracture, occurs when the porous bone is compressed, resulting in a bulging projection at the fracture site. A greenstick fracture, the most frequently seen type in children, occurs when the bone is angulated beyond the limits of bending. The fracture is incomplete, and there is a break through the periosteum on the compressed side only. A spiral, or transverse, fracture occurs from a sudden, twisting, and violent exertion upon an extremity, resulting in a fracture line across the bone.

The Salter-Harris system is used to categorize fractures by 5 fracture types. Type I involves a fracture along the growth plate, rather than across it, that separates the epiphysis and the metaphysis. The X-ray appears normal and the diagnosis is based on clinical information. Type II involves a fracture along the growth plate, with an oblique extension through a piece of the metaphysis. This type is the most common growth plate fracture. Type I and II fractures usually do not require surgery for a good prognosis. Type III is a fracture through the growth plate that extends into the epiphysis and joint space. Type IV is a fracture through the growth plate that extends into both the metaphysis and epiphysis and into the joint space. Type III and Type IV fractures both require surgery and can threaten growth potential and joint function. Type V is a compression of the growth plate, usually recognized only after the fact, when failure of growth is noted. This crush injury is the rarest type of fracture.

Diagnosis of fractures can be made from clinical evaluation and/or X-ray films of the injured area. An older child may be able to describe their injury and localize the area of pain. A young child may present with irritability, pseudoparalysis of the injured area, or refusal to walk or bear weight. There may be changes in the skin, tenderness, swelling, or deformity of the injured area. Once the injury has been localized, the appropriate radiographs should be obtained.

The management and treatment of fractures involves bringing the fracture fragments into proper alignment and maintaining the alignment through immobilization. This can be accomplished by open or closed reduction. Closed reduction, the most common method used in children, consists of a combination of manual manipulation and force applied with the hands to push the bone ends into position. Some overriding of the fracture fragments (1 cm) is sometimes desirable in children to allow for the overgrowth that may occur in the injured extremity. After manual manipulation, the fragments are held in place with a cast. When the pull or spasms of muscles close to the fracture make setting difficult, traction or internal or external fixation devices are used to hold the fragments in place. Open reduction, used when alignment cannot be obtained by the closed method, is a surgical procedure and requires general anesthesia. Some type of internal fixation device, such as a rod, screw, or plate, is used to stabilize the fracture.

Complications of fractures include malunion as healing occurs, compartment syndrome (progressive interference of blood flow to an extremity), pulmonary emboli, nonunion, nerve compression syndrome, circulatory impairment, epiphyseal damage, infection, and growth disturbance.

Primary Nursing Diagnosis   Acute Pain

Definition	Condition in which an individual experiences acute mild to severe pain
Possibly Related to	• Break in the continuity of the tissue of the bone
	• Muscle spasms
	• Injury

Primary Nursing Diagnosis: Acute pain related to break in the continuity of the tissue of the bone, muscle spasms, injury

Assessment/Defining Characteristics of Child and/or Family (Subjective & Objective Data):

- Crying or moaning
- Facial grimacing
- Verbal communication of pain
- Restlessness
- Guarding or protection behavior of injured site
- Rating of pain on pain-assessment tool
- Physical signs/symptoms (tachycardia, tachypnea, increased blood pressure, diaphoresis)

Expected Outcomes	Possible Nursing Interventions	Rationale	Evaluation for Charting
Child will have decreased pain or be free of severe and/or constant pain as evidenced by • verbal communication of comfort • lack of 1. constant crying or moaning 2. facial grimacing 3. extreme restlessness 4. diaphoresis • decreased guarding or protective behavior of the injured site • heart rate within acceptable range (state specific range)	Assess and record HR, RR, T, BP, and any signs/symptoms of pain (such as those listed under Assessment) every 2 to 4 hours and PRN. Use age-appropriate pain-assessment tool.	Provides data regarding the level of pain child is experiencing.	Document range of HR, RR, T, BP, and degree of pain child was experiencing. Describe any successful measures used to decrease pain.
	Assess and record neurovascular status of extremity every 1 to 2 hours and PRN.	Provides information about compromised circulation or feeling to the injured area.	Describe neurovascular assessment of extremity.
	Administer analgesics and/or narcotics on schedule. Assess and record effectiveness and any side effects (e.g., constipation, nausea).	Analgesics and narcotics are administered to decrease pain.	Document whether analgesics and/or narcotics were administered on schedule. Describe effectiveness and any side effects noted.

(continued)

Primary Nursing Diagnosis: Acute Pain *(continued)*

Expected Outcomes	Possible Nursing Interventions	Rationale	Evaluation for Charting
• respiratory rate within acceptable range (state specific range) • blood pressure within acceptable range (state specific range) • rating of decreased pain or no pain on pain-assessment tool • lack of signs/symptoms of pain (such as those listed under Assessment)	Handle injured area with extreme care. Avoid bumping or jarring the bed if the child is in traction. Maintain correct alignment of injured area.	These measures will help prevent pain caused by movement. Correct alignment is needed to assist in healing of the injured area.	Document if child was handled with care and if correct alignment was maintained. Describe effectiveness of measures.
	Encourage family members to stay and comfort child when possible.	Helps to comfort and support the child.	Document whether family was able to remain with child and describe effectiveness of their presence.
	Allow family members to participate in care of child when possible.	This may increase the comfort level of the child and thus help child in managing pain.	Document whether family participated in care and if this was successful in helping child with pain management.
	Use diversional activities (e.g., music, television, playing games, relaxation) when appropriate.	Diversional activities can distract child and may help to decrease pain.	Document whether diversional activities were successful in helping to manage pain.
	If age appropriate, explain all procedures beforehand.	Allowing child some control can assist child with pain management.	Describe if this measure was effective in helping child to manage pain.
	If age appropriate, allow the child to participate in planning his or her care. Encourage the child to practice self-care (e.g., bathing, removing dressing).	Allowing child some control can assist child with pain management.	Describe if this measure was effective in helping child to manage pain.
	When indicated, institute additional pain relief measures, such as hypnosis and guided imagery. Assess and record effectiveness.	These nonpharmacologic measures may help decrease pain.	Document whether these measures were successful in helping to manage pain.
TEACHING GOALS Child and/or family will be able to verbalize at least 4 characteristics of pain such as • verbal communication of pain or tenderness • restlessness • facial grimacing • guarding or protective behavior of the injured site • rapid heart rate	Teach child/family about characteristics of pain. Assess and record results.	Increased knowledge will assist the child/family in recognizing and reporting changes in the child's condition.	Document whether teaching was done and describe results.

Primary Nursing Diagnosis: Acute Pain *(continued)*			
Expected Outcomes	**Possible Nursing Interventions**	**Rationale**	**Evaluation for Charting**
Child and/or family will be able to verbalize knowledge of care such as • medication administration • correct alignment of injured area • gentle handling of child • identification of any signs/symptoms of pain (such as those listed under Assessment) • when to contact health-care provider	Teach child/family about care. Assess and record child's/family's knowledge of and participation in care regarding medication administration, etc.	Education of child/family will allow for accurate care.	Document whether teaching was done and describe results.

Nursing Diagnosis   Impaired Physical Mobility

Definition   Limited ability of movement

Possibly Related to
- Break in continuity of the tissue of the bone
- Cast
- Traction

Nursing Diagnosis: Impaired physical mobility related to break in continuity of the tissue of the bone; cast; traction			
Assessment/Defining Characteristics of Child and/or Family (Subjective & Objective Data): • Restricted movement of part of the body • Inability to ambulate • Decreased range of motion of part of the body • Muscle pull and/or spasms			
Expected Outcomes	**Possible Nursing Interventions**	**Rationale**	**Evaluation for Charting**
Child will return to preinjury mobility level	Assess and record any signs/symptom of impaired physical mobility (such as those listed under Assessment) once/shift and PRN.	Provides information that can assist when planning nursing care for the child.	Describe any signs/symptoms of impaired physical mobility noted.
	Ensure that child keeps scheduled appointments with occupational therapy and physical therapy as indicated.	Therapy will help maximize ability of movement.	Describe any therapeutic measures used to improve physical mobility. State their effectiveness.

(continued)

Nursing Diagnosis: Impaired Physical Mobility *(continued)*			
Expected Outcomes	**Possible Nursing Interventions**	**Rationale**	**Evaluation for Charting**
	Encourage child to participate as much as possible in self-care. Provide apparatus, such as overhead trapeze, when indicated.	Promotes autonomy.	Document child's ability to participate in self-care.
	Make available activities within child's limitations (state specific examples for each child).	Decreases anxiety and frustration while allowing child to accomplish activities.	Describe any activities in which the child was able to participate.
	Allow adequate rest periods (state specific amount of rest needed for each child).	Maintains ability to participate in usual activities.	Document effectiveness of rest periods.
	Perform scheduled active and passive range-of-motion exercises every 4 hours and PRN.	Helps preserve muscle and joint function.	Document whether range-of-motion exercises were done and their effectiveness.
	Ensure that injured area remains in proper alignment at all times. Use appropriate adaptive equipment (e.g., molded splints or boots) when indicated.	Proper alignment allows for proper healing of the injured area and prevents complications.	Document if proper alignment was maintained and effectiveness of any adaptive equipment used.
	If child is in a cast, assess and record the following every 2 to 4 hours and PRN • neurovascular status of affected area • warm area on the cast • swelling • bleeding on cast. Mark bleeding and record date and time on cast with a ballpoint pen.	Neurovascular assessment provides information about compromised circulation or feeling to the injured area. Warm spots on the cast may indicate the presence of an infection. Assessment of the amount of swelling and bleeding provides information on the healing process. Increased amounts can indicate need for intervention.	If child is casted, describe neurovascular assessment, amount of any bleeding or swelling present, and any warm spots noted.
	Pedal cast when indicated.	Pedaling the cast decreases skin irritation and prevents skin breakdown.	Describe effectiveness of pedaling cast.

Nursing Diagnosis: Impaired Physical Mobility *(continued)*

Expected Outcomes	Possible Nursing Interventions	Rationale	Evaluation for Charting
TEACHING GOALS Child and/or family will be able to verbalize at least 4 characteristics of impaired mobility such as • restricted movement of part of the body • decreased range of motion of part of the body • inability to ambulate • muscle pull and/or spasms	Teach child/family about characteristics of impaired mobility. Assess and record results.	Increased knowledge will assist the child/family in recognizing and reporting changes in the child's condition.	Document whether teaching was done and describe results.
Child and/or family will be able to verbalize knowledge of care such as • monitoring of activity and rest periods • activity restrictions as indicated • drying, cleaning, and care of cast (assessment for hot spots) • neurovascular assessment of injured area • correct use of crutches when indicated • monitoring for bleeding, swelling, pain, or discoloration of exposed portion of injured area • monitoring of casted extremity for "hot spots" • assistance with activities of daily living (may need bedpan and/or urinal if child is in a hip spica) • appropriate use of resources • identification of any signs/symptoms of impaired mobility (such as those listed under Assessment) • when to contact health-care provider	Teach child/family about care. Assess and record child's/family's knowledge of and participation in care regarding monitoring of activity and rest periods, cast care, etc.	Education of child/family will allow for accurate care.	Document whether teaching was done and describe results.

Related Nursing Diagnoses

Impaired Skin Integrity *related to*
a. immobility
b. traction
c. internal or external fixation devices
d. cast

Fear: Child *related to*
a. discomfort
b. procedures and equipment
c. forced contact with strangers
d. hospital environment

Self-Care Deficit: (Specify) *related to*
a. immobility
b. traction
c. cast

THREE

JUVENILE RHEUMATOID ARTHRITIS/ JUVENILE IDIOPATHIC ARTHRITIS
MEDICAL DIAGNOSIS

PATHOPHYSIOLOGY The American classification of juvenile rheumatoid arthritis (JRA) is being replaced by a new classification developed by the International League Against Rheumatism. The term juvenile rheumatoid arthritis, JRA, is being replaced with juvenile idiopathic arthritis, JIA. JIA is defined as the presence of objective signs of arthritis in at least one joint for more than 6 weeks, in a child younger than 16 years, after other types of childhood arthritis have been excluded. Arthritis is defined as the presence of swelling of the joint or two or more of the following: limitation of motion, tenderness, pain with motion, or joint warmth. These symptoms are caused by a chronic inflammation of the synovium with joint effusion. Eventually, there is erosion, destruction, and fibrosis (scar tissue formation) of the articular cartilage. Adhesions and joint ankylosis can also occur. The cause of JIA is unknown, but there is evidence to suggest that it is a multifactorial auto-immune response, involving both T- and B- cells, as well as the body's inflammatory response.

There are eight categories of JIA, each designated by the clinical manifestations present during the first 6 months of illness. The categories are: 1) systemic, 2) oligoarthritis persistent, 3) oligoarthritis extended, 4) polyarthritis rheumatoid factor (RF)-negative, 5) polyarthritis RF-positive, 6) enthesitis-related arthritis, 7) psoriatic arthritis, and 8) other.

Systemic JIA (10% of all JIA cases) is characterized by high intermittent fevers and accompanied by a variety of other extra-articular manifestations. These can include rheumatoid rash, hepatomegaly, splenomegaly, lymphadenopathy, pleuritis, pericarditis, abdominal pain, leukocytosis, severe anemia, and disseminated intravascular coagulation syndrome. The disease may present at any time during childhood, and there is a slight male preponderance.

Oligoarthritis JIA (40% of all cases) usually involves four or fewer joints in the first 6 months of the disease. There are two subgroups of oligo JIA, persistent and extended. In persistent oligo JIA, no more than four joints are affected throughout the disease. In extended oligo JIA, more than four joints become involved throughout the disease. Oligo JIA predominantly affects girls (4:1), and the age of onset is between the first and

fifth birthday. Many of these children have antinuclear antibody (ANA) positive serum (75 to 85% of the time), and those who are ANA positive are at greatest risk for developing uveitis (a nongranulomatous chronic inflammatory process in the anterior chamber of the eye). They also have minimal systemic complaints. Large joints are affected, especially the knees and ankles, and these children often present with a warm, swollen joint and a limp that is worse after resting.

Polyarthritis JIA (poly JIA) (25% of all cases) is defined as JIA involving five or more joints within the first 6 months of the disease. It may occur at anytime during childhood and is more common in girls. Poly JIA cases can be further divided into those who have a positive serum rheumatoid factor (RF) and those who are RF negative. Rheumatoid factor-negative poly JIA may have its onset any time during childhood, whereas rheumatoid factor-positive poly JIA rarely begins before the eighth birthday. Children with RF-positive poly JIA usually have symmetric, small-joint arthritis and are at greater risk for developing erosive joint disease, rheumatoid nodules, and a poor functional outcome. RF-negative poly JIA often involves fewer joints and may not be symmetrical. Morning stiffness, joint swelling, and limited joint mobility are characteristic of poly JIA. Other symptoms can include fatigue, delayed growth, and anemia.

The last three categories of JIA are enthesitis-related arthritis, psoriatic arthritis, and other. Enthesitis-related arthritis is characterized by inflammation of the enthesitis (where the tendon attaches to the bone) and arthritis. Psoriatic arthritis is diagnosed when the children have chronic arthritis and definite psoriasis. Two of the following criteria may replace the definite psoriasis criteria: dactylitis, nail pitting or onycholysis, or a family history of psoriasis.

Juvenile idiopathic arthritis is one of the most common chronic illnesses in children. It is characterized by spontaneous exacerbations and remissions, with the prognosis depending on the subtype. Treatment involves attempts to reduce inflammation, relieve pain, and prevent joint contractures and other complications in an attempt to preserve the joint and its function. Pharmacological management includes nonsteroidal anti-inflammatory drugs (NSAIDs), disease-modifying antirheumatic drugs (DMARDs), biologics (e.g., Etanercept) and corticosteroids (oral, intravenous, or intra-articular). Methotrexate is the most commonly prescribed DMARD for JIA, with approximately 70% of children having a positive response. Folic acid is administered daily to decrease the side effects of methotrexate. The side effects can include abdominal pain, mouth ulcers, and decreased appetite.

A multidisciplinary team is needed to address all the needs of the child and family with JIA. The child and family need the involvement of a pediatric rheumatologist and nurses, as well as a social worker and primary physician. Occupational therapy and physical therapy are important in helping the child maintain strength and mobility and make adaptations to function independently in the activities of daily living. Exercise and splints help maintain good joint position and prevent the development of contractures. Total joint replacement is a surgical option for those whose joint cartilage is destroyed. If all other therapies fail, an autologous stem cell transplant can be considered.

Primary Nursing Diagnosis   Impaired Physical Mobility

Definition	Limited ability of movement
Possibly Related to	• Pain
	• Joint inflammation
	• Synovitis
	• Erosion of the articular cartilage
	• Destruction of the articular cartilage
	• Fibrosis of the articular cartilage
	• Adhesions
	• Joint ankylosis
	• Multifactorial autoimmune response

Primary Nursing Diagnosis: Impaired physical mobility related to pain, joint inflammation, synovitis, erosion of the articular cartilage, destruction of the articular cartilage, fibrosis of the articular cartilage, adhesions, joint ankylosis, multifactorial autoimmune response

Assessment/Defining Characteristics of Child and/or Family (Subjective & Objective Data):

- Decreased range of motion
- Contractures
- Arthralgia
- Myalgia
- Fatigue
- Swelling
- Joint stiffness
- Joint destruction

Expected Outcomes	Possible Nursing Interventions	Rationale	Evaluation for Charting
Child will maximize ability of movement as evidenced by (state specific for each child)	Assess and record child's activity level at least once/shift.	Provides a mobility base-line, which can be used to describe increased or decreased activity.	Describe child's level of mobility.
	Assess and record any signs/symptoms of impaired physical mobil-ity (such as those listed under Assessment) once/shift and PRN.	Provides information that can assist when planning nursing care for the child.	Describe any signs/symptoms of impaired physical mobility noted.

Primary Nursing Diagnosis: Impaired Physical Mobility *(continued)*

Expected Outcomes	Possible Nursing Interventions	Rationale	Evaluation for Charting
	Ensure that child keeps scheduled appointments with occupational therapy and physical therapy as indicated.	Therapy will help maximize ability of movement.	Describe any therapeutic measures used to improve physical mobility. Document their effectiveness.
	Encourage child to participate as much as possible in self-care.	Promotes autonomy.	Document child's ability to participate in self-care.
	Make available activities within child's limitations (state specific examples for each child).	Decreases anxiety and frustration while allowing child to accomplish activities.	Describe any activities in which the child was able to participate.
	Allow adequate rest periods (state specific amount of rest needed for each child).	Maintains ability to participate in usual activities.	Document effectiveness of rest periods.
	Perform scheduled active and passive range-of-motion exercises every 4 hours and PRN.	Helps preserve muscle and joint function.	Document whether range-of-motion exercises were done and their effectiveness.
	Reposition child every 1 to 2 hours.	Helps to prevent skin breakdown.	Document whether child was repositioned on schedule.
	Ensure that child's body stays in proper alignment, whether in bed, chair, or wheelchair.	Maintains position and helps to prevent deformities.	Document whether child's body was kept in proper alignment.
	Assist child as necessary with use of splints and other appliances.	Used to increase mobility.	Describe any therapeutic measures used to improve physical mobility. Document their effectiveness.
	Administer analgesics on schedule as well as 30 to 60 minutes prior to activity, exercise, and getting up in the morning. Assess and record effectiveness.	Analgesics are administered to decrease pain.	Document whether analgesics were administered on schedule. Describe effectiveness.
	Administer nonsteroidal anti-inflammatory (NSAIDs) on schedule as well as 30 to 60 minutes prior to activity, exercise, and getting up in the	NSAIDs are administered to decrease inflammation, which will help to relieve pain.	Document whether NSAIDs were administered on schedule. Describe effectiveness and any side effects noted.

(continued)

Primary Nursing Diagnosis: Impaired Physical Mobility *(continued)*

Expected Outcomes	Possible Nursing Interventions	Rationale	Evaluation for Charting
	morning. Assess and record effectiveness and any side effects (e.g., dizziness, headache, mood changes).		
	If indicated, administer disease-modifying antirheumatic drugs (DMARDs) on schedule. Assess and record any side effects (e.g., vomiting, diarrhea, dermatitis).	DMARDs are administered to decrease inflammation and slow disease process.	Document whether DMARDs were administered on schedule. Describe any side effects noted.
	If indicated, administer biologics (e.g., Etanercept) on schedule. Assess and record any side effects (e.g., liver injury, infections, blood disorders).	Biologics are administered to decrease inflammation in patients with autoimmune disease.	Document if biologics were administered on schedule. Describe any side effects noted.
TEACHING GOALS Child and/or family will be able to verbalize at least 4 characteristics of impaired mobility such as • decreased range of motion • contractures • fatigue • joint stiffness	Teach child/family about characteristics of impaired mobility. Assess and record results.	Increased knowledge will assist the child/family in recognizing and reporting changes in the child's condition.	Document whether teaching was done and describe results.
Child and/or family will be able to verbalize knowledge of care such as • correct use of adaptive devices and home modifications • monitoring handling and positioning • appropriate use of resources and referrals; visiting nurses, social services • identification of any signs/symptoms of impaired mobility (such as those listed under Assessment) • when to contact health-care provider	Teach child/family about care. Assess and record child's/family's knowledge of and participation in care regarding correct use of adaptive devices and home modifications, etc.	Education of child/family will allow for accurate care.	Document whether teaching was done and describe results.

Nursing Diagnosis   Self-Care Deficit: (Specify)

Definition   State in which the individual has decreased ability to complete the activities of daily living for his/her age, such as feeding, hygiene/bathing, dressing/grooming, and toileting

Possibly Related to
- Pain
- Joint contractures
- Immobility
- Decreased range of motion
- Visual impairment

Nursing Diagnosis: Self-care deficit (specify) related to pain, joint contractures, immobility, decreased range of motion, visual impairment

Assessment/Defining Characteristics of Child and/or Family (Subjective & Objective Data):

- Feeding self-care deficits (e.g., inability to hold utensils or cut food)
- Bathing self-care deficits (e.g., inability to get in and out of the tub)
- Toileting self-care deficits (e.g., inability to sit on and rise from the toilet seat)
- Dressing self-care deficits (e.g., inability to fasten or unfasten clothing or shoes)
- Hygiene self-care deficits (e.g., inability to hold toothbrush)

Expected Outcomes	Possible Nursing Interventions	Rationale	Evaluation for Charting
Child will demonstrate no self-care deficit or will have increased ability to accomplish usual activities of daily living for age (state specific examples for each child). Child will demonstrate correct use of adaptive devices to accomplish activities of daily living (state specific examples for each child).	Assess and record child's current level of self-care.	Provides a database for current activities and helps to monitor progress.	Document child's current level of self-care.
	Encourage child to have maximum independence in performing activities of daily living. Provide assistance when necessary. Record results.	Promotes autonomy and independence.	Describe any therapeutic measures used to promote self-care. Document their effectiveness.
	Initiate consultations with physical therapist and occupational therapist to assist in establishment of a self-care program. Be sure to include child when establishing plans and goals.	Allows child some control in decision making about needed care.	Describe any therapeutic measures used to promote self-care. Document their effectiveness.

(continued)

Nursing Diagnosis: Self-Care Deficit (Specify) *(continued)*			
Expected Outcomes	**Possible Nursing Interventions**	**Rationale**	**Evaluation for Charting**
	Advise child/family to allow extra time for activities. Assist in obtaining articles or devising methods to facilitate independent functioning, such as • utensils for eating with large, graspable handles • toothbrush, comb, and brush with large, graspable handles • chair or stool in tub or shower • elevate toilet seat • handrails in the home (especially in hallways and bathrooms) • clothes that are easy to put on and remove • dressing aides as needed, such as Velcro fasteners	Allows child more autonomy and independence.	Describe any therapeutic measures used to promote self-care. Document their effectiveness.
	Initiate referrals to home health-care agencies, visiting nurses, social services, local or national arthritis foundations, and clearinghouses.	Provides child and family access to resources that can promote child's independence in self-care activities.	Describe any therapeutic measures used to promote self-care. Document their effectiveness.
TEACHING GOALS Child and/or family will be able to verbalize at least 4 characteristics of self-care deficit such as • pain • joint contractures • immobility • decreased range of motion • visual impairment	Teach child/family about characteristics of self-care deficit. Assess and record results.	Increased knowledge will assist the child/family in recognizing and reporting changes in the child's condition.	Document whether teaching was done and describe results.

Nursing Diagnosis: Self-Care Deficit (Specify) *(continued)*

Expected Outcomes	Possible Nursing Interventions	Rationale	Evaluation for Charting
Child and/or family will be able to verbalize knowledge of care such as • correct use of adaptive devices and home modifications • appropriate use of resources and referrals; visiting nurses, social services • identification of any signs/symptoms of self-care deficit (such as those listed under Assessment) • when to contact health-care provider	Teach child/family about care. Assess and record child's/family's knowledge of and participation in care regarding correct use of adaptive devices and home modifications, etc.	Education of child/family will allow for accurate care.	Document whether teaching was done and describe results.

Related Nursing Diagnoses

Chronic Pain   *related to*
a. inflamed joints
b. joint immobility and stiffness
c. gastric irritation secondary to aspirin use

Disturbed Body Image   *related to*
a. chronic illness
b. disabling features of illness
c. side effects of medications

Delayed Growth and Development   *related to*
a. physical limitations of illness
b. weight loss or inadequate weight gain due to increased metabolic needs
c. weight gain due to decreased mobility
d. irregular school attendance
e. parents with overprotective behavior
f. side effects of medications

Compromised Family Coping   *related to*
a. child's debilitating chronic illness
b. knowledge deficit

| FOUR |

OSTEOMYELITIS
MEDICAL DIAGNOSIS

PATHOPHYSIOLOGY Osteomyelitis is an infection of the bone. Approximately half of all pediatric osteomyelitis cases occur in children younger than 5 years of age. Boys are approximately twice as likely to be affected as girls. In immunocompromised children, such as those with sickle cell disease, higher rates of osteomyelitis are seen. Most cases of osteomyelitis occur in a long bone, such as the femur, tibia, or humerus. Osteomyelitis is usually limited to a single site.

The most common etiology of osteomyelitis is a blood-borne infection secondary to an infection elsewhere in the body, referred to as hematogenous sources. In this type of osteomyelitis, the sources of foci can include boils, skin abrasions, impetigo, upper respiratory tract infection, acute otitis media, tonsillitis, abscessed teeth, pyelonephritis, and infected burns. Osteomyelitis can also be acquired from exogenous sources, as when it results from an extension of a local infectious process, a contamination of a compound fracture, or introduction of infection during a surgical procedure. Group B streptococci and *Escherichia coli* are the causative organism in cases involving neonates. *Staphylococcus aureus*, group A streptococci, and *Haemophilus influenzae* type b, are the predominate causative organisms in children beyond the neonatal period. In children with sickle cell disease who have osteomyelitis, it is often caused by *Salmonella* organisms.

The infection usually localizes in the bone metaphysis. The infectious process leads to accumulation of pus under the periosteum, causing elevation of the periosteum and compression of medullary circulation, resulting in local bone destruction. In children, the site of infection is often near the epiphyseal plate, which acts to contain the infection by forming new bone (involucrum). The abscess formed exerts pressure because of the rigid, unyielding nature of the bone, resulting in further vascular compromise and necrosis. Eventually the abscess can cause the periosteum to rupture, leading to the release of purulent matter, which can infect the nearest joint. Necrotic bone that is not absorbed continues to produce more intraosseous tension and necrosis, with eventual formation of a sequestrum (granulation around dead bone). Sinuses that occasionally develop between the sequestra and the skin surface or into a joint can lead to septic arthritis. If large areas of sequestrum are present, multiple sinuses can retain infective material and result in chronic osteomyelitis.

The clinical presentation of osteomyelitis is variable. Older children and adolescents often present after days or weeks of symptoms, such as pain at the site and fever. Infants and younger children may be irritable, limping, and refusing to bear weight or use the affected extremity. Children with hematogenous osteomyelitis usually present with pain and redness and swelling over the infected area. The child may also exhibit decreased movement of the affected limb and adjacent joint. Systemic signs and symptoms can be nonspecific. They can include fever, malaise, and irritability. In osteomyelitis following trauma, systemic symptoms may be absent. In chronic osteomyelitis, local signs may be absent or intermittent and often systemic symptoms are absent.

The child with osteomyelitis will have either a normal or elevated leukocyte count, an elevated erythrocyte sedimentation rate, and an elevated C-reactive protein concentration. A blood culture is positive in about 50% of all cases. A needle aspiration, with or without bone biopsy, may be necessary to direct treatment. Imaging can be very useful in diagnosing and managing osteomyelitis. Radiographs, bone scans, and magnetic resonance imaging (MRI) with intravenous gadolinium-based contrast are often used.

Treatment consists of prompt and vigorous antibiotic therapy for the appropriate duration to avoid recurrence and chronicity of the osteomyelitis. Surgical intervention may be indicated to decrease pressure within the metaphyseal space and allow drainage of the pus. Recurrence is the most common complication of osteomyelitis.

Primary Nursing Diagnosis   Actual Infection*

Definition   Condition in which microorganisms have invaded the body

Possibly Related to   • Bacterial invasion of the bone via a hematogenous or exogenous source
                                  (specify when possible)

*Non-DANDA diagnosis.

Primary Nursing Diagnosis: Actual infection related to bacterial invasion of the bone via a hematogenous or exogenous source (specify when possible)

Assessment/Defining Characteristics of Child and/or Family (Subjective & Objective Data):

- Fever
- Tachycardia
- Tachypnea
- Hypotension
- Localized tenderness, redness, and swelling over involved area
- Increased warmth over involved area

- Irritability
- Restlessness
- Pain on movement of involved area
- Leukocytosis
- Elevated erythrocyte sedimentation rate
- Elevated C-reactive protein concentration
- Positive blood culture

Expected Outcomes	Possible Nursing Interventions	Rationale	Evaluation for Charting

Child will be free of infection as evidenced by
 	
• body temperature within acceptable range of 36.5°C to 37.2°C
• heart rate within acceptable range (state specific range)
• respiratory rate within acceptable range (state specific range)
• blood pressure within acceptable range (state specific range)
• lack of extreme irritability and restlessness
• lack of the following in the infected area
  1. tenderness
  2. redness
  3. swelling
  4. increased warmth
• freedom from pain on movement of the involved area
	Assess and record T, HR, RR, BP, and any signs/symptoms of infection (such as those listed under Assessment) every 4 hours and PRN.	If infection is present, the T, HR, and RR will increase and the BP may decrease.	Document range of T, HR, RR, and BP. Describe any signs/symptoms of infection noted.

	Assess and record IV fluids and condition of IV site every hour.	It is necessary to record the amount of IV fluids every hour to make sure the child is not being over or under hydrated. The IV site needs to be assessed every hour for signs of redness or swelling.	Document amount of IV fluids and describe condition of IV site along with any interventions needed.
	Keep accurate record of intake and output. If wound is draining, record amount and characteristics of drainage.	Provides information on child's hydration status. Also provides a baseline for description of wound drainage, which will help in recognition of changes that occur.	Document intake and output. Describe characteristics of wound site and any drainage.
	Administer antibiotics on schedule. Assess and record any side effects (e.g., rash, diarrhea).	Antibiotics are given to combat infection.	Document whether antibiotics were administered on schedule. Describe any side effects noted.

(continued)

Primary Nursing Diagnosis: Actual Infection *(continued)*

Expected Outcomes	Possible Nursing Interventions	Rationale	Evaluation for Charting
• WBC within acceptable range (state specific range) • erythrocyte sedimentation rate within acceptable range (state specific range) • negative blood culture • C-reactive protein (CRP) within acceptable range (state specific range • lack of signs/symptoms of infection (such as those listed under Assessment)	Administer antipyretics on schedule. Assess and record effectiveness.	Antipyretics are used to reduce fever.	Document whether an antipyretic was needed and describe effectiveness.
	Administer analgesics on schedule. Assess and record effectiveness and any side effects (e.g., constipation, nausea).	Analgesics are administered to decrease pain.	Document whether analgesics were administered on schedule. Describe effectiveness and any side effects noted.
	Maintain good hand-washing technique. If an open wound is present, maintain wound isolation precautions in accordance with institutional policy.	Good hand-washing is the single most important measure in decreasing infection. Following institutional policy for open wound care will decrease spread of infection and prevent wound contamination.	Document whether good hand-washing technique was used. State whether institutional policy for open wound care was followed.
	If surgical drainage has been performed, make sure that antibiotic solution is draining properly into involved area and that suction is properly applied to remove drainage.	Antibiotic solution is used to treat the infection. Suction is used to remove drainage.	Document any therapeutic measures used to treat the infection. Describe their effectiveness.
	When indicated, change the dressing on schedule according to institutional protocol. Assess and record characteristics of drainage and wound site every shift and PRN.	Prevents spread of infection and provides a way to assess the progress of the wound.	Describe characteristics of wound site and any drainage.
	When indicated, keep involved area immobilized. Assess and record area for sensation, circulation, pain, color, swelling, heat, and tenderness every shift and PRN. If indicated, ensure that bed rest is maintained.	Immobilization prevents pain caused by movement of the involved area. Assessment for sensation, circulation, pain, color, swelling, heat, and tenderness provides information about status of involved area.	Document any therapeutic measures used to treat the infection. Describe their effectiveness.
	Check and record results of any blood cultures and/or laboratory work. Notify physician if results are out of the normal range.	Blood cultures identify the infectious organisms and provide a guide for treatment. Elevated WBC, erythrocyte sedimentation rate, and C-reactive protein can indicate the presence of an infection.	Document current results of any blood cultures and/or any laboratory work.

Primary Nursing Diagnosis: Actual Infection (*continued*)

Expected Outcomes	Possible Nursing Interventions	Rationale	Evaluation for Charting
TEACHING GOALS Child and/or family will be able to verbalize at least 4 characteristics of infection such as • fever • localized tenderness, redness, swelling over involved area • increased warmth over involved area • irritability • restlessness • pain on movement of involved area	Teach child/family about characteristics of infection. Assess and record results.	Increased knowledge will assist the child/family in recognizing and reporting changes in the child's condition.	Document whether teaching was done and describe results.
Child and/or family will be able to verbalize knowledge of care such as • good hand-washing technique • fever control • medication administration • dressing change and wound assessment • activity restrictions, including avoidance of falls and jerky movements, quiet play activities, and immobilization and bed rest when indicated • preventive factors, including adequate nutrition, rest, and maintenance of skin integrity • identification of any signs/symptoms of infection (such as those listed under Assessment) • when to contact health-care provider	Teach child/family about care. Assess and record child's/family's knowledge of and participation in care regarding good hand-washing technique, medication administration, dressing change, wound assessment, etc.	Education of child/family will allow for accurate care.	Document whether teaching was done and describe results.

Nursing Diagnosis   Acute Pain

Definition   Condition in which an individual experiences acute mild to severe pain

Possibly Related to   • Inflammatory process secondary to bacterial invasion of the bone

---

Nursing Diagnosis: Acute pain related to inflammatory process secondary to bacterial invasion of the bone

Assessment/Defining Characteristics of Child and/or Family (Subjective & Objective Data):

- Verbal communication of pain
- Crying unrelieved by usual comfort measures
- Hesitation or refusal to use limb
- Decreased activity, self-imposed
- Severe discomfort on movement of involved area
- Physical signs/symptoms (tachycardia, tachypnea, increased blood pressure, diaphoresis)

Expected Outcomes	Possible Nursing Interventions	Rationale	Evaluation for Charting

Child will have decreased pain or be free of severe and/or constant pain as evidenced by
 	
• verbal communication of comfort
• lack of
  1. constant crying
  2. hesitation or refusal to use limb
  3. self-imposed decreased activity
  4. discomfort on movement of involved area
• heart rate within acceptable range (state specific range)
• respiratory rate within acceptable range (state specific range)
• blood pressure within acceptable range (state specific range)
• decrease in or lack of diaphoresis
• rating of decreased pain or no pain on pain-assessment tool
• lack of signs/symptoms of pain (such as those listed under Assessment)
	Assess and record HR, RR, BP, and any signs/symptoms of pain (such as those listed under Assessment) every 2 to 4 hours and PRN. Use age-appropriate pain-assessment tool.	Provides data regarding the level of pain child is experiencing.	Document range of HR, RR, BP, and degree of pain child was experiencing. Describe any successful measures used to decrease pain.

	Administer analgesics on schedule. Assess and record effectiveness and any side effects (e.g., constipation, nausea).	Analgesics are administered to decrease pain.	Document whether analgesics were administered on schedule. Describe effectiveness and any side effects noted.
	Handle injured area with extreme care. Support and protect involved area when the child is moved. Have two individuals move child if necessary. When indicated, keep involved area immobilized.	These measures will help prevent pain caused by movement.	Document if child was handled with care. Describe effectiveness.
	Encourage family members to stay and comfort child when possible.	Helps to comfort and support the child.	Document whether family was able to remain with child and describe effectiveness of their presence.
	Allow family members to participate in care of child when possible.	This may increase the comfort level of the child and thus help child in managing pain.	Document whether family participated in care and if this was successful in helping child with pain management.

Nursing Diagnosis: Acute Pain *(continued)*

Expected Outcomes	Possible Nursing Interventions	Rationale	Evaluation for Charting
	Use diversional activities (e.g., music, television, playing games, relaxation) when appropriate.	Diversional activities can distract child and may help to decrease pain.	Document whether diversional activities were successful in helping to manage pain.
	If age appropriate, explain all procedures beforehand.	Allow child some control, which can assist child with pain management.	Describe if this measure was effective in helping child to manage pain.
	If age appropriate, allow the child to participate in planning his or her care. Encourage the child to practice self-care (e.g., bathing, removing dressing).	Allowing child some control can assist child with pain management.	Describe if this measure was effective in helping child to manage pain.
	When indicated, institute additional pain relief measures, such as hypnosis, and guided imagery. Assess and record effectiveness.	These nonpharmacologic measures may help decrease pain.	Document whether these measures were successful in helping to manage pain.
TEACHING GOALS Child and/or family will be able to verbalize at least 4 characteristics of pain such as • verbal communication of pain • crying unrelieved by usual comfort measures • hesitation or refusal to use limb • decreased activity, self-imposed • rapid heart rate	Teach child/family about characteristics of pain. Assess and record results.	Increased knowledge will assist the child/family in recognizing and reporting changes in the child's condition.	Document whether teaching was done and describe results.
Child and/or family will be able to verbalize knowledge of care such as • medication administration • gentle handling of child • identification of any signs/symptoms of pain (such as those listed under Assessment) • when to contact health-care provider	Teach child/family about care. Assess and record child's/family's knowledge of and participation in care regarding medication administration, etc.	Education of child/family will allow for accurate care.	Document whether teaching was done and describe results.

Related Nursing Diagnoses

Impaired Physical Mobility	*related to* pain on movement of involved area secondary to bacterial invasion of the bone
Deficient Knowledge: Child/Family	*related to* a. disease process and treatment b. prevention of complications c. activity restrictions
Noncompliance	*related to* a. bed rest b. non-weight-bearing on lower extremities
Compromised Family Coping	*related to* a. prolonged hospitalization of child (antibiotic therapy needed for 4 to 6 weeks) b. complicated home care (if child is sent home with a heparin lock for IV therapy at home) c. financial considerations d. interruption of parental work schedule

FIVE

SCOLIOSIS
MEDICAL DIAGNOSIS

PATHOPHYSIOLOGY Scoliosis is defined as curvature of the spine greater than 10 degrees from the midline usually associated with rotation of a series of vertebrae. This curvature of the spine can be visualized on a standing posterior-anterior (PA) spine radiograph. Scoliosis is an inflexible curve that cannot be voluntarily corrected and is further classified as congenital, neuromuscular, or idiopathic.

Congenital scoliosis is an embryonic malformation of the bony vertebral column that occurs during the third to fifth week of gestation. It is not unusual for children with this type of scoliosis to have other anomalies, such as urinary tract and cardiac defects. Congenital scoliosis may be seen at any age and the curves may worsen slowly, rapidly, or not at all.

Neuromuscular or paralytic scoliosis is secondary to neuropathic and myopathic diseases such as poliomyelitis, cerebral palsy, myelomeningocele, and muscular dystrophy or traumatic neuromuscular conditions. Scoliosis is believed to occur as a result of paralysis of the paraspinal and trunk muscles or of alteration of balance mechanisms. The curves associated with neuromuscular scoliosis usually worsen significantly as time passes.

Idiopathic scoliosis, the most common form of scoliosis, accounts for 80% of all structural curves. The etiology is unknown. Individual types of idiopathic scoliosis include infantile, juvenile, and adolescent. Infantile scoliosis, which occurs in the first 3 years of life, can resolve spontaneously or may progress and require intervention. The onset of juvenile idiopathic scoliosis is between 3 and 10 years of age. Adolescent idiopathic scoliosis occurs after 10 years of age and is more common in girls than boys. Curves associated with idiopathic scoliosis can worsen at approximately 1 degree per month until the child reaches skeletal maturity. Skeletal maturity usually occurs during the adolescent growth spurt. The patient's age, skeletal maturity, menarchal status, curve size, and curve pattern are all related to the risk of the curve progressing. Young, premenarchal girls with large curves experience the highest risk of progression. Back pain, cosmetic issues, and pulmonary problems are the primary sequelae of untreated idiopathic scoliosis. Thoracic curves as small as 20 degrees can decrease the child's exercise tolerance due to impaired pulmonary function, while lumbar and thoracolumbar curves have no impact on lung function. Children who have infantile or juvenile idiopathic scoliosis experience a large increase in mortality from cardiac and pulmonary causes later in life, so treatment focuses on the chest wall deformity. With adolescent idiopathic scoliosis, there is no evidence of increased mortality.

Overall, adolescent idiopathic scoliosis is the most common form of scoliosis. Since adolescent idiopathic scoliosis is the most prevalent type, the remainder of this discussion will refer to this type of scoliosis.

Diagnosis of scoliosis should include a thorough history and physical examination, focusing on the neurologic assessment to rule out any underlying neurological deficit that might be associated with the scoliosis. During the physical examination, the child is observed walking, standing erect, and bending forward at the waist (the Adams position). Positive findings include scapular prominence, thoracic rib hump or lumbar asymmetry, shoulder asymmetry, hip asymmetry, uneven waistline, torso malalignment when standing erect, and anterior rib and breast asymmetry. The diagnosis is confirmed by radiographs, which also establish the degree of spinal curvature. Magnetic resonance imaging (MRI) is usually indicated if the child is younger than 10 years of age to assess for intraspinal disease or anomalies. An MRI may also be indicated to rule out a nonidiopathic process, if the curve is progressing more rapidly than 1 degree per month.

Treatment for adolescent idiopathic scoliosis includes observation, bracing, and surgery. Small curves should be observed. Mild to moderate curves (20 to 30 degrees) in skeletally immature children can usually be treated with bracing. This requires a great deal of compliance from the child and family. The brace is used to prevent or minimize curve progression, not for correction of the curve. Some consider the use of bracing for scoliosis controversial. A procedure called Vertebral Body Stapling (VBS) is available at some centers for those children who have an idiopathic spine curvature between 25 and 45 degrees. With this procedure, staples are implanted on the outside curve of the spine to help immediately correct some of the bend and prevent curve progression. VBS is another option for the child, especially if he/she does not want to wear a brace. For severe or progressive curves (thoracic curves greater than 50 degrees or thoracolumbar curves greater than 40 to 45 degrees), surgical management is usually indicated. Without intervention, these curves can continue to worsen into adulthood. Surgery consists of a spinal fusion (arthrodesis) with instrumentation (rods or implants). The most common surgical procedure is a posterior spinal fusion with instrumentation.

Postoperative Nursing Care Plan

Primary Nursing Diagnosis   Acute Pain

Definition   Condition in which an individual experiences acute mild to severe pain

Possibly Related to   • Surgical incision and manipulation

Primary Nursing Diagnosis: Acute pain related to surgical incision and manipulation			
Assessment/Defining Characteristics of Child and/or Family (Subjective & Objective Data):			
• Verbal communication of pain • Crying • Moaning • Facial grimacing		• Restlessness • Rating of pain on pain-assessment tool • Physical signs/symptoms (tachycardia, tachypnea, increased blood pressure, diaphoresis)	
Expected Outcomes	**Possible Nursing Interventions**	**Rationale**	**Evaluation for Charting**

Child will have decreased pain or be free of severe and/or constant pain as evidenced by
 	
• verbal communication of comfort
• lack of
  1. constant crying or moaning
  2. grimacing
  3. extreme restlessness
  4. diaphoresis
• heart rate within acceptable range (state specific range)
• respiratory rate within acceptable range (state specific range)
• blood pressure within acceptable range (state specific range)
• rating of decreased pain or no pain on pain-assessment tool
	Assess and record HR, RR, BP, and any signs/symptoms of pain (such as those listed under Assessment) every 2 to 4 hours and PRN. Use age-appropriate pain-assessment tool.	Provides data regarding the level of pain child is experiencing.	Document range of HR, RR, BP, and degree of pain child was experiencing. Describe any successful measures used to decrease pain.

	Log-roll on schedule (every 2 to 4 hours) and handle child gently.	Log rolling keeps the body in proper alignment. Gentle handling helps to decrease pain.	Document if child was handled with care and if log rolling was done on schedule. Describe effectiveness.
	Administer analgesics and/or narcotics on schedule. Assess and record effectiveness and any side effects (e.g., constipation, nausea).	Analgesics and narcotics are administered to decrease pain.	Document whether analgesics and/or narcotics were administered on schedule. Describe effectiveness and any side effects noted.
	Monitor patient-controlled analgesia (PCA). Record findings according to hospital protocol.	PCA is used to decrease pain.	Describe effectiveness of PCA pump.
	Assess and record neurovascular status of extremity every 1 to 2 hours and PRN.	Provides information about compromised circulation or feeling to the injured area.	Describe neurovascular assessment of extremity.

Primary Nursing Diagnosis: Acute Pain *(continued)*

Expected Outcomes	Possible Nursing Interventions	Rationale	Evaluation for Charting
	Encourage family members to stay and comfort child when possible.	Helps to comfort and support the child.	Document whether family was able to remain with child and describe effectiveness of their presence.
	Allow family members to participate in care of child when possible.	This may increase the comfort level of the child and thus help child in managing pain.	Document whether family participated in care and if this was successful in helping child with pain management.
	Use diversional activities (e.g., music, television, playing games, relaxation) when appropriate.	Diversional activities can distract child and may help to decrease pain.	Document whether diversional activities were successful in helping to manage pain.
	If age appropriate, explain all procedures beforehand.	Allowing child some control can assist child with pain management.	Describe if this measure was effective in helping child to manage pain.
	If age appropriate, allow the child to participate in planning his or her care. Encourage the child to practice self-care (e.g., brushing teeth, grooming).	Allowing child some control can assist child with pain management.	Describe if this measure was effective in helping child to manage pain.
	When indicated, institute additional pain relief measures, such as hypnosis, and guided imagery. Assess and record effectiveness.	These nonpharmacologic measures may help decrease pain.	Document whether these measures were successful in helping to manage pain.
TEACHING GOALS Child and/or family will be able to verbalize at least 4 characteristics of pain such as • verbal communication of pain • restlessness • facial grimacing • rapid heart rate	Teach child/family about characteristics of pain. Assess and record results.	Increased knowledge will assist the child/family in recognizing and reporting changes in the child's condition.	Document whether teaching was done and describe results.

(continued)

Primary Nursing Diagnosis: Acute Pain *(continued)*			
Expected Outcomes	**Possible Nursing Interventions**	**Rationale**	**Evaluation for Charting**
Child and/or family will be able to verbalize knowledge of care such as • medication administration • activity progression • identification of any signs/symptoms of pain (such as those listed under Assessment) • when to contact health-care provider	Teach child/family about care. Assess and record child's/family's knowledge of and participation in care regarding medication administration, activity progression, etc.	Education of child/family will allow for accurate care.	Document whether teaching was done and describe results.

Nursing Diagnosis   Deficient Fluid Volume

Definition   Decrease in the amount of circulating fluid volume

Possibly Related to   • Blood loss secondary to surgical procedure

Nursing Diagnosis: Deficient fluid volume related to blood loss secondary to surgical procedure			
Assessment/Defining Characteristics of Child and/or Family (Subjective & Objective Data):			

- Dry mucous membranes
- Decreased skin turgor (skin recoil greater than 2 to 3 seconds)
- Decreased urine output
- Increased urine specific gravity
- Tachycardia
- Tachypnea
- Hypotension
- Diminished or absent bowel sounds

Expected Outcomes	**Possible Nursing Interventions**	**Rationale**	**Evaluation for Charting**
Child will have adequate fluid volume as evidenced by • adequate fluid intake, IV and oral (state specific amount of intake needed for each child) • heart rate, respiratory rate, and blood pressure	Keep accurate record of intake and output. Child will have an indwelling urinary catheter, a nasogastric tube, and possibly a Hemovac wound drain in the immediate postoperative period. Measure the output from each and record characteristics of the drainage.	Provides information on child's hydration status.	Document intake and output. Describe amount and characteristics of nasogastric and Hemovac drainage.

Nursing Diagnosis: Deficient Fluid Volume *(continued)*

Expected Outcomes	Possible Nursing Interventions	Rationale	Evaluation for Charting
within acceptable range (state specific range) • presence of bowel sounds • moist mucous membranes • adequate urine output (state specific range; 1 to 2 ml/kg/hr) • rapid skin recoil (less than 2 to 3 seconds) • urine specific gravity from 1.008 to 1.020 • lack of signs/ symptoms of deficient fluid volume (such as those listed under Assessment)	Ensure that nasogastric tube is patent and connected to low intermittent suction. Measure and record drainage. Irrigate as indicated.	A nasogastric tube is used to provide gastric drainage. It is irrigated to maintain patency.	Document if nasogastric tube was irrigated and its patency status. Describe amount and characteristics of nasogastric drainage.
	If indicated, keep NPO in the immediate postoperative period. When indicated, offer oral fluids when bowel sounds are present.	Oral fluids need to be restricted until peristalsis has returned postoperatively in order to prevent abdominal distention.	Describe tolerance of oral fluids.
	Assess and record • IV fluids and condition of IV site every hour • HR, RR, and BP every 4 hours and PRN • bowel sounds every 4 hours and PRN • any signs/symptoms of deficient fluid volume every 4 hours and PRN	Provides information about fluid status of patient. If patient has deficient fluid volume, the HR will increase at first, and eventually decrease. The RR will increase. The BP will eventually decrease. The bowel sounds will be hypoactive in the postoperative period until peristalsis returns. It is necessary to record the amount of IV fluids every hour to make sure the child is not being over or under hydrated. The IV site needs to be assessed every hour for signs of redness or swelling.	Document range of HR, RR, and BP. Document amount of IV fluids and describe condition of IV site along with any interventions needed. Describe bowel sounds and any signs/ symptoms of deficient fluid volume noted.
	Check and record urine specific gravity with every void or as indicated.	Urine specific gravity provides information about hydration status.	Document range of urine specific gravity.
	Assess and record condition of mucous membranes and skin turgor every shift and PRN.	Provides information on hydration status.	Describe status of mucous membranes and skin turgor.

(continued)

	Possible Nursing		Evaluation for
Nursing Diagnosis: Deficient Fluid Volume *(continued)*			
Expected Outcomes	**Possible Nursing Interventions**	**Rationale**	**Evaluation for Charting**
TEACHING GOALS Child and/or family will be able to verbalize at least 4 characteristics of deficient fluid volume such as • dry mucous membranes • decreased skin turgor (skin recoil greater than 2 to 3 seconds) • decreased urine output • rapid heart rate	Teach child/family about characteristics of deficient fluid volume. Assess and record results.	Increased knowledge will assist the child/family in recognizing and reporting changes in the child's condition.	Document whether teaching was done and describe results.
Child and/or family will be able to verbalize knowledge of care such as • child's need for appropriate fluids • monitoring intake and output • identification of any signs/symptoms of deficient fluid volume (such as those listed under Assessment) • when to contact health-care provider	Teach child/family about care. Assess and record child's/family's knowledge of and participation in care regarding child's need for appropriate fluids, monitoring intake and output, etc.	Education of child/family will allow for accurate care.	Document whether teaching was done and describe results.

Related Nursing Diagnoses

Deficient Knowledge: Child/Family	*related to* a. surgical procedure b. immediate postoperative care c. home care
Disturbed Body Image	*related to* wearing of a cast and/or brace
Self-Care Deficit (Specify Bathing/Hygiene, Dressing/Grooming, and/or Toileting)	*related to* mobility restrictions and pain
Compromised Family Coping	*related to* a. assisting child in accepting a postoperative period of casting and/or bracing and activity restriction b. assisting child in choosing appropriate clothing to wear over cast and/or brace c. long-term follow-up care (may need assistance from home health agencies)

SIX

SEPTIC ARTHRITIS
MEDICAL DIAGNOSIS

PATHOPHYSIOLOGY Septic arthritis, also called suppurative, pyogenic, or purulent arthritis, is an infection of the joint and the subsequent inflammatory response. Approximately half of all the cases of septic arthritis occur in patients younger than 20 years of age with the peak incidence being in children younger than 3 years of age. Boys are affected twice as often as girls. Septic arthritis occurs more commonly in children who also have sickle cell disease, diabetes mellitus, and immunodeficiencies.

There are several ways bacteria can enter into the synovial fluid. The usual introduction of infection is by hematogenous dissemination. It can also occur by direct extension of a soft tissue infection, such as osteomyelitis, or a direct inoculation from organisms into the joint space via a wound. The synovial membrane of the joint produces increased amounts of synovial fluid in response to the presence of infection. Pus begins to accumulate, leading to destructive and degenerative changes in the articular cartilage. The increased amounts of fluids and pus cause distention, and the joint can eventually dislocate. The usual causative organisms are *Staphylococcus aureus*, group A beta-hemolytic streptococci, and *S. pneumoniae*. Before an effective vaccine, *Haemophilus influenzae* type b was a common cause of septic arthritis. *Salmonella* organisms are often the cause of bone and joint infections in children with sickle cell disease. Joints of the lower extremities and large joints, such as the hip, knee, ankle, elbow, and shoulder, are most commonly affected. Usually only one joint is involved.

The signs and symptoms of septic arthritis include a warm, swollen, red, and tender joint, which is painful even to gentle pressure or passive movement. The child will want to keep the affected joint in a position that maximizes intracapsular volume and comfort, such as keeping the knees moderately flexed. The child may exhibit pseudoparalysis (refusal to move the joint). Systemic symptoms will include fever, malaise, and poor appetite. Most children have symptoms for no more than 72 hours before diagnosis, as the disease progression is rapid. Leukocytosis and an increased erythrocyte sedimentation rate are present.

Diagnosis is made mainly upon the findings of the joint aspiration fluid. Radiographic studies (which will indicate joint swelling) and blood cultures are also helpful.

Treatment consists of joint immobilization, vigorous antibiotic therapy (initially intravenously then orally), needle aspiration of the joint for decompression in order to avoid interference with blood supply, and, sometimes, surgical opening and drainage of the joint. Septic arthritis of the hip is considered a medical emergency, requiring immediate surgical drainage. Physical therapy may be indicated for some children. Complications of septic arthritis include recurrence of infection and degeneration of the affected joint.

Primary Nursing Diagnosis   Actual Infection*

Definition   Condition in which microorganisms have invaded the body

Possibly Related to   • Bacterial invasion of the joint

*Non-NANDA diagnosis.

Primary Nursing Diagnosis: Actual infection related to bacterial invasion of the joint

Assessment/Defining Characteristics of Child and/or Family (Subjective & Objective Data):

- Fever
- Tachycardia
- Tachypnea
- Hypotension
- Localized tenderness, redness, swelling, and increased warmth over involved joint
- Pain on movement of affected joint
- Limited range of motion of affected joint
- Muscular rigidity
- Limping or refusal to walk (if lower extremities are affected)
- Leukocytosis
- Elevated erythrocyte sedimentation rate
- Joint swelling revealed on X-ray
- Increased uptake of radioisotope in the infected areas, as shown on a bone scan
- Joint aspiration containing pus

Expected Outcomes	Possible Nursing Interventions	Rationale	Evaluation for Charting

Child will be free of infection as evidenced by
 	
• body temperature within acceptable range of 36.5°C to 37.2°C
• heart rate within acceptable range (state specific range)
• respiratory rate within acceptable range (state specific range)
• blood pressure within acceptable range (state specific range)
• lack of the following in the infected area
  1. tenderness
  2. redness
  3. swelling
  4. increased warmth
  5. muscular rigidity
  6. limping or refusal to walk
• freedom from pain on movement of the involved area
• adequate range of motion of affected joint
• WBC within acceptable range (state specific range)
• erythrocyte sedimentation rate within acceptable range (state specific range)
• lack of signs/symptoms of joint infection (such as those listed under Assessment)
	Assess and record T, HR, RR, BP, and any signs/symptoms of infection (such as those listed under Assessment) every 4 hours and PRN.	If infection is present, the T, HR, and RR will increase and the BP may decrease.	Document range of T, HR, RR, and BP. Describe any signs/symptoms of infection noted.

	Assess and record IV fluids and condition of IV site every hour.	It is necessary to record the amount of IV fluids every hour to make sure the child is not being over or under hydrated. The IV site needs to be assessed every hour for signs of redness or swelling.	Document amount of IV fluids and describe condition of IV site along with any interventions needed.
	Keep accurate record of intake and output.	Provides information on child's hydration status.	Document intake and output.
	Administer antibiotics on schedule. Assess and record any side effects (e.g., rash, diarrhea).	Antibiotics are given to combat infection.	Document whether antibiotics were administered on schedule. Describe any side effects noted.
	Administer antipyretics on schedule. Assess and record effectiveness.	Antipyretics are used to reduce fever.	Document whether an antipyretic was needed and describe effectiveness.
	Administer analgesics on schedule. Assess and record effectiveness and any side effects (e.g., constipation, nausea).	Analgesics are administered to decrease pain.	Document whether analgesics were administered on schedule. Describe effectiveness and any side effects noted.
	Maintain good hand-washing technique. If an open wound is present, maintain wound isolation precautions in accordance with institutional policy.	Good hand washing is the single most important measure in decreasing infection. Following institutional policy for open wound care will decrease spread of infection and prevent wound contamination.	Document whether good hand-washing technique was used. Document whether institutional policy for open wound care was followed.

Primary Nursing Diagnosis: Actual Infection *(continued)*

Expected Outcomes	Possible Nursing Interventions	Rationale	Evaluation for Charting
	If surgical drainage has been performed, make sure that antibiotic solution is draining properly into involved area and that suction is properly applied to remove drainage.	Antibiotic solution is used to treat the infection. Suction is used to remove drainage.	Document any therapeutic measures used to treat the infection. Describe their effectiveness.
	When indicated, change the dressing on schedule according to institutional protocol. Assess and record characteristics of drainage and wound site every shift and PRN.	Prevents spread of infection and provides a way to assess the progress of the wound.	Describe characteristics of wound site and any drainage.
	When indicated, keep involved area immobilized. Begin range-of-motion exercises when indicated. Protect weight-bearing joints from pressure. Assess and record area for sensation, circulation, pain, color, swelling, heat, and tenderness every shift and PRN. If indicated, ensure that bed rest is maintained.	Immobilization and decreased pressure on the affected joint prevents pain caused by movement of the involved area. When indicated, range-of-motion exercises will help prevent contractures to the affected joint. Assessment for sensation, circulation, pain, color, swelling, heat, and tenderness provides information about status of involved area.	Document any therapeutic measures used to treat the infection. Describe their effectiveness.
	Check and record results of any laboratory work or X-rays. Notify physician if results are out of the normal range.	Elevated WBC and erythrocyte sedimentation rate can indicate the presence of an infection. X-ray can reveal joint swelling of the affected joint.	Document current results of any laboratory work or X-rays.
TEACHING GOALS Child and/or family will be able to verbalize at least 4 characteristics of infection such as • fever • localized tenderness, redness, swelling over involved joint • limping or refusal to walk • pain on movement of involved joint	Teach child/family about characteristics of infection. Assess and record results.	Increased knowledge will assist the child/family in recognizing and reporting changes in the child's condition.	Document whether teaching was done and describe results.

(continued)

	Possible Nursing		Evaluation for
Expected Outcomes	**Interventions**	**Rationale**	**Charting**
Child and/or family will be able to verbalize knowledge of care such as • good hand-washing technique • fever control • medication administration • dressing change and wound assessment • identification of any signs/symptoms of infection (such as those listed under Assessment) • when to contact health-care provider	Teach child/family about care. Assess and record child's/family's knowledge of and participation in care regarding good hand-washing technique, fever control, medication administration, dressing change, wound assessment, etc.	Education of child/family will allow for accurate care.	Document whether teaching was done and describe results.

Primary Nursing Diagnosis: Actual Infection *(continued)*

Nursing Diagnosis   Acute Pain

Definition   Condition in which an individual experiences acute mild to severe pain

Possibly Related to   • Inflammation and swelling secondary to bacterial invasion of the joint
                        • Treatment methods (e.g., surgery, exercise)

Nursing Diagnosis: Acute pain related to inflammation and swelling secondary to bacterial invasion of the joint, treatment methods (e.g., surgery, exercise)

Assessment/Defining Characteristics of Child and/or Family (Subjective & Objective Data):

• Verbal communication of pain
• Crying unrelieved by usual comfort measures
• Hesitation or refusal to bear weight on limb
• Decreased activity, self-imposed

• Severe discomfort on movement of affected joint
• Rating of pain on pain-assessment tool
• Physical signs/symptoms (tachycardia, tachypnea, increased blood pressure, diaphoresis)

	Possible Nursing		Evaluation for
Expected Outcomes	**Interventions**	**Rationale**	**Charting**
Child will have decreased pain or be free of severe and/or constant pain as evidenced by • verbal communication of comfort • lack of constant crying	Assess and record HR, RR, BP, and any signs/symptoms of pain (such as those listed under Assessment) every 2 to 4 hours and PRN. Use age-appropriate pain-assessment tool.	Provides data regarding the level of pain child is experiencing.	Document range of HR, R, BP, and degree of pain child was experienceing. Describe any successful measures used to decrease pain.

Nursing Diagnosis: Acute Pain *(continued)*

Expected Outcomes	Possible Nursing Interventions	Rationale	Evaluation for Charting
• decrease in or lack of diaphoresis • ability to bear weight on joint without pain • heart rate within acceptable range (state specific range) • respiratory rate within acceptable range (state specific range) • blood pressure within acceptable range (state specific range) • rating of decreased pain or no pain on pain-assessment tool • lack of signs/ symptoms of acute pain (such as those listed under Assessment)	Administer analgesics on schedule. Assess and record effectiveness and any side effects (e.g., constipation, nausea).	Analgesics are administered to decrease pain.	Document whether analgesics were administered on schedule. Describe effectiveness and any side effects noted.
	Handle injured area with extreme care. Support and protect involved area when the child is moved. Have two individuals move child if necessary. When indicated, keep involved area immobilized.	These measures will help prevent pain caused by movement.	Document if child was handled with care. Describe effectiveness.
	Encourage family members to stay and comfort child when possible.	Helps to comfort and support the child.	Document whether family was able to remain with child and describe effectiveness of their presence.
	Allow family members to participate in care of child when possible.	This may increase the comfort level of the child and thus help child in managing pain.	Document whether family participated in care and if this was successful in helping child with pain management.
	Use diversional activities (e.g., music, television, playing games, relaxation) when appropriate.	Diversional activities can distract child and may help to decrease pain.	Document whether diversional activities were successful in helping to manage pain.
	If age appropriate, explain all procedures beforehand.	Allow child some control which can assist child with pain management.	Describe if this measure was effective in helping child to manage pain.
	If age appropriate, allow the child to participate in planning his or her care. Encourage the child to practice self-care (e.g., bathing, removing dressing).	Allowing child some control can assist child with pain management.	Describe if this measure was effective in helping child to manage pain.
	When indicated, institute additional pain relief measures, such as hypnosis, and guided imagery. Assess and record effectiveness.	These nonpharmacologic measures may help decrease pain.	Document whether these measures were successful in helping to manage pain.

(continued)

	Possible Nursing		Evaluation for
Expected Outcomes	**Interventions**	**Rationale**	**Charting**
TEACHING GOALS Child and/or family will be able to verbalize at least 4 characteristics of pain such as • verbal communication of pain • crying unrelieved by usual comfort measures • hesitation or refusal to use limb • decreased activity, self-imposed • rapid heart rate	Teach child/family about characteristics of pain. Assess and record results.	Increased knowledge will assist the child/family in recognizing and reporting changes in the child's condition.	Document whether teaching was done and describe results.
Child and/or family will be able to verbalize knowledge of care such as • medication administration • gentle handling of child • identification of any signs/symptoms of pain (such as those listed under Assessment) • when to contact health-care provider	Teach child/family about care. Assess and record child's/family's knowledge of and participation in care regarding medication administration, etc.	Education of child/family will allow for accurate care.	Document whether teaching was done and describe results.

Nursing Diagnosis: Acute Pain *(continued)*

Related Nursing Diagnoses

Impaired Physical Mobility	*related to* pain on movement of involved area secondary to bacterial invasion of the joint
Deficient Knowledge: Child/Family	*related to* a. disease process and treatment b. prevention of complications c. activity restrictions
Impaired Skin Integrity	*related to* a. bed rest b. surgical wound
Compromised Family Coping	*related to* a. prolonged hospitalization of child (antibiotic therapy needed for 2 to 4 weeks) b. financial considerations c. interruption of parental work schedule

CARE OF CHILDREN WITH NEUROLOGIC/ NEUROMUSCULAR DYSFUNCTION

9

ONE

CEREBRAL PALSY
MEDICAL DIAGNOSIS

PATHOPHYSIOLOGY Cerebral palsy (CP) is defined as any nonprogressive central motor deficit linked to events in the prenatal, perinatal, or postnatal period that resulted in damage to or dysfunction of the central nervous system. Intrauterine insults (infarcts, hemorrhage, infection, anoxia) or structural abnormalities of the central nervous system are the cause of most cases of CP. This central nervous system injury manifests itself as abnormal muscle tone and coordination in the child, who then exhibits impaired movement and posture. The types of movement exhibited by the child differ for the varieties of cerebral palsy and are influenced by muscle tone. Hypertonic muscles have a high degree of tension and can severely limit movement. Hypotonic muscles have low tone and feel limp. A child with cerebral palsy can have both extremes of muscle tone. Cerebral palsy is the most common cause of spasticity and physical disability of children and it is the most common chronic disorder of childhood. Since the 1960s, the prevalence of cerebral palsy has risen approximately 20%, and it is thought that this rise is due to the increase in the survival rate of low and very-low-birth-weight infants.

The four types of cerebral palsy are classified by the nature and distribution of neuromuscular dysfunction exhibited, which corresponds to the injured area of the brain. The 4 types of CP are spastic, dyskinetic/athetoid, ataxic, and mixed. Spastic cerebral palsy is the most common and accounts for 75% of all CP cases. The limb and trunk muscles of a child with spastic cerebral palsy are tight and contract strongly with sudden attempted movements or stretching. The spasticity may involve one or both sides of the body; posture, coordination and balance are poor; and both fine and gross motor skills can be impaired. Injuries to the cerebral cortex or pyramidal tract can result in this type of cerebral palsy. Spastic cerebral palsy can be further classified by what part of the body is involved or the number of extremities involved (hemiplegia, quadriparesis or tetraparesis, diplegia, monoplegia, triplegia, paraplegia).

A child with dyskinetic (athetoid) cerebral palsy has uncontrolled and involuntary movements; the limbs have involuntary, purposeless movements and purposeful movements that are contorted. Athetoid movements are characterized by slow, worm-like writhering motion. These children can have speech and articulation

problems or drooling if the pharyngeal and oral muscles are involved. Damage to cells in the basal ganglia can result in dyskinesia. Ten to 15% of all CP cases are dyskinetic.

Children with ataxic cerebral palsy have a disturbance in the coordination of voluntary movements. Damage to the cerebellum, which controls balance, equilibrium, and kinesthetic sense, results in ataxia. Five to 10% of all CP cases are ataxic. Children with mixed cerebral palsy exhibit more than one movement disorder due to injuries in multiple areas of the brain.

In addition to nonprogressive motor disability, the child with cerebral palsy may exhibit other manifestations of cerebral dysfunction, such as epilepsy, mental retardation, learning disabilities, poor attention span, easy distractibility, hyperactivity, hearing or vision loss, and/or emotional problems. Additionally, due to oropharyngeal and respiratory muscle impairment, these children are at risk for nutritional deficiencies and respiratory disease. Presentation and clinical manifestations for each child vary depending on limb involvement, type of movement, and other accompanying conditions. A child with severe cerebral palsy can be exceptionally adept in learning, while some mildly physically involved children can be severely mentally retarded and others can be both mentally and physically debilitated.

Diagnosis of cerebral palsy is usually based on clinical findings. Once CP is suspected the infant may undergo a number of tests to help confirm the diagnosis. Ultrasonography, computed tomography (CT) scan, and magnetic resonance imaging (MRI) can provide information about anatomical structures and detect abnormalities of the brain. Positron emission tomography (PET) can provide additional information. Neuromotor testing is helpful in evaluating the child's movement patterns, reflexes, and tone.

The treatment goals for children with cerebral palsy include improving motor function and preventing further disabilities. Comprehensive care can best be provided by a multidisciplinary team. Orthopedic management may include surgery and/or the use of braces, casts, and corrective or adaptive appliances. Neurosurgical procedures have been essential in the treatment of cerebral palsy and can include one or more of the following: chemical or surgical neurotomies, botulinum toxin injections, selective dorsal rhizotomy, or chronic intrathecal baclofen therapy. Physical therapy, occupational therapy, speech therapy, and special educational programming are integral to the child's management.

Oral medications are often used to reduce spasticity. All treatments should work together to promote the maximum level of functioning and independence of the child and family.

Primary Nursing Diagnosis Impaired Physical Mobility

Definition Limited ability of movement

Possibly Related to
- Nonprogressive motor deficits secondary to central nervous system injury
- Status/postorthopedic surgery
- Status/postneurosurgery
- Status/postcasting

Primary Nursing Diagnosis: Impaired physical mobility related to nonprogressive motor deficits secondary to central nervous system injury, status/postorthopedic surgery, status/postneurosurgery, status/postcasting

Assessment/Defining Characteristics of Child and/or Family (Subjective & Objective Data):
- Muscle weakness
- Muscle dysfunction
- Problems with coordination, balance, and kinesthetic sense
- Hypertonic and/or hypotonic muscles
- Uncontrolled movements
- Involuntary movements
- Decreased range of motion
- Monoplegia, hemiplegia, paraplegia, diplegia, triplegia, or quadriplegia
- Contractures

Expected Outcomes	Possible Nursing Interventions	Rationale	Evaluation for Charting
Child will maximize ability of movement as evidenced by (state specific examples for each child).	Assess and record child's activity level at least once/shift.	Provides a mobility baseline, which can be used to describe increased or decreased activity.	Describe child's level of mobility.
	Assess and record any signs/symptoms of impaired physical mobility (such as those listed under Assessment) once/shift and PRN.	Provides information that can assist when planning nursing care for the child.	Describe any signs/symptoms of impaired physical mobility.
	Ensure that child keeps scheduled appointments with occupational therapist and physical therapist as indicated.	Therapy will help maximize ability of movement.	Describe any therapeutic measures used to improve physical mobility. State their effectiveness.
	Encourage child to participate as much as possible in self-care.	Promotes autonomy.	Document child's ability to participate in self-care.

(continued)

Primary Nursing Diagnosis: Impaired Physical Mobility (*continued*)

Expected Outcomes	Possible Nursing Interventions	Rationale	Evaluation for Charting
	Make available activities within child's limitations (state specific examples for each child).	Decreases anxiety and frustration while allowing child to accomplish activities.	Describe any activities in which the child was able to participate.
	Perform scheduled active and passive range-of-motion exercises every 4 hours and PRN.	Helps preserve muscle and joint function.	Document whether range-of-motion exercises were done and their effectiveness.
	Reposition child every 1 to 2 hours.	Helps to prevent skin breakdown.	Document whether child was repositioned on schedule.
	Ensure that child's body stays in proper alignment, whether in bed, chair, or wheelchair.	Maintains position and helps to prevent deformities.	Document whether child was kept in proper alignment.
	Assist child as necessary in using splints, braces, and other appliances.	Provides support in meeting mobility goals.	Describe any therapeutic measures used to improve physical mobility. Document their effectiveness.
	When indicated, use Hoyer lift for totally dependent transfers. Use pivot or two-person transfer as indicated.	Provides safe support when transferring the child who is unable to transfer by other means.	Describe any therapeutic measures used to improve physical mobility. State their effectiveness.
TEACHING GOALS Child and/or family will be able to verbalize at least 4 characteristics of impaired mobility such as • muscle weakness and/or dysfunction • problems with coordination, balance and kinesthetic sense • uncontrolled movements • involuntary movements	Teach child/family about characteristics of impaired mobility. Assess and record results.	Increased knowledge will assist the child/family in recognizing and reporting changes in the child's condition.	Document whether teaching was done and describe results.
Child and/or family will be able to verbalize knowledge of care such as • correct use of adaptive devices and home modifications • correct handling and positioning technique	Teach child/family about care. Assess and record child's/family's knowledge of and participation in care regarding correct use of adaptive devices and home modifications, etc.	Education of child/family will allow for accurate care.	Document whether teaching was done and describe results.

Primary Nursing Diagnosis: Impaired Physical Mobility *(continued)*

Expected Outcomes	Possible Nursing Interventions	Rationale	Evaluation for Charting
• appropriate use of resources • identification of any signs/symptoms of impaired mobility (such as those listed under Assessment) • when to contact health-care provider			

Nursing Diagnosis Disturbed Body Image

Definition Condition in which the child has a negative self-view

Possibly Related to
- Spastic or athetoid movements
- Physical deformities secondary to spasticity
- Delayed growth and development
- Personal frustration with difficulty in speech, feeding, eating, and motor behaviors

Nursing Diagnosis: Disturbed body image related to spastic or athetoid movements; physical deformities secondary to spasticity; delayed growth and development; personal frustration with difficulty in speech, feeding, eating, and motor behaviors

Assessment/Defining Characteristics of Child and/or Family (Subjective & Objective Data):
- Verbalization about displeasure with body
- Refusal to look in mirror
- Refusal to participate in care or play and social activities
- Decreased interest in appearance

Expected Outcomes	Possible Nursing Interventions	Rationale	Evaluation for Charting
Child will indicate acceptance of body image as evidenced by • ability to verbally describe self positively • ability to look in mirror • willingness to participate in care • willingness to participate in play and social activities • developmentally appropriate interest in appearance	Assess and record child's/family's ability to accept body image.	Provides a baseline, which can be used to describe increased or decreased acceptance of body image.	Describe child's/family's ability to accept body image.
	Encourage child to express feelings, fears, or concerns regarding cerebral palsy and appearance.	Provides information about child's feelings, fears, and concerns related to their appearance.	Describe any feelings, fears, or concerns that child expressed.
	Clarify any misconceptions child may express regarding cerebral palsy and appearance.	Provides an opportunity for health-care team to correct any misinformation.	Document any misinformation stated by child and measures used to dispel misinformation.

(continued)

Nursing Diagnosis: Disturbed Body Image *(continued)*

Expected Outcomes	Possible Nursing Interventions	Rationale	Evaluation for Charting
	Provide child with opportunities for age-appropriate therapeutic play.	Provides an outlet for child to express their feelings.	Describe any therapeutic play measures used to help child express his/her feelings.
	Encourage child to maintain usual state of grooming and appearance.	Helps to increase child's body image.	Describe any therapeutic measures used to help child improve his/her body image.
	Encourage child to attend camp and participate in additional activities with other children with cerebral palsy.	Provides an opportunity for positive experiences for the child.	Describe any additional activities in which the child agreed to participate.
	When indicated, consult with social services for appropriate counseling.	Provides resources to help the child deal with body image issues.	Describe any therapeutic measures used to help child improve his/her body image.
TEACHING GOALS Child and/or family will be able to verbalize at least 4 characteristics of disturbed body image such as • verbalization about displeasure with body • refusal to look in mirror • refusal to participate in care or play and social activities • decreased interest in appearance	Teach child/family about characteristics of disturbed body image. Assess and record results.	Increased knowledge will assist the child/family in recognizing and reporting changes in the child's condition.	Document whether teaching was done and describe results.
Child and/or family will be able to verbalize knowledge of care such as • participating in care regarding promoting a positive body image. • identification of any signs/symptoms of impaired body image (such as those listed under Assessment) • when to contact health-care provider	Teach child/family about care. Assess and record child's/family's knowledge of and participation in care regarding ways to promote a positive body image (see previous Nursing Interventions).	Education of child/family will allow for accurate care.	Document whether teaching was done and describe results.

Related Nursing Diagnoses

Imbalanced Nutrition: Less than Body Requirements	*related to* a. increased caloric needs secondary to increased muscle tension and movements b. difficulty with chewing and swallowing secondary to muscle weakness and/or dental irregularities c. inability to feed self secondary to motor deficits d. distractibility
Impaired Parenting	*related to* a. child with a physical dysfunction and possible intellectual impairment b. inability of infant to cuddle or mold to caregiver for comfort c. frequent hospitalizations of child
Delayed Growth and Development	*related to* a. inadequate caloric intake b. lack of muscle strength and coordination to achieve motor milestones and perform skills or activities of daily living c. limited social interaction secondary to speech and motor deficits d. lack of appropriate stimulation in environment
Impaired Home Maintenance	*related to* a. child's need for assistance with hygiene, feeding, toileting, ambulation, and communication b. child's need for equipment c. inadequate resources, including relief from caregiving d. need to change and adapt home environment

TWO

GUILLAIN-BARRÉ SYNDROME
MEDICAL DIAGNOSIS

PATHOPHYSIOLOGY Guillain-Barré syndrome (GBS), in its classic form, is an acute inflammatory demyelinating polyneuropathy. It is characterized by progressive symmetric muscle weakness, paralysis, and hyporeflexia with or without autonomic or sensory symptoms. The exact cause is unknown, although it is thought to be an autoimmune response to a viral or bacterial agent. In GBS, sensitized lymphocytes migrate to the peripheral nerves and spinal roots (and at times cranial nerves), causing inflammation and demyelinization. In some instances, axonal injury can also occur. As a result, peripheral, spinal, and/or cranial nerve conduction becomes slower and less intense. This leads to a gradual, but progressive, paresis or paralysis, accompanied by loss of sensation. In the pediatric population, GBS most commonly occurs in children ages 4 to 10 years, and both genders are affected with equal frequency.

There are four subtypes of acute peripheral neuropathy of GBS. The most common subtype is acute inflammatory demyelinating polyradiculoneuropathy (AIDP), which resembles an autoimmune neuritis. In AIDP, the myelin sheaths are invaded by macrophages, which also denude the axons. In acute motor axonal neuropathy (AMAN) the neurological deficit is purely motor. Acute motor and sensory axonal neuropathy (AMSAN) has both motor and sensory fiber deficits. In AMAN and AMSAN, the pathogenesis is consistent with an antibody-mediated inflammatory response involving the ventral (AMAN) or ventral and dorsal (AMSAN) roots where the macrophages invade the perinodal space of Ranvier, leaving the myelin sheath intact. The last subtype, Fisher's syndrome, involves the triad of acute ophthalmoplegia, ataxia, and areflexia. The pathology of Fisher's syndrome is unclear.

Approximately 50 to 70% of patients with GBS have a history of an antecedent illness (usually a flulike illness, an upper respiratory infection, or gastroenteritis) within the previous 4 weeks. Approximately one quarter of all cases had a recent *Campylobacter jejuni* infection. The progression of muscle weakness and paralysis in GBS may be rapid, but most often it continues for several weeks before reaching a plateau (usually after 2 to 4 weeks). Symmetrical motor weakness and loss of deep tendon reflexes begin in the lower extremities and advance rapidly upward to the upper extremities, trunk, chest, neck, face, and head. These processes are characterized by a prickling sensation in the hands and feet, accompanied by pain, with the eventual development of paralysis. Often the respiratory muscles are affected, resulting in respiratory insufficiency. Severe respiratory insufficiency or failure can progress to the point where the child requires a tracheostomy and/or mechanical ventilation. Cranial nerve paralysis may also appear, presenting as impaired swallowing, impaired gag reflex, and/or facial weakness. Sensory impairment, manifested as paresthesia (numbness or tingling) and/or loss of position sense, may occur as well but is less common. Autonomic involvement is common, causing hypertension, diaphoresis, pupillary changes, postural hypotension, cardiac arrhythmias, ileus, and/or urinary retention. In severe cases, the muscles can become wasted after 2 weeks. Recovery (with remyelination) begins after a variable plateau phase and can take weeks or months. Initially, proximal muscle strength returns, followed by distal muscle strength. Children usually recover rapidly and completely. Children with a rapid onset phase or severe disease are more likely to do poorly or retain disability.

Neurophysiological studies are important in diagnosing and classifying Guillain-Barré syndrome. Electrodiagnostic studies of motor conduction (usually of 3 motor nerves) to identify demyelination are done and then sensory conduction (usually of 3 sensory nerves) can provide additional details. A lumbar puncture is almost always indicated and 80% show an elevated cerebral spinal protein, after the first few days of illness.

The most significant advances in the management of GBS have been the development of specific therapies that favorably alter the course of the disease, namely plasma exchange and intravenous immune globulin (IVIG). Otherwise, treatment is usually supportive, and recovery is generally complete. Physiotherapy and occupational therapy are helpful during the recovery period. Persistent fatigue can be a common problem. The GBS/CIDP Foundation International provides information and resources for these children and their families. (CIDP is chronic inflammatory demyelinating polyradiculoneuropathy.)

Primary Nursing Diagnosis   Ineffective Breathing Pattern

Definition   Breathing pattern that results in inadequate oxygen consumption (failure to meet the cellular requirements of the body)

Possibly Related to   • Respiratory insufficiency secondary to intercostal and phrenic nerve paralysis

Primary Nursing Diagnosis: Ineffective breathing pattern related to respiratory insufficiency secondary to intercostal and phrenic nerve paralysis

Assessment/Defining Characteristics of Child and/or Family (Subjective & Objective Data):

- Shallow, irregular respirations
- Diminished breath sounds
- Decreased chest expansion
- Pallor or cyanosis
- Restlessness in vocalizations
- Inability to swallow
- Inability to clear secretions due to weak cough
- Tachypnea
- Tachycardia
- Hypoxia
- Hypercarbia
- Drowsiness
- Confusion
- Restlessness

Expected Outcomes	Possible Nursing Interventions	Rationale	Evaluation for Charting

Child will have effective breathing pattern as evidenced by
 	
• respiratory rate within acceptable range (state specific range)
• heart rate within acceptable range (state specific range)
• strong, clear, and equal breath sounds bilaterally A & P
• adequate and equal bilateral chest expansion
• pink/tan color
• clear, audible vocalizations
• ability to swallow secretions
• ability to clear secretions
• absence of
  1. pallor or cyanosis
  2. hpercarbia
  3. drowsiness
  4. confusion
  5. restlessness
	Assess and record the following every 2 to 4 hours and PRN
	
	• RR, rhythm, and depth
	• HR
	• breath sounds
	• chest expansion
	• color
	• status of speech
	• ability to swallow or cough
	• any signs/symptoms of ineffective breathing pattern (such as those listed under Assessment)
		If child experiences ineffective breathing pattern the RR and HR will increase and the child will work harder to breathe, exhibiting some of the characteristics of ineffective breathing pattern.	Document RR, HR, and breath sounds. Describe any signs/symptoms of ineffective breathing pattern noted.

	When indicated, administer humidified oxygen in correct amount and route of delivery. Record percent of oxygen and route of delivery. Assess and record effectiveness of therapy.	Humidified oxygen will dilate the pulmonary vasculature, which increases surface area available for gas exchange. Extra source oxygen will also allow for better oxygenation to body tissues and thus help combat ineffective breathing pattern.	Document amount and route of oxygen delivery. Describe effectiveness.

(continued)

Primary Nursing Diagnosis: Ineffective Breathing Pattern *(continued)*

Expected Outcomes	Possible Nursing Interventions	Rationale	Evaluation for Charting
• oxygen saturation (via pulse oximeter) from 94 to 100% on room air • lack of signs/symptoms of ineffective breathing pattern (such as listed under Assessment)	Keep head of bed elevated at a 30° to 45° angle.	Elevating the head of the bed to a 30° to 45° angle causes a shift of the abdominal contents downward and this in turn will allow for increased lung expansion in order to help improve breathing pattern.	Document whether head of bed was kept elevated.
	When indicated, ensure that chest physiotherapy is done on schedule. Record effectiveness and child's response to treatment.	Chest percussion loosens secretions and positioning can help to assist the flow of secretions out of the lungs by gravity. This will aid in effective breathing pattern.	Document whether chest physiotherapy was done on schedule. Describe effectiveness and child's response to treatment.
	When using a pulse oximeter, record reading every 2 to 4 hours and PRN.	Pulse oximetry detects the oxygen saturation in the bloodstream. It is important to detect small changes in oxygen saturation before the child starts displaying overt characteristics of ineffective breathing pattern.	Document range of oxygen saturation.
	When indicated, assess and record arterial blood gases. Report any abnormalities to the physician.	An arterial blood gas detects the oxygen saturation in the blood. It is important to detect small changes in oxygen saturation before the child starts displaying overt characteristics of ineffective breathing pattern.	When indicated, document range of arterial blood gas values. Document ongoing physiological process (e.g., respiratory acidosis).
	Assist child with deep breathing and use of incentive spirometry.	Helps to promote lung expansion that inflates alveoli and helps to prevent atelectasis.	Describe any therapeutic measures used to improve ineffective breathing pattern. Document their effectiveness.
	Provide gentle oropharyngeal and/or nasotracheal suctioning as needed.	Assists with removal of secretions.	Document whether child needed suctioning. If so, document frequency and describe amount and characteristics of secretions.

Primary Nursing Diagnosis: Ineffective Breathing Pattern *(continued)*			
Expected Outcomes	**Possible Nursing Interventions**	**Rationale**	**Evaluation for Charting**
	Administer IVIG on schedule. Assess and record any side effects such as tightness in the chest, vomiting, or hypotension. Assess and record blood pressure every 15 to 30 minutes during infusion (or according to institutional protocol).	Administered for its anti-inflammatory and passive immunity effects.	Document whether IVIG was administered on schedule. Describe any side effects noted.
TEACHING GOALS Child and/or family will be able to verbalize 4 signs/symptoms of ineffective breathing pattern such as • color change from pink/tan to gray or blue • rapid respirations • status of speech • ability to swallow or clear secretions	Teach child/family about characteristics of ineffective breathing pattern. Assess and record results.	Increased knowledge will assist the child/family in recognizing and reporting changes in the child's condition.	Document whether teaching was done and describe results.
Child and/or family will be able to verbalize knowledge of care such as • treatments such as chest physiotherapy • positioning • identification of any signs/symptoms of ineffective breathing pattern (such as those listed under Assessment) • when to contact health-care provider	Teach child/family about care. Assess and record child's/family's knowledge of and participation in care regarding chest physiotherapy treatments, etc.	Education of child/family will allow for accurate care.	Document whether teaching was done and describe results.

Nursing Diagnosis   Impaired Physical Mobility

Definition   Limited ability of movement

Possibly Related to
• Weakness
• Paralysis secondary to demyelinization

Nursing Diagnosis: Impaired physical mobility related to weakness, paralysis secondary to demyelination			
Assessment/Defining Characteristics of Child and/or Family (Subjective & Objective Data): • Inability to move part or all of body • Decreased range of motion • Limited or decreased coordination • Hesitation to walk or run • Reduced muscle tone • Decreased muscle strength, control, and/or mass • Paraparesis • Quadriplegia • Complete areflexia • Contractures			
Expected Outcomes	**Possible Nursing Interventions**	**Rationale**	**Evaluation for Charting**
Child will maximize ability of movement as evidenced by (state specific examples for each child)	Assess and record child's activity level at least once/shift and PRN.	Provides a mobility baseline, which can be used to describe increased or decreased activity.	Describe child's level of mobility.
	Assess and record any signs/symptom of impaired physical mobility (such as those listed under Assessment) once/shift and PRN.	Provides information that can assist when planning nursing care for the child.	Describe any signs/symptoms of impaired physical mobility noted.
	Ensure that child keeps scheduled appointments with occupational therapy and physical therapy as indicated.	Therapy will help maximize ability of movement.	Describe any therapeutic measures used to improve physical mobility. Document their effectiveness.
	Encourage child to participate as much as possible in self-care.	Promotes autonomy.	Document child's ability to participate in self-care.
	Make available activities within child's limitations (state specific examples for each child).	Decreases anxiety and frustration while allowing child to accomplish activities.	Describe any activities in which the child was able to participate.
	Allow adequate rest periods (state specific amount of rest needed for each child).	Maintains ability to participate in usual activities.	Document effectiveness of rest periods.
	Perform scheduled active and passive range-of-motion exercises every 4 hours and PRN.	Helps preserve muscle and joint function.	Document whether range-of-motion exercises were done and their effectiveness.
	Reposition child every 1 to 2 hours.	Helps to prevent skin breakdown.	Document whether child was repositioned on schedule.
	Ensure that child's body stays in proper alignment, whether in bed, chair, or wheelchair.	Maintains position and helps to prevent deformities.	Document whether child's body was kept in proper alignment.

Nursing Diagnosis: Impaired Physical Mobility *(continued)*

Expected Outcomes	Possible Nursing Interventions	Rationale	Evaluation for Charting
	Arrange for therapeutic play, occupational therapy, and physical therapy as indicated.	Promotes child's coping skills. Assists with mobility and promotes independence.	Describe any activities in which the child was able to participate. Describe any therapeutic measures used to improve physical mobility. Document their effectiveness.
	Use footboard, splints, braces, and/or high top shoes when indicated.	Assists in preventing foot drop and in facilitating activities of daily living.	Document whether devices were used and their effectiveness in preventing foot drop and in facilitating activities of daily living.
	Administer IVIG on schedule. Assess and record any side effects such as tightness in the chest, vomiting, or hypotension. Assess and record blood pressure every 15 to 30 minutes during infusion (or according to institutional protocol).	Administered for its anti-inflammatory and passive immunity effects.	Document whether IVIG was administered on schedule. Describe any side effects noted.
TEACHING GOALS Child and/or family will be able to verbalize at least 4 characteristics of impaired mobility such as • inability to move parts of all of the body • decreased range of motion • limited or decreased coordination • hesitation to walk or run • reduced muscle tone • decreased muscle strength, control, and/or mass	Teach child/family about characteristics of impaired mobility. Assess and record results.	Increased knowledge will assist the child/family in recognizing and reporting changes in the child's condition.	Document whether teaching was done and describe results.

(continued)

Nursing Diagnosis: Impaired Physical Mobility *(continued)*			
Expected Outcomes	**Possible Nursing Interventions**	**Rationale**	**Evaluation for Charting**
Child and/or family will be able to verbalize knowledge of care such as • correct use of adaptive devices and home modifications • correct handling and positioning technique • appropriate use of resources • identification of any signs/symptoms of impaired mobility (such as those listed under Assessment) • when to contact health-care provider	Teach child/family about care. Assess and record child's/family's knowledge of and participation in care regarding correct use of adaptive devices and home modifications, etc.	Education of child/family will allow for accurate care.	Document whether teaching was done and describe results.

Related Nursing Diagnoses

Decreased Cardiac Output	*related to* cardiac arrhythmias, hypotension, or hypertension secondary to autonomic instability
Acute Pain	*related to* a. sensitivity to touch b. cramping muscles c. prickling sensations d. paresthesia
Impaired Nutrition: Less than Body Requirements	*related to* a. paralysis b. anorexia c. diarrhea and/or steatorrhea
Fear: Child	*related to* a. paralysis b. uncertain prognosis c. procedures/treatments d. loss of control

THREE

HYDROCEPHALUS
MEDICAL DIAGNOSIS

PATHOPHYSIOLOGY Hydrocephalus results from an increased accumulation of cerebrospinal fluid (CSF) within the ventricles of the brain due to an imbalance between the production and absorption of CSF. Cerebrospinal fluid protects the brain from the normal movements of the head, assists in the maintenance of the blood-brain barrier, and helps maintain normal chemical balance. Cerebrospinal fluid, primarily produced in the choroid plexus, normally circulates through the ventricular cavities and subarachnoid space. Subarachnoid villi, located in the dural sinuses, reabsorb the CSF.

Congenital hydrocephalus occurs in 3 to 4 out of every 1,000 live births and is usually a result of a maldevelopment or an intrauterine infection. Aqueductal stenosis, Chiari I and II malformation, and Dandy-Walker malformation are some of the congenital anomalies that can cause hydrocephalus. Hydrocephalus may also be acquired. Causes of acquired hydrocephalus can include hematoma secondary to trauma, tumors, infection, and vascular malformations or cysts.

Hydrocephalus occurs either when reabsorption of CSF in the subarachnoid space is impaired (also called communicating hydrocephalus) or when the flow of CSF from the ventricles of the brain to the subarachnoid space is obstructed (also called noncommunicating or obstructive hydrocephalus). A less common cause is increased CSF production resulting from a choroid plexus tumor. With an increased amount of CSF, the fluid accumulates in the ventricles, which then begin to dilate and compress the brain against the bony cranium. When this occurs prior to the fusion of the cranial sutures, enlargement of the skull results. As the CSF continues to accumulate, intracranial pressure increases. In communicating hydrocephalus, the CSF pathways are open, but reabsorption is impaired because of occlusion of the subarachnoid cisterns, obliteration of the subarachnoid spaces, or fibrosis of the arachnoid villa (often the result of hemorrhage or infection). Noncommunicating hydrocephalus most often results from developmental malformations such as aqueduct stenosis (narrowing or obstruction of the aqueduct of Sylvius between the third and fourth ventricles), Chiari malformations

(defects in the lower brain stem, cerebellum, or fourth ventricle), and Dandy-Walker syndrome (congenital atresia of the fourth ventricle that resembles a cyst). Other causes of noncommunicating hydrocephalus include neoplasms, infection, and trauma.

The age of the child at the onset of hydrocephalus and the degree of increased CSF determine the signs and symptoms. Visible characteristics of children from infancy through 2 years of age include an enlarging head size, bulging fontanels, a prominent forehead, and "sunset sign" (downward rotation of the eyes with sclera visible above the iris). They may exhibit irritability and a high-pitched cry. Older children commonly show signs and symptoms of increased intracranial pressure, such as headache, lethargy or irritability, nausea and vomiting, gait disturbances, and diplopia.

Definitive treatment of hydrocephalus is usually surgical intervention to correct an obstruction to CSF and/or to implant a shunting device to divert CSF. When a shunt is implanted, CSF drains from the ventricle into an extracranial body compartment such as the peritoneal cavity (ventriculoperitoneal [VP] shunt) or the right atrium (ventriculoatrial [VA] shunt). Once fluid reaches the extracranial body compartment, it is reabsorbed or excreted in a normal fashion. If the initial shunt is on a young infant, shunt revisions may be planned for specific times during development. These planned revisions are to accommodate the normal growth of the child. Infection and malfunction are the major complications associated with shunts and the usual reasons for shunt replacement.

A small group of children with obstructive hydrocephalus may be candidates for a procedure called endoscopic third ventriulostomy (ETV). With this procedure an endoscope is used to visualize the floor of the ventricle and a fenestration is made that allows CSF to flow around the obstruction. Some complications of ETV include hemorrhage, CSF leak, and injury to the periventricular structures.

Children treated for hydrocephalus are encouraged to live as normal a life as possible. Contact sports that may cause head trauma are to be avoided and helmets should be worn for other sports where head injury may occur. These children will need lifelong neurosurgical follow-up.

Postoperative Nursing Care Plan

Primary Nursing Diagnosis   Impaired Level of Consciousness*

Definition	Reduced or impaired state of awareness, ranging from mild to complete impairment (coma)
Possibly Related to	• Increased intracranial pressure secondary to increased amount of cerebrospinal fluid in the cerebrum as a consequence of obstruction, impaired reabsorption, or increased production

*Non-NANDA diagnosis.

Primary Nursing Diagnosis: Impaired level of consciousness related to increased intracranial pressure secondary to amount of cerebrospinal fluid in the cerebrum as a consequence of obstruction, impaired reabsorption, or increased production

Assessment/Defining Characteristics of Child and/or Family (Subjective & Objective Data):

FOR INFANTS

- Increasing head circumference
- Dilated scalp veins; shiny skin on scalp
- Widening of cranial sutures
- Full or bulging fontanels
- "Sunset sign" of the eyes
- High-pitched cry
- Vomiting
- Decreased oral intake
- Lethargy or irritability
- Change in level of consciousness
- Seizures
- Pupillary changes

FOR OLDER CHILDREN

- Headache
- Vomiting
- Lethargy
- Diplopia
- Ataxia
- Irritability
- Decline in school work
- Change in level of consciousness
- Seizures

Expected Outcomes	Possible Nursing Interventions	Rationale	Evaluation for Charting
Child will have appropriate level of consciousness and be free of increased intracranial pressure as evidenced by • stable head circumference • alertness when awake • if age appropriate, orientation to person, place, and time (oriented X3) • if age appropriate, recognition of family members	Assess and record the following every 4 hours and PRN • neurological vital signs (e.g., changes in level of consciousness, orientation to time and place, pupillary changes, equal movements of extremities, Glasgow Coma Scale, if available) • operative site for bleeding, drainage, swelling, and/or redness	Provides data on child's neurological status, level of consciousness, and operative site.	Describe neurological signs. Describe any signs/symptoms of decreasing level of consciousness noted. Describe condition of operative site. Document amount and characteristics of any bleeding, drainage, swelling, or redness.

Primary Nursing Diagnosis: Impaired Level of Consciousness *(continued)*

Expected Outcomes	Possible Nursing Interventions	Rationale	Evaluation for Charting
• age-appropriate response to pain • normal-pitched cry • strong, equal movements of all extremities • pupils that are equal and react to light • absence of signs/symptoms of impaired level of consciousness (such as those listed under Assessment)	• signs/symptoms of impaired level of consciousness and increased intracranial pressure (such as those listed under Assessment)		
	Measure the head circumference daily (measure the FOC, frontal occipital circumference).	Increasing FOC can indicate increased intracranial pressure secondary to accumulation of cerebrospinal fluid (CSF).	Document current head circumference and determine whether it has increased or decreased since previous measurement.
	Position child on the nonoperative side. When indicated, use sheepskin under the head. Keep child's head flat or in a slightly elevated position.	Nonoperative side positioning is done to prevent pressure on the operative site. Sheepskin is used to prevent skin breakdown. Keeping the child's head flat or only slightly elevated prevents too rapid reduction in CSF.	Describe any therapeutic measures used to increase level of consciousness and/or decrease intracranial pressure. Document their effectiveness.
	Organize nursing care to allow child uninterrupted rest periods.	Promotes comfort and aids in decreasing intracranial pressure.	Describe any therapeutic measures used to increase level of consciousness and/or decrease intracranial pressure. Document their effectiveness.
	Keep accurate record of intake (IV and/or PO) and output.	Overhydration can cause an increase in intracranial pressure.	Document intake and output.
	Administer antibiotics on schedule. Assess and record any side effects (e.g., rash, diarrhea).	Antibiotics are administered to prevent infection.	Document whether antibiotics were administered on schedule. Describe any side effects noted.
TEACHING GOALS Child and/or family will be able to verbalize at least 4 characteristics of impaired level of consciousness such as • full or bulging fontanels • high-pitched cry • vomiting • decreased oral intake	Teach child/family about characteristics of impaired level of consciousness. Assess and record results.	Increased knowledge will assist the child/family in recognizing and reporting changes in the child's condition.	Document whether teaching was done and describe results.

(continued)

| | Possible Nursing | | Evaluation for |
Expected Outcomes	**Interventions**	**Rationale**	**Charting**
• headache • lethargy or irritability • change in level of consciousness • seizures			
Child and/or family will be able to verbalize knowledge of care such as • assessment of surgical incision for redness, swelling, and/or drainage • palpation of the shunt and valve to denote normal activity • if indicated, "pumping" of the shunt to check for patency • avoidance of contact sports • use of helmet with any sport where head injury may occur. • administration of prophylactic antibiotic therapy prior to dental treatment to reduce the risk of bacteremia. • identification of any signs/symptoms of impaired level of consciousness and/or increased intracranial pressure (such as those listed under Assessment) that might be present if the shunt becomes obstructed or infected. • when to contact health-care provider	Teach child/family about care. Assess and record child's/family's knowledge of and participation in care regarding incision care, shunt care, prophylactic medication administration, avoidance of contact sports, etc.	Education of child/family will allow for accurate care.	Document whether teaching was done and describe results.

Primary Nursing Diagnosis: Impaired Level of Consciousness (*continued*)

Nursing Diagnosis   Acute Pain

Definition   Condition in which an individual experiences acute mild to severe pain

Possibly Related to   • Surgical incision and manipulation
• Headache

Nursing Diagnosis: Acute pain related to surgical incision and manipulation, headache

Assessment/Defining Characteristics of Child and/or Family (Subjective & Objective Data):

- Verbal communication of pain
- Facial grimacing
- Crying unrelieved by usual comfort measures
- Decreased activity, self-imposed
- Restlessness
- Rating of pain on pain-assessment tool
- Physical signs/symptoms (tachycardia, tachypnea, increased blood pressure, diaphoresis)

Expected Outcomes	Possible Nursing Interventions	Rationale	Evaluation for Charting

Child will have decreased pain or be free of severe and/or constant pain as evidenced by
• verbal communication of comfort
• lack of
  1. constant crying
  2. facial grimacing
  3. restlessness
• heart rate within acceptable range (state specific range)
• respiratory rate within acceptable range (state specific range)
• blood pressure within acceptable range (state specific range)
• rating of decreased pain or no pain on pain-assessment tool
• lack of signs/symptoms of pain (such as those listed under Assessment)
	Assess and record HR, RR, BP, and any signs/symptoms of pain (such as those listed under Assessment) every 2 to 4 hours and PRN. Use age-appropriate pain-assessment tool.	Provides data regarding the level of pain child is experiencing.	Document range of HR, RR, BP, and degree of pain child was experiencing. Discuss any successful measures used to decrease pain.

	Administer analgesics (carefully titrated in order to relieve pain and still allow for adequate neurological assessment) on schedule. Assess and record effectiveness and any side effects (e.g., constipation, nausea).	Analgesics are administered to decrease pain.	Document whether analgesics were administered on schedule. Describe effectiveness and any side effects noted.
	Handle child gently.	Helps to increase comfort.	Document if child was handled gently. Describe effectiveness.
	Encourage family members to stay and comfort child when possible.	Helps to comfort and support the child.	Document whether family was able to remain with child and describe effectiveness of their presence.
	Allow family members to participate in care of child when possible.	This may increase the comfort level of the child and thus help child in managing pain.	Document whether family participated in care and if this was successful in helping child with pain management.
	Use diversional activities (e.g., music, television, playing games, relaxation) when appropriate.	Diversional activities can distract child and may help to decrease pain.	Document whether diversional activities were successful in helping to manage pain.
	If age appropriate, explain all procedures beforehand.	Allowing child some control can assist child with pain management.	Describe if this measure was effective in helping child to manage pain.

(continued)

Nursing Diagnosis: Acute Pain *(continued)*

Expected Outcomes	Possible Nursing Interventions	Rationale	Evaluation for Charting
	If age appropriate, allow the child to participate in planning his or her care. Encourage the child to practice self-care (e.g., bathing, dressing).	Allowing child some control can assist child with pain management.	Describe if this measure was effective in helping child to manage pain.
	When indicated, institute additional pain relief measures, such as hypnosis, and guided imagery. Assess and record effectiveness.	These nonpharmacologic measures may help decrease pain.	Document whether these measures were successful in helping to manage pain.
TEACHING GOALS Child and/or family will be able to verbalize at least 4 characteristics of pain such as • verbal communication of pain • crying unrelieved by usual comfort measures • decreased activity, self-imposed • rapid heart rate	Teach child/family about characteristics of pain. Assess and record results.	Increased knowledge will assist the child/family in recognizing and reporting changes in the child's condition.	Document whether teaching was done and describe results.
Child and/or family will be able to verbalize knowledge of care such as • medication administration • gentle handling of child • identification of any signs/symptoms of pain (such as those listed under Assessment) • when to contact health-care provider	Teach child/family about care. Assess and record child's/family's knowledge of and participation in care regarding medication administration, etc.	Education of child/family will allow for accurate care.	Document whether teaching was done and describe results.

Related Nursing Diagnoses

Risk for Infection	*related to* a. surgical incision b. foreign body (shunt and catheters) inserted into cranium
Impaired Skin Integrity	*related to* a. thin and fragile skin of the head b. pressure and weight of the head c. child's inability to move head
Fluid Volume Deficit	*related to* a. vomiting b. lethargy c. decreased level of consciousness
Fear: Family	*related to* a. long term outcome of surgery b. possible recurrence of child's neurological symptoms
Ineffective Tissue Perfusion: Cerebral	*related to* possibility of subdural hematoma secondary to shunt complications
Compromised Family Coping	*related to* a. need for repeated surgical procedures in the future b. possible recurrence of child's neurological symptoms c. home care of shunt d. seriousness of illness e. possibility of long-term developmental problems of child f. child's physical appearance

FOUR

BACTERIAL MENINGITIS
MEDICAL DIAGNOSIS

PATHOPHYSIOLOGY Meningitis is defined as inflammation of the meninges (the protective membrane covering the brain and spinal cord). Bacterial meningitis results when bacteria invade the meninges via the bloodstream from various possible foci of infection. For example, the pathogens responsible for pneumonia, otitis media, and sinusitis can disseminate into the meninges via the bloodstream. Bacterial organisms can also directly invade the meninges after head trauma, penetrating wounds, and neurosurgical procedures.

Neisseria meningitidis (meningococcus), and *Streptococcus pneumoniae* are currently the bacterial organisms most likely to cause meningitis in children. Prior to the use of the *Haemophilus* conjugate vaccines, *H influenzae* type b accounted for the majority of all meningitis cases in children ages 0 to 12 months. In the United States, disease caused by this organism has been markedly reduced. In neonates, group B streptococci (GBS) and gram-negative enteric bacilli (*Escherichia coli*, *Klebsiella*, *Enterobacter*, and *Salmonella*) are the most common etiologic agents of meningitis. Other pathogens that occasionally cause meningitis in this age group include *Listeria monocytogenes*, *Enterobacter sakazaki*, and *Citrobacter koseri*.

Bacterial invasion and the spread of the pathogen into the cerebrospinal fluid (CSF) and to the brain parenchyma lead to inflammation. The brain becomes hyperemic and edematous as a purulent exudate forms and cerebral perfusion is compromised. Obstruction of CSF by clumps of purulent exudate at the base of the brain can result in hydrocephalus and cranial nerve palsies. Vasculitis with associated thrombosis can cause infarctions, seizures, and focal deficits. Two of the classic signs of meningitis, headache and stiff neck, are caused by inflammation of the spinal nerves and roots. Cerebral edema and increased intracranial pressure contribute to damage or necrosis of brain cells. Increased intracranial pressure and cardiovascular collapse can be seen in the late stages of meningitis and can lead to permanent neurological damage or death.

The child with meningitis usually presents with signs of generalized infection, since bacteremia often precedes the meningitis. The child also exhibits signs and symptoms of meningeal irritation such as headache, photophobia, stiff neck, positive Kernig's sign, positive Brudzinski's sign, and a change in level of consciousness. A petechial rash and purpura may occur with any bacterial meningitis, but are most common in meningococcal meningitis (*N. meningitides*). In infants, the signs and symptoms are less specific and can include poor feeding, vomiting, bulging fontanel, high-pitched cry, apnea, irritability or lethargy, and either hypothermia or hyperthermia.

For the definitive diagnosis of bacterial meningitis, a lumbar puncture is necessary to evaluate the CSF for white blood cells, protein levels, and glucose levels. To determine the causative organism, a Gram stain and culture is done on the CSF. Neuroimaging should be done instead of the lumbar puncture if signs and symptoms of increased intracranial pressure are present, to avoid possible herniation.

Therapeutic management consists of the prompt initiation of antibiotic therapy. The administration of corticosteroids (given prior to or with the first dose of antibiotic) is recommended for infants and children with Hib meningitis (*H. influenza* type b). Corticosteroid use should be considered in other types of bacterial meningitis after weighing the potential risks and benefits. Corticosteroids can reduce the meningeal inflammation of meningitis and decrease the auditory and neurological sequelae. Additionally, antipyretics and anticonvulsants may be given, ventilation and hydration must be maintained, and acute complications treated.

Long-term complications of meningitis can include hearing impairment (most common), chronic seizure disorders, hydrocephalus, and developmental delay. The administration of prophylactic antibiotics to close contacts of children with *H. influenzae* and *N. meningitidis* is recommended to prevent spread of the disease.

Primary Nursing Diagnosis Impaired Level of Consciousness*

Definition   Reduced or impaired state of awareness, ranging from mild to complete impairment (coma)

Possibly Related to   • Inflammation of the meninges secondary to invasion by a bacterial agent (state specific organism, if known)

*Non-NANDA diagnosis.

Primary Nursing Diagnosis: Impaired level of consciousness related to inflammation of the meninges secondary to invasion by a bacterial agent (state specific organism, if known)

Assessment/Defining Characteristics of Child and/or Family (Subjective & Objective Data):

- Fever
- Tachycardia
- Tachypnea
- Headache
- Irritability
- Lethargy
- Vomiting
- Bulging fontanel
- Photophobia

- Nuchal rigidity
- Decreased feeding
- High-pitched cry
- Pupillary changes
- Positive Kernig's and Brudzinski's signs
- Seizures
- Apnea
- Increased head circumference
- Change in level of consciousness

Expected Outcomes	Possible Nursing Interventions	Rationale	Evaluation for Charting
Child will have appropriate level of consciousness and be free of increased intracranial pressure as evidenced by • alertness when awake • if age appropriate, orientation to person, place, and time (oriented X3) • age-appropriate response to pain • normal-pitched cry • strong, equal movements of all extremities • pupils that are equal and react to light • age-appropriate reflexes • recognition of family members (if age appropriate) • head circumference appropriate for age (per growth chart)	Assess and record the following every 2 to 4 hours and PRN • neurological vital signs (e.g., changes in level of consciousness, orientation to time and place, pupillary changes, equal movements of extremities, Glasgow Coma Scale, if available) • RR, HR, and T • signs/symptoms of impaired level of consciousness and increased intracranial pressure (such as those listed under Assessment)	Provides data on child's neurological status, level of consciousness, RR, HR, and T. If T is elevated, the RR and HR will increase.	Describe neurological signs. Describe any signs/symptoms of decreasing level of consciousness noted. Document range of RR, HR, and T.
	Measure the head circumference daily (measure the FOC, frontal occipital circumference).	Increasing FOC can indicate increased intracranial pressure secondary to bacterial invasion of meninges causing inflammation.	Document current head circumference and determine whether it has increased or decreased since previous measurement.

(continued)

Primary Nursing Diagnosis: Impaired Level of Consciousness *(continued)*

Expected Outcomes	Possible Nursing Interventions	Rationale	Evaluation for Charting
• temperature within acceptable range of 36.5°C to 37.2°C • heart rate within acceptable range (state specific range) • respiratory rate within acceptable range (state specific range) • spontaneous respirations within acceptable range (state specific range) • lack of signs/ symptoms of impaired level of consciousness (such as those listed under Assessment)	Elevate head of bed at a 30° angle.	Helps to decrease intracranial pressure using gravity.	Document if head of bed was maintained at a 30° angle.
	Organize nursing care to minimize disturbance and stimulation of child.	Promotes comfort and aids in decreasing intracranial pressure.	Describe any therapeutic measures used to increase level of consciousness and/or decrease intracranial pressure. Document their effectiveness.
	Keep child's environment as quiet as possible.	Helps to decrease intracranial pressure.	Describe any therapeutic measures used to increase level of consciousness and/or decrease intracranial pressure. Document their effectiveness.
	Keep child's body temperature between 36.5°C to 37.2°C.	Increased body temperature increases metabolic demands and this in turn increases intracranial pressure.	Document range of child's temperature.
	Keep accurate record of intake and output. Restrict fluid intake as indicated (usually two thirds of maintenance).	Overhydration can result in increase intracranial pressure.	Document intake and output.
	Administer antibiotics on schedule. Assess and record any side effects (e.g., rash, diarrhea).	Antibiotics are given to combat the bacterial infection.	Document whether antibiotics were administered on schedule. Describe any side effects noted.
	When indicated, administer antipyretics on schedule. Assess and record effectiveness.	Antipyretics are used to reduce fever.	Document whether an antipyretic was needed and describe effectiveness.
	When indicated, administer corticosteroids on schedule. Assess and record any side effects (e.g., leukocytosis, moon faces, acne).	Used to decrease inflammation of the brain and meninges.	Document whether corticosteroids were administered on schedule. Describe any side effects noted.
	When indicated, administer anticonvulsants on schedule. Assess and record any side effects (e.g., sedation, ataxia).	Used to prevent seizures.	Document whether anticonvulsants were administered on schedule. Describe any side effects noted.

	Possible Nursing Interventions	Rationale	Evaluation for Charting
Primary Nursing Diagnosis: Impaired Level of Consciousness *(continued)*			
Expected Outcomes	**Possible Nursing Interventions**	**Rationale**	**Evaluation for Charting**
TEACHING GOALS Child and/or family will be able to verbalize at least 4 characteristics of impaired level of consciousness such as • full or bulging fontanels • high-pitched cry • vomiting • decreased feeding • headache • lethargy or irritability • change in level of consciousness • seizures	Teach child/family about characteristics of impaired level of consciousness. Assess and record results.	Increased knowledge will assist the child/family in recognizing and reporting changes in the child's condition.	Document whether teaching was done and describe results.
Child and/or family will be able to verbalize knowledge of care such as • fever control • medication administration • identification of any signs/symptoms of impaired level of consciousness and/or increased intracranial pressure (such as those listed under Assessment). • when to contact health-care provider	Teach child/family about care. Assess and record child's/family's knowledge of and participation in care regarding fever control, medication administration, etc.	Education of child/family will allow for accurate care.	Document whether teaching was done and describe results.

Nursing Diagnosis Acute Pain

Definition Condition in which an individual experiences acute mild to severe pain

Possibly Related to
- Headache, nuchal rigidity, and/or fever secondary to inflammation and/or irritation of the meninges
- Head trauma
- Earache
- Invasive procedures (such as blood drawing and lumbar puncture)

Nursing Diagnosis: Acute pain related to headache, nuchal rigidity, and/or fever secondary to inflammation and/or irritation of the meninges; head trauma; earache; invasive procedures (such as blood drawing and lumbar puncture)

Assessment/Defining Characteristics of Child and/or Family (Subjective & Objective Data):

- Verbal communication of pain
- Facial grimacing
- Crying unrelieved by usual comfort measures
- Decreased activity, self-imposed
- Restlessness
- Rating of pain on pain-assessment tool
- Physical signs/symptoms (tachycardia, tachypnea, increased blood pressure, diaphoresis)

Expected Outcomes	Possible Nursing Interventions	Rationale	Evaluation for Charting

Child will have decreased pain or be free of severe and/or constant pain as evidenced by
 	
• verbal communication of comfort
• lack of
  1. constant crying
  2. facial grimacing
  3. restlessness
• heart rate within acceptable range (state specific range)
• respiratory rate within acceptable range (state specific range)
• blood pressure within acceptable range (state specific range)
• rating of decreased pain or no pain on pain-assessment tool
• lack of signs/symptoms of pain (such as those listed under Assessment)
	Assess and record HR, RR, BP, and any signs/symptoms of pain (such as those listed under Assessment) every 2 to 4 hours and PRN. Use age-appropriate pain-assessment tool.	Provides data regarding the level of pain child is experiencing.	Document range of HR, RR, BP, and degree of pain child was experiencing. Discuss any successful measures used to decrease pain.

	Administer analgesics (carefully titrated in order to relieve pain and still allow for adequate neurological assessment) on schedule. Assess and record effectiveness and any side effects (e.g., constipation, nausea).	Analgesics are administered to decrease pain.	Document whether analgesics were administered on schedule. Describe effectiveness and any side effects noted.
	Handle child gently.	Helps to increase comfort.	Document if child was handled gently. Describe effectiveness.
	Encourage family members to stay and comfort child when possible.	Helps to comfort and support the child.	Document whether family was able to remain with child and describe effectiveness of their presence.
	Allow family members to participate in care of child when possible.	This may increase the comfort level of the child and thus help child in managing pain.	Document whether family participated in care and if this was successful in helping child with pain management.
	Use diversional activities (e.g., music, television, playing games, relaxation) when appropriate.	Diversional activities can distract child and may help to decrease pain.	Document whether diversional activities were successful in helping to manage pain.
	If age appropriate, explain all procedures beforehand.	Allowing child some control can assist child with pain management.	Describe if this measure was effective in helping child to manage pain.

Nursing Diagnosis: Acute Pain *(continued)*

Expected Outcomes	Possible Nursing Interventions	Rationale	Evaluation for Charting
	If age appropriate, allow the child to participate in planning his or her care. Encourage the child to practice self-care (e.g., bathing, dressing).	Allowing child some control can assist child with pain management.	Describe if this measure was effective in helping child to manage pain.
	When indicated, institute additional pain relief measures, such as hypnosis, and guided imagery. Assess and record effectiveness.	These nonpharmacologic measures may help decrease pain.	Document whether these measures were successful in helping to manage pain.
TEACHING GOALS Child and/or family will be able to verbalize at least 4 characteristics of pain such as • verbal communication of pain • crying unrelieved by usual comfort measures • decreased activity, self-imposed • rapid heart rate	Teach child/family about characteristics of pain. Assess and record results.	Increased knowledge will assist the child/family in recognizing and reporting changes in the child's condition.	Document whether teaching was done and describe results.
Child and/or family will be able to verbalize knowledge of care such as • medication administration • gentle handling of child • identification of any signs/symptoms of pain (such as those listed under Assessment) • when to contact health-care provider	Teach child/family about care. Assess and record child's/family's knowledge of and participation in care regarding medication administration, etc.	Education of child/family will allow for accurate care.	Document whether teaching was done and describe results.

Related Nursing Diagnoses

Fluid Volume Deficit

related to
a. poor feeding
b. vomiting
c. fever

Actual Infection*

related to the invasion of the meninges by bacterial organisms

Compromised Family Coping

related to
a. seriousness of illness
b. hospitalization
c. potential for neurological or sensory sequelae

Risk for Injury

related to
a. increased intracranial pressure
b. infectious process
c. seizure activity

*Non-NANDA diagnosis.

FIVE

NEURAL TUBE DEFECTS (SPINA BIFIDA AND MYELOMENINGOCELE)
MEDICAL DIAGNOSIS

PATHOPHYSIOLOGY Congenital malformations of the neural tube that occur during embryonic development are referred to as neural tube defects. During the initial formation of the central nervous system (within 1 month of conception), the neural groove folds over to become the neural tube. The spinal cord and vertebral arches develop from the neural tube. A neural tube defect forms if the neural tube does not close or fuse completely at some point along its length. The cause of neural tube defects is unknown. Genetic and environmental factors, as well as maternal health conditions, have all been implicated. Per year, neural tube defects occur in approximately 0.7 to 1 per 1,000 births in the United States.

There are several types of neural tube defects. Anencephaly (little or no development of brain tissue) or encephalocele (protrusion of part of the cranial contents through a midline defect in the skull) result if there is defective closure in the area of the developing embryonic head. The terms myelodysplasia, spinal dysraphism, and spina bifida are used interchangeably to describe conditions in which there are vertebral arch fusion defects and abnormalities of the spinal cord and its coverings. Spina bifida results if the defective closure occurs lower in the spinal column. Per year, spina bifida occurs in approximately 1 per 2,000 births in the United States.

Spina bifida occulta is the incomplete fusion of the vertebrae at a level in which the meninges or neural tissues are not exposed. An overlying dimple or tuft of hair may be the only indication of a spina bifida occulta. Neurologic or musculoskeletal disorders rarely accompany this condition. The lumbosacral area is the most common site for spina bifida occulta.

Spina bifida cystica is the incomplete fusion of one or more of the vertebral laminae, resulting in an external protrusion of the spinal tissue. When the sac contains meninges, spinal fluid, and neural tissue, the defect is called a myelomeningocele. Motor and sensory functions below the sac are usually affected as the spinal nerve roots end in the sac. Myelomeningoceles most often occur in the lumbar or lumbosacral area of the spinal cord. Lesions at L3 or above result in total paraplegia, sensory loss, and bowel and bladder incontinence. The lower the myelomeningocele, the less severe the neurologic deficit. Abnormalities in brain development, including Chiari Type II malformation and hydrocephalus, often accompany myelomeningocele. Skeletal deformities, such as scoliosis, hip dislocation, and foot deformities, are also common, as well as skin lesions. Neurologic impairment and urinary retention also affect kidney function. Children with these malformations can also have a number of associated disabilities, such as cognitive impairment, visual impairment, seizure disorders, and mobility problems. A meningocele, the other form of spina bifida cystica, contains meninges and spinal fluid that have protruded through the unfused vertebral arches. Neurological complications are less severe than with myelomeningocele, as the spinal cord is not involved and the spinal nerve roots retain their function even if displaced. Meningoceles also occur less commonly than myelomeningoceles. Clinically, the term spina bifida is used to refer to myelomeningocele.

Prenatally, elevated maternal alpha-fetoprotein and a high resolution fetal ultrasound may aid in the diagnosis of neural tube defects. After birth, to pinpoint the bony defect a variety of imaging tests can be done, such as flat films of the spinal column, computed tomography (CT) scan, and magnetic resonance imaging (MRI), as well as ultrasonography.

Recently, there have been two important findings in the area of neural tube defects. First, the supplementation of folic acid during pregnancy has significantly reduced the incidence of neural tube defects. Secondly, between 18 and 40% of children with spina bifida have a latex allergy. A latex-safe environment in the hospital and at home is essential for these children.

Comprehensive care for the child with spina bifida is best provided by a multidisciplinary health-care team. Surgical repair of these anomalies is usually performed soon after diagnosis to preserve neural tissue and to provide an anatomic barrier. When necessary, a ventriculoperitoneal shunt is placed to control progressive hydrocephalus. Surgical management of shunt malfunctions, Chiari II malformation, spinal cord tethering, and syringomyelia can stabilize or improve the status of these children. As the child grows, orthopedic care involving exercise, braces, casts, and surgery may be

271

needed to promote mobility and prevent deformities. The goals of urological management are to promote urinary continence and to prevent infections, reflux, and renal damage. The child and family are often taught to perform clean, intermittent catheterizations and to monitor for urinary tract infections. Bowel management often involves methods to help the child achieve continence. Dietary measures to alter stool consistency are also used. Families can be referred to the Spina Bifida Association of America for support and resources.

Primary Nursing Diagnosis   Impaired Physical Mobility

Definition   Limited ability of movement

Possibly Related to   • Neuromuscular and sensory deficits secondary to congenital malformations of the neural tube

Primary Nursing Diagnosis: Impaired physical mobility related to neuromuscular and sensory deficits secondary to congenital malformations of the neural tube

Assessment/Defining Characteristics of Child and/or Family (Subjective & Objective Data):

- Lower extremity motor weakness
- Paraplegia
- Flaccid paralysis of the lower extremities
- Weakened abdominal and trunk musculature
- Hip flexion
- Knee extension
- Scoliosis
- Foot deformities
- Dislocated joints
- Small muscle bulk
- Contractures
- Fractures

Expected Outcomes	Possible Nursing Interventions	Rationale	Evaluation for Charting
Child will maximize ability of movement as evidenced by (state specific examples for each child)	Assess and record child's activity level at least once/shift and PRN.	Provides a mobility baseline, which can be used to describe increased or decreased activity.	Describe child's level of mobility.
	Assess and record any signs/symptom of impaired physical mobility (such as those listed under Assessment) once/shift and PRN.	Provides information that can assist when planning nursing care for the child.	Describe any signs/symptoms of impaired physical mobility noted.
	Ensure that child keeps scheduled appointments with occupational therapy and physical therapy as indicated.	Therapy will help maximize ability of movement.	Describe any therapeutic measures used to improve physical mobility. Document their effectiveness.
	Encourage child to participate as much as possible in self-care.	Promotes autonomy.	Document child's ability to participate in self-care.
	Make available activities within child's limitations (state specific examples for each child).	Decreases anxiety and frustration while allowing child to accomplish activities.	Describe any activities in which the child was able to participate.

Primary Nursing Diagnosis: Impaired Physical Mobility *(continued)*

Expected Outcomes	Possible Nursing Interventions	Rationale	Evaluation for Charting
	Allow adequate rest periods (state specific amount of rest needed for each child).	Maintains ability to participate in usual activities.	Document effectiveness of rest periods.
	Perform scheduled active and passive range-of-motion exercises every 4 hours and PRN.	Helps preserve muscle and joint function.	Document whether range-of-motion exercises were done and their effectiveness.
	Reposition child every 1 to 2 hours.	Helps to prevent skin breakdown.	Document whether child was repositioned on schedule.
	Ensure that child's body stays in proper alignment, whether in bed, chair, or wheelchair.	Maintains position and helps to prevent deformities.	Document whether child's body was kept in proper alignment.
	Assist child as necessary in using splints, braces, and other appliances.	Provides support in meeting mobility goals.	Describe any therapeutic measures used to improve physical mobility. Document their effectiveness.
	When indicated, use Hoyer lift for totally dependent transfers. Use pivot or two-person transfer as indicated.	Provides safe support when transferring the child who is unable to transfer by other means.	Describe any therapeutic measures used to improve physical mobility. Document their effectiveness.
TEACHING GOALS Child and/or family will be able to verbalize at least 4 characteristics of impaired mobility such as • lower extremity weakness • flaccid paralysis of lower extremities • weakened abdominal and trunk musculature • scoliosis • foot deformities	Teach child/family about characteristics of impaired mobility. Assess and record results.	Increased knowledge will assist the child/family in recognizing and reporting changes in the child's condition.	Document whether teaching was done and describe results.

(continued)

Primary Nursing Diagnosis: Impaired Physical Mobility *(continued)*			
Expected Outcomes	**Possible Nursing Interventions**	**Rationale**	**Evaluation for Charting**
Child and/or family will be able to verbalize knowledge of care such as • correct use of adaptive devices and home modifications • correct handling and positioning technique • appropriate use of resources • identification of any signs/symptoms of impaired mobility (such as those listed under Assessment) • when to contact health-care provider	Teach child/family about care. Assess and record child's/family's knowledge of and participation in care regarding correct use of adaptive devices and home modifications etc.	Education of child/family will allow for accurate care.	Document whether teaching was done and describe results.

Nursing Diagnosis   Impaired Skin Integrity

Definition   Interruption in integrity of the skin

Possibly Related to
- Altered patterns of urinary and/or bowel elimination
- Impaired mobility
- Irritation from casts or braces

Nursing Diagnosis: Impaired skin integrity related to altered patterns of urinary and/or bowel elimination, impaired mobility, irritation from casts or braces			
Assessment/Defining Characteristics of Child and/or Family (Subjective & Objective Data):			
• Perineal skin breakdown or excoriation • Pressure sores		• Reddened areas of skin • Incontinence (bladder and/or bowel)	
Expected Outcomes	**Possible Nursing Interventions**	**Rationale**	**Evaluation for Charting**

Child will be free of signs/symptoms of impaired skin integrity as evidenced by
 	
• clean, intact skin
• natural skin color
• lack of
  1. redness
  2. excoriation
  3. lesions
	Assess and record skin condition every shift and PRN.	Provides a baseline on the condition of the child's skin, which can be used to describe any areas of potential or actual skin breakdown.	Describe any areas of potential or actual skin breakdown.

	Handle child gently.	Helps to minimize pain and promote comfort.	Document if child was handled gently and effectiveness of measure.

Nursing Diagnosis: Impaired Skin Integrity *(continued)*

Expected Outcomes	Possible Nursing Interventions	Rationale	Evaluation for Charting
	Bathe child daily (or as indicated) with water and a nonirritating soap.	Provides additional assistance with skin assessment and reveals any potential or actual areas of skin breakdown.	Describe any areas of potential or actual skin breakdown.
	Keep the perineal area clean and dry by • changing diapers/linens as soon as possible after elimination or soiling • using cotton under-wear • keeping area open to air when indicated	Helps to prevent skin breakdown in the perineal area.	Describe any therapeutic measures used to prevent or correct impaired skin integrity.
	Apply any topical medications on schedule. Assess and record effectiveness.	Used to prevent infection and promote healing.	Document whether topical medications were used and their effectiveness.
	Use a barrier cream/ointment on schedule as indicated.	Helps to prevent skin breakdown.	Document whether barrier creams/ointments were used and their effectiveness.
	Reposition child every 2 hours.	Helps to prevent skin breakdown.	Document whether child was repositioned on schedule.
	When indicated, use sheepskin surfaces, waterbeds, or egg-crate mattresses.	Helps to prevent skin breakdown.	Describe any therapeutic measures used to prevent or correct impaired skin integrity.
	Use lotion to moisturize skin when indicated.	Helps to prevent skin breakdown.	Describe any therapeutic measures used to prevent or correct impaired skin integrity.
	Massage pressure points as indicated.	Helps to prevent skin breakdown.	Describe any therapeutic measures used to prevent or correct impaired skin integrity.
	Encourage compliance with bladder and/or bowel continence programs.	Helps to prevent skin breakdown in the perineal area.	Describe any therapeutic measures used to prevent or correct impaired skin integrity.

(continued)

Nursing Diagnosis: Impaired Skin Integrity (continued)

Expected Outcomes	Possible Nursing Interventions	Rationale	Evaluation for Charting
TEACHING GOALS Child and/or family will be able to verbalize at least 4 characteristics of impaired skin integrity such as • perineal skin breakdown or excoriation • pressure sores • reddened areas of skin • incontinence (bladder and/or bowel)	Teach child/family about characteristics of impaired skin integrity. Assess and record results.	Increased knowledge will assist the child/family in recognizing and reporting changes in the child's condition.	Document whether teaching was done and describe results.
Child and/or family will be able to verbalize knowledge of care such as • measures related to preventing or correcting impaired skin integrity • topical medication administration • compliance with bladder and/or bowel continence programs • identification of any signs/symptoms of impaired mobility (such as those listed under Assessment) • when to contact health-care provider	Teach child/family about care. Assess and record child's/family's knowledge of and participation in care regarding preventing or correcting impaired skin integrity, topical medication administration, etc.	Education of child/family will allow for accurate care.	Document whether teaching was done and describe results.

Nursing Diagnosis Impaired Home Maintenance

Definition Inability to provide and maintain a safe home environment to promote optimal growth for the individual or family

Possibly Related to
- Child's need for special equipment (e.g., wheelchair, crutches, braces, casts)
- Child's need for assistance with hygiene, feeding, catheterizations, and/or mobility
- Inadequate resources or use of resources, including lack of relief from caretaking, transportation problems, cleaning, and meals
- Financial difficulties
- Need to adapt or change home environment
- Insufficient family organization and/or time management
- Lack of knowledge

Nursing Diagnosis: Impaired home maintenance related to child's need for special equipment (e.g., wheelchair, crutches, braces, casts); child's need for assistance with hygiene, feeding, catheterizations, and/or mobility; inadequate resources or use of resources, including lack of relief from caretaking, transportation, problems, cleaning, and meals; financial difficulties; need to adapt or change home environment; insufficient family organization and/or time management; lack of knowledge

Assessment/Defining Characteristics of Child and/or Family (Subjective & Objective Data):

- Overtaxed caregiver
- Child and/or family with poor hygiene
- Report or verbalization of
    1. unclean and/or unsafe home environment
    2. offensive home environmental odors
    3. misuse or lack of use of special equipment
- Offensive body odor of child/family

- Unkempt child upon admission
- Injured child upon admission
- Misuse or lack of use of resources, special services, and support
- Verbalization of inability to manage care of the child and/or home

Expected Outcomes	Possible Nursing Interventions	Rationale	Evaluation for Charting
Child and/or primary caregiver will indicate that home maintenance is improved as evidenced by • identification of factors that make the child's home care difficult and possible ways to deal with these factors • identification of factors that facilitate the child's home care • demonstration of proper use of equipment and skills needed to care for the child at home (state specific examples for each child) • expression of satisfaction with the home situation • demonstration of correct use of resources, special services, and supports • lack of signs/symptoms of impaired home maintenance (such as those listed under Assessment)	Assess and record any signs/symptoms of impaired home maintenance (such as those listed under Assessment) upon child's admission and PRN.	Provides a baseline assessment, which can be used to improve home maintenance.	Describe any signs/symptoms of impaired home maintenance noted.
	Assess and record causative or contributing factors of impaired home maintenance.	Identifying contributing factors can assist with planning interventions for improving home maintenance.	Document any causative or contributing factors identified and describe measures used to improve home maintenance.
	Assist child/family in reducing or eliminating causative or contributing factors when possible (be specific).	Promotes autonomy for child/family and assists with problem solving.	Describe any therapeutic measures used to improve home maintenance.
	When indicated, consult with social services for assistance in obtaining equipment, funds, respite care, transportation, and other supports.	Provides resources that help to facilitate child's care and can help to reduce the anxiety and stress of the child and caregiver.	Describe any therapeutic measures used to improve home maintenance.
	When indicated, consult with service organizations and community agencies for assistance and support.	Provides resources that help to facilitate child's care and can help to reduce the anxiety and stress of the child and caregiver.	Describe any therapeutic measures used to improve home maintenance.
	Encourage child and caregiver to verbalize concerns, problems, and feelings.	Promotes open lines of communication and provides a database for improving child's care.	Describe any feelings, problems, and concerns expressed by child/caregiver.

(continued)

	Nursing Diagnosis: Impaired Home Maintenance *(continued)*		
Expected Outcomes	**Possible Nursing Interventions**	**Rationale**	**Evaluation for Charting**
TEACHING GOALS Child and/or family will be able to verbalize at least 4 characteristics of impaired home maintenance such as • overtaxed caregiver • misuse of lack of resources, special services, and supports • inability to demonstrate correct use of equipment and skills • verbalization of inability to manage care of the child and/or home	Teach child/family about characteristics of impaired home maintenance. Assess and record results.	Increased knowledge will assist the child/ family in recognizing and reporting changes in the child's condition.	Document whether teaching was done and describe results.
Child and/or family will be able to verbalize knowledge of care such as • correct utilization of resources • correct use of equipment • proper skills in caring for child • identification of any signs/symptoms of impaired home maintenance (such as those listed under Assessment) • when to contact health-care provider	Teach child/family about care. Assess and record child's/family's knowledge of and participation in care regarding correct use of resources, etc.	Education of child/ family will allow for accurate care.	Document whether teaching was done and describe results.

Related Nursing Diagnoses

Disturbed Body Image   *related to*
a. bladder/bowel incontinence
b. reduced muscle mass
c. limited physical mobility secondary to neuromuscular deficit

Risk for Infection   *related to*
a. chronic retention of urine
b. repeated catheterizations
c. ventriculoperitoneal shunt

Compromised Family Coping   *related to*
a. child's chronic illness
b. demands of child's care

SIX

SEIZURES
MEDICAL DIAGNOSIS

PATHOPHYSIOLOGY A seizure can be defined as a paroxysmal, uncontrolled episode of behavior that results from an alteration in brain function caused by abnormal electrical discharges from neuronal tissue (hyperexcited brain cells). During a seizure, groups of neurons are activated all at once, disrupting normal brain function. This excessive discharge of electrical energy may remain localized in one part of the brain, may start in a focal area and spread to the rest of the brain, or may be generalized over the entire cortex without localized onset. Alterations of consciousness and/or motor, sensory, perceptual, and autonomic function characterize seizure activity. The behavior exhibited reflects the type of abnormal electrical activity and the area of brain involvement. Seizure activity can occur as a single episode or recur intermittently.

Seizures can result from a number of conditions affecting the nervous system or from various systemic disorders. These conditions can include meningitis, encephalitis, brain tumors, head trauma, asphyxia, hypoglycemia, hypo- and hypernatremia, hypocalcemia, and degenerative neurological disorders. Seizures are one of the three most common neurological conditions in children (the other two being headaches and school problems).

Seizures are classified on the basis of clinical event and electroencephalographic abnormalities. Partial (focal) or generalized are the two broad categories into which seizures can be grouped.

Partial (focal) seizures originate in a localized area of the cortex of the brain. The area of the brain involved and how extensively the discharge spreads from the "focus" determines the child's clinical presentation. There are three types of partial seizures: simple, complex, and simple or complex secondarily generalized. A simple partial seizure does not impair consciousness, but a complex one does. The clinical presentation of simple partial seizures depends on what part of the brain is affected. Localized motor (twitching of the face or an extremity or weakness of a muscle group), sensory (tingling, numbness, or feeling of warmth), visual, olfactory, auditory, gustatory, or affective disturbances are characteristic of simple partial seizures. Complex partial seizures have widely varying manifestations. They usually begin with some impairment of consciousness, followed by automatisms (automatic uncontrolled behaviors such as repetitive lip smacking or gesturing, repeated words or

phrases, and purposeless body movements or wandering). Partial seizures can rapidly spread to involve the entire brain and therefore appear generalized. This makes accurate diagnosis and treatment difficult.

Generalized seizures arise from the whole brain. The electroencephalogram (EEG) does not indicate one distinct area of where the seizure originated. Consciousness is always lost and is the initial clinical symptom. Generalized seizures include generalized tonic-clonic seizures (formerly called grand mal seizures), absence seizures (formerly called petit mal seizures), myoclonic seizures, and atonic seizures (formerly called drop attacks). Generalized tonic-clonic seizures usually have five identifiable phases: flexion, extension or tonic (stiffening of the muscle groups), tremor, clonic (rapid succession of alternating involuntary muscle contraction and relaxation), and postictal. Absence seizures are characterized by a brief, sudden cessation of all motor activity, accompanied by a blank stare and loss of awareness, followed by a rapid return to consciousness and no memory of the seizure. Myoclonic seizures are characterized by sudden, brief contractures of a muscle or muscle groups (sudden jerks of body or limbs). Atonic seizures are characterized by a sudden decrease in muscle tone and a loss of consciousness.

When a child has two or more unprovoked seizures (not triggered by infection, trauma, illicit drugs, alcohol intake, or sleep deprivation, etc.), the diagnosis of epilepsy is made. Epilepsy is a chronic seizure disorder and can have a genetic or acquired cause. In many children the cause of recurrent seizures cannot be determined. This is referred to as idiopathic epilepsy. The median age for the development of epilepsy is between 5 and 6 years of age. One in 100 people have epilepsy. Associated learning, emotional, and behavioral problems are higher in children with epilepsy and present additional challenges for the child and family.

Infantile spasms are a rare disorder whose pathophysiology is unknown. It appears within the first 4 to 7 months of life. The child presents with salaam or jackknife movements (head drop and extension of the upper extremities). Infantile spasms occur in 1 child out of 2,000 to 6,000 live births. Most of these cases occur in children with tuberous sclerosis, congenital infectious diseases, inborn errors of metabolism, malformations of cortical development, and genetic or chromosomal abnormalities. Adrenalcorticotropic hormone (ACTH) given intramuscularly is usually the treatment for infantile spasms. Children with infantile spasms are at high risk for developing other types of epilepsy or intractable seizures, and their long-term prognosis is poor.

Febrile seizures are a common disorder of early childhood, characterized by generalized tonic-clonic seizures associated with fever but without evidence of any known central nervous system infection or disorder. The peak incidence of febrile seizures is at age 18 months, and onset is uncommon after age 7. Treatment involves fever reduction and management of the illness causing the fever.

The diagnosis of a seizure is made after a thorough history and physical. Laboratory studies will vary, and can include a lumbar puncture (if the child is febrile) and anticonvulsant medication levels. An electroencephalogram (EEG) may be done. Radiologic tests such as computed tomography (CT) scan or magnetic resonance imaging (MRI) may also be performed.

The treatment goal for seizures is to prevent recurrent episodes. This can be accomplished through management of the specific cause of the seizures and the use of anticonvulsants. Other therapies may include vagus nerve stimulation, surgery, and ketogenic diet.

Primary Nursing Diagnosis   Impaired Level of Consciousness*

Definition	Reduced or impaired state of awareness, ranging from mild to complete impairment (coma)
Possibly Related to	• Metabolic disorders
	• Head trauma
	• Central nervous system infections
	• Asphyxia
	• Degenerative neurological disorder
	• Drug intoxication
	• Neoplasms
	• Genetic disorders
	• Fever
	• Unknown etiology

*Non-NANDA diagnosis.

Primary Nursing Diagnosis: Impaired level of consciousness related to metabolic disorders, head trauma, central nervous system infections, asphyxia, degenerative neurological disorder, drug intoxication, neoplasms, genetic disorders, fever, unknown etiology

Assessment/Defining Characteristics of Child and/or Family (Subjective & Objective Data):

- Change in level of consciousness and/or responsiveness
- Fever
- Tachypnea
- Tachycardia
- Tonic-clonic movements
- Jerking
- Twitching
- Pupillary changes
- Apnea
- Grunting
- Increased salivation
- Eye rolling
- Eye or head deviation to one side

- Staring into space
- Confusion
- Cyanosis
- Flushed appearance
- Incontinence of urine/stool
- Auras: unusual sensations (smells, flashing lights, buzzing sounds), abdominal pain, fear, and/or changes in behavior
- Lip smacking
- Plucking at clothes
- Agitation
- Wandering
- Drowsiness and/or lethargy
- Frothing from the mouth

	Primary Nursing Diagnosis: Impaired Level of Consciousness *(continued)*		
Expected Outcomes	**Possible Nursing Interventions**	**Rationale**	**Evaluation for Charting**
Child will have appropriate level of consciousness and be free of increased intracranial pressure as evidenced by • lack of seizure activity • alertness when awake • if age appropriate, orientation to person, place, and time (oriented X3) • age-appropriate response to pain • strong, equal movements of all extremities • pupils that are equal and react to light • age-appropriate reflexes • recognition of family members (if age appropriate) • head circumference appropriate for age (per growth chart) • body temperature between 36.5°C to 37.2°C • spontaneous respirations within acceptable range (state specific range) • heart rate within acceptable range (state specific range) • lack of signs/symptoms of impaired level of consciousness (such as those listed under Assessment)	Maintain seizure precautions per institutional policy, which may include any or all of the following • keeping oxygen, suction, and airway equipment at bedside • padding sides of bed or crib • monitoring axillary temperatures • supervising ambulation • supervising mealtime • using chest restraint when child is in a chair • having child wear protective helmet • keeping child away from sharp toys and furniture	Provides safety and support for child and helps to prevent unsafe environment by taking precautions.	Document whether seizure precautions were maintained and describe precautions used to prevent an unsafe environment.
	Assess and record all seizure activity, including • precipitating event • occurrence of an aura • beginning and progression sequence • duration • type of movements • eye movements • tongue or lip biting • apnea or color changes • incontinence • level of consciousness • falls • frequency	Provides data on child's seizure activity.	Describe any seizure activity noted.
	If seizure does occur • stay with child • protect child from injury • keep side rails padded and up if child is in a bed or crib • place child on soft, flat surface	Provides support and safety for child and allows for accurate documentation of event.	Describe any seizure activity noted and any therapeutic measures needed.

(continued)

Primary Nursing Diagnosis: Impaired Level of Consciousness *(continued)*

Expected Outcomes	Possible Nursing Interventions	Rationale	Evaluation for Charting
	• move sharp objects away from child • loosen any restrictive clothing • position child to prevent upper airway obstruction and to facilitate drainage of secretions • administer oxygen as indicated		
	Assess and record postictal state. Reorient child.	Allows for accurate documentation of event and assists in restoring appropriate level of consciousness.	Describe postictal state and any measures used to restore appropriate level of consciousness.
	Assess and record the following every 2 to 4 hours and PRN • neurological vital signs (e.g., changes in level of consciousness, orientation to time and place, pupillary changes, equal movements of extremities, Glasgow Coma Scale, if available) • RR, HR, and T • signs/symptoms of impaired level of consciousness and increased intracranial pressure (such as those listed under Assessment)	Provides data on child's neurological status, level of consciousness, respiratory rate, and temperature. If T is elevated, the RR and HR will increase.	Describe neurological signs. Describe any signs/symptoms of decreasing level of consciousness noted. Document range of RR, HR, and T.
	Measure the head circumference daily (measure the FOC, frontal occipital circumference).	Increasing FOC can indicate increased intracranial pressure.	Document current head circumference and determine whether it has increased or decreased since previous measurement.
	Organize nursing care to minimize disturbance and stimulation of child.	Promotes comfort and aids in decreasing intracranial pressure.	Describe any therapeutic measures used to increase level of consciousness and/or decrease intracranial pressure. Document their effectiveness.

Primary Nursing Diagnosis: Impaired Level of Consciousness *(continued)*

Expected Outcomes	Possible Nursing Interventions	Rationale	Evaluation for Charting
	Keep child's body temperature between 36.5°C to 37.2°C.	Increased temperature can be an etiology for seizure activity and can result in increased intracranial pressure.	Document range of child's temperature.
	When indicated, administer antipyretics on schedule. Assess and record effectiveness.	Antipyretics are used to reduce fever.	Document whether an antipyretic was needed and describe effectiveness.
	Keep accurate record of intake and output.	Overhydration can be an etiology for seizure activity and can result in increased intracranial pressure.	Document intake and output.
	Administer anticonvulsants on schedule. Assess and record effectiveness and side effects (e.g., gingival hyperplasia, rash, sedation). When indicated, check and record serum drug levels. Report any abnormalities to the physician.	Anticonvulsants are administered to combat seizure activity.	Document whether anticonvulsants were administered on schedule. Describe any side effects noted.
TEACHING GOALS Child and/or family will be able to verbalize at least 4 characteristics of impaired level of consciousness such as • change in level of consciousness • seizure activity • fever • eye or head deviated to one side • confusion	Teach child/family about characteristics of impaired level of consciousness. Assess and record results.	Increased knowledge will assist the child/family in recognizing and reporting changes in the child's condition.	Document whether teaching was done and describe results.
Child and/or family will be able to verbalize knowledge of care such as • fever control • medication administration	Teach child/family about care. Assess and record child's/family's knowledge of and participation in care regarding fever control, medication administration, etc.	Education of child/family will allow for accurate care.	Document whether teaching was done and describe results.

(continued)

Primary Nursing Diagnosis: Impaired Level of Consciousness *(continued)*			
Expected Outcomes	**Possible Nursing Interventions**	**Rationale**	**Evaluation for Charting**
• identification of any signs/symptoms of impaired level of consciousness and/or increased intracranial pressure (such as those listed under Assessment). • when to contact health-care provider			

Nursing Diagnosis   Risk for Injury

Definition   Situation in which the child is at risk for sustaining damage or harm

Possibly Related to   • Seizure activity

Nursing Diagnosis: Risk for injury related to seizure activity			
Assessment/Defining Characteristics of Child and/or Family (Subjective & Objective Data):			
• Pain • Hematoma	• Edema • Open wounds		
Expected Outcomes	**Possible Nursing Interventions**	**Rationale**	**Evaluation for Charting**
Child will be free of injury during seizure activity	Maintain seizure precautions per institutional policy, which may include any or all of the following • keeping oxygen, suction, and airway equipment at bedside • padding sides of bed or crib • monitoring axillary temperatures • supervising ambulation • supervising mealtime • using chest restraint when child is in a chair • having child wear protective helmet • keeping child away from sharp toys and furniture	Provides safety and support for child and helps to prevent unsafe environment by taking precautions.	Describe any interventions implemented to prevent injury, and state their effectiveness.

Nursing Diagnosis: Risk for Injury *(continued)*

Expected Outcomes	Possible Nursing Interventions	Rationale	Evaluation for Charting
	During seizure activity, • do not attempt to restrain child or use force • do not attempt to put anything in child's mouth • stay with child • protect child's head from injury • loosen any restrictive clothing • ease child onto a soft, flat surface	Provides safety and support for child and helps to prevent unsafe environment by taking precautions.	Describe any interventions implemented to prevent injury, and state their effectiveness.
TEACHING GOALS Child and/or family will be able to verbalize at least 4 characteristics of risk for injury such as • pain • hematoma • edema • open wounds	Teach child/family about characteristics of risk for injury. Assess and record results.	Increased knowledge will assist the child/family in recognizing and reporting changes in the child's condition.	Document whether teaching was done and describe results.
Child and/or family will be able to verbalize knowledge of care such as • care of child during seizure activity • identification of any signs/symptoms of impaired level of consciousness and/or increased intracranial pressure (such as those listed under Assessment). • when to contact health-care provider	Teach child/family about care. Assess and record child's/family's knowledge of and participation in care regarding prevention of injury during seizure activity, etc.	Education of child/family will allow for accurate care.	Document whether teaching was done and describe results.

Related Nursing Diagnoses

Ineffective Breathing Pattern	*related to* airway obstruction secondary to seizure activity
Deficient Knowledge: Child/Family	*related to* a. disease state b. medications c. seizure precautions
Compromised Family Coping	*related to* a. anxiety/fear secondary to unpredictable nature of seizures b. fear of injury to child secondary to seizures c. overprotection by family
Disturbed Body Image	*related to* a. unpredictable nature of seizures b. safety/activity restrictions that may be placed on child c. potential social stigmas

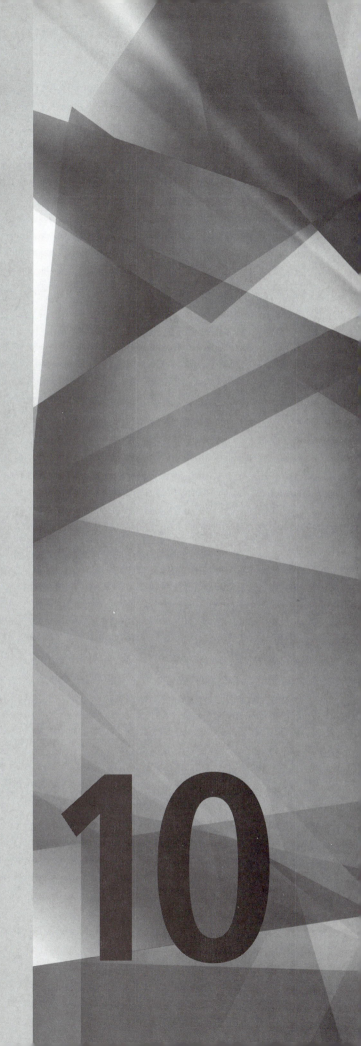

CARE OF
CHILDREN WITH
PULMONARY
DYSFUNCTION

10

ONE

APNEA OF INFANCY (AOI)
MEDICAL DIAGNOSIS

PATHOPHYSIOLOGY   The most common disorder of breathing control in neonates is apnea (the cessation of breathing). Apnea in neonates can be central, obstructive, or mixed. There is an absence of breathing effort and absence of airflow with central apnea. Central apnea can occur normally with no physiological consequences. Central nervous system abnormalities (either structural or functional) can cause central apnea associated with acute physiologic consequences such as desaturation or an apparent life-threatening event (ALTE). Obstructive apnea is characterized by the presence of breathing effort with no airflow. Infants are predisposed to upper airway obstruction for many anatomical or physiological reasons. For example, infants have a large tongue; small, under developed maxilla, mandible, and face; hypotonia of the upper airway; and poor integration of neuromuscular responses. Mixed apnea involves a combination of central and obstructive features.

Apnea of prematurity (AOP) occurs in preterm infants secondary to their prematurity. The incidence of AOP increases with lower gestational age. AOP usually presents between 2 and 7 days of life, and resolves in most infants by 40 weeks postconceptional age.

Apnea of infancy (AOI) occurs in infants of more than 37 weeks gestation. Apnea of infancy presents as an apparent life-threatening event (ALTE) with a combination of the following symptoms: cessation of breathing for 20 seconds or more, color change (visible pallor or cyanosis), limp muscle tone, and choking or gagging. Apnea of infancy may also be accompanied by bradycardia. Analysis of arterial blood gases reveals the presence of acidosis.

Since AOI can be a symptom of many disorders, extensive testing needs to be done to rule out specific and treatable causes such as airway obstruction, cardiac anomalies, seizures, gastroesophageal reflux, infection, and electrolyte imbalance. To confirm the diagnosis, a pneumocardiogram or polysomography is done. Unfortunately, these tests do not predict risk. When no identifiable cause for the ALTE is found, the diagnosis of AOI is made. Apnea of infancy should not be confused with sudden infant death syndrome (SIDS). ALTE is experienced by about 5% of children who die of SIDS.

The treatment for AOI includes respiratory stimulant drugs (methylxanthines such as theophylline or caffeine) and home cardiorespiratory monitoring. Monitoring is usually discontinued after a specified amount of time passes during which the infant has not needed intervention. Family support is essential as parents and guardians are presented with a great deal of detailed information regarding their child's condition and care.

Primary Nursing Diagnosis   Ineffective Breathing Pattern

Definition   Breathing pattern that results in inadequate oxygen consumption (failure to meet the cellular requirements of the body)

Possibly Related to
- Specific conditions such as
  - airway obstruction secondary to pulmonary pathology
  - central nervous system alteration
  - infection
  - dehydration
  - cardiac anomaly
  - electrolyte imbalance
  - immature or incompetent gastroesophageal sphincter
- Unknown cause

Primary Nursing Diagnosis: Ineffective breathing pattern related to specific condition such as: airway obstruction secondary to pulmonary pathology, central nervous system alteration, infection, dehydration, cardiac anomaly, electrolyte imbalance, immature or incompetent gastroesophageal sphincter, or unknown cause

Assessment/Defining Characteristics of Child and/or Family (Subjective & Objective Data):
- Cessation of breathing for 20 seconds or more
- Bradycardia
- Pallor
- Cyanosis
- Hypotonia
- Choking or gagging

Expected Outcomes	Possible Nursing Interventions	Rationale	Evaluation for Charting
Infant will have an effective breathing pattern as evidenced by • respiratory rate within acceptable range (state specific range) • heart rate within acceptable range (state specific range) • clear and equal breath sounds bilaterally A & P • oxygen saturation (via pulse oximeter) from 94 to 100% on room air • absence of 1. pallor 2. cyanosis 3. hypotonia 4. choking or gagging • lack of signs/symptoms of ineffective breathing pattern (such as those listed under Assessment)	Assess and record the following every 2 to 4 hours and PRN: • RR and HR • breath sounds • infant's color • infant's muscle tone • any signs/symptoms of ineffective breathing pattern (such as those listed under Assessment)	If the infant experiences an ineffective breathing pattern the RR and HR will change, the infant's color may change, the infant may become hypotonic, and the infant will work harder to breathe.	Document range of RR and HR. Describe breath sounds, infant's color, muscle tone, and any signs/symptoms of ineffective breathing pattern noted.
	When using a pulse oximeter, record reading every 1 to 2 hours and PRN.	Indirectly measures oxygen saturation and can be used to determine if treatment is effective or to indicate need for change in treatment.	Document range of oxygen saturation.
	Ensure that sleeping infant remains on apnea monitor with alarms appropriately set. Record frequency and duration of any apneic episodes. Record type and duration of stimulation needed.	Detects infant's heart rate and respirations. If either falls below the set parameters the monitor will alarm.	Describe any apneic episodes and type and effectiveness of stimulation.
	Assist with pneumogram, pneumocardiogram, or polysomnogram as needed.	Confirms the diagnosis.	Document results of any tests performed.
	Administer methylxanthines (e.g., theophylline or caffeine) on schedule. Assess and record effectiveness and any side effects (e.g., tachycardia, irritability, vomiting).	Helps to stimulate the respiratory drive.	Document whether medications were administered on schedule. Describe effectiveness and any side effects noted.

(continued)

	Primary Nursing Diagnosis: Ineffective Breathing Pattern *(continued)*		
Expected Outcomes	**Possible Nursing Interventions**	**Rationale**	**Evaluation for Charting**
TEACHING GOALS Family will be able to verbalize 4 signs/symptoms of ineffective breathing pattern such as • apneic episodes • color change from pink/tan to gray or blue • choking or gagging • decreased muscle tone	Teach family about characteristics of ineffective breathing pattern. Assess and record results.	Increased knowledge will assist the family in recognizing and reporting changes in the infant's condition.	Document whether teaching was done and describe results.
Family will be able to verbalize knowledge of care such as • correct use of apnea monitor • medication administration • identification of any signs/symptoms of ineffective breathing pattern (such as those listed under Assessment) • when to contact health-care provider	Teach family about care. Assess and record family's knowledge of and participation in care regarding correct use of apnea monitor, etc.	Education of family will allow for accurate care.	Document whether teaching was done and describe results.

Nursing Diagnosis Compromised Family Coping

Definition Decreased ability of family members to manage problems and concerns effectively

Possibly Related to
- Unknown cause of illness
- Hospitalization of infant
- Fear secondary to responsibility for infant's survival when infant is discharged from the hospital
- Stress, anxiety, and fatigue from having to respond to apnea monitor alarms

Nursing Diagnosis: Compromised family coping related to unknown cause of illness; hospitalization of infant; fear secondary to responsibility for infant's survival when infant is discharged from the hospital; stress, anxiety, and fatigue from having to respond to apnea monitor alarms

Assessment/Defining Characteristics of Child and/or Family (Subjective & Objective Data):

- Inability to leave infant's bedside
- Inappropriate emotions (e.g., anger) toward members of the health-care team
- Inability to meet own basic needs such as eating and resting

- Inability to ask for and accept outside help
- Failure to understand repeated explanations regarding illness, treatments, and procedures

Expected Outcomes	Possible Nursing Interventions	Rationale	Evaluation for Charting
Family will be able to cope effectively as evidenced by • ability to leave infant's bedside for short periods, especially to care for own basic needs such as eating meals and getting rest • appropriate expression of emotions toward staff or others • ability to express fears and concerns to members of the health-care team • ability to accept outside help when appropriate • verbalized understanding of explanations regarding the illness, treatments, and procedures • participation in infant's care	Assess and record family's stress level and ability to cope once a shift and PRN.	Provides information about family's coping ability.	Describe family's stress level.
	Communicate with family concerning infant's condition at least once/shift and PRN. This may require telephoning the family when members are not able to come to the hospital.	Helps to provide family with up-to-date, accurate information and can assist family with coping ability.	Document whether family received communication from the health-care team once/shift and if this was effective in helping family to cope.
	Encourage family to express feelings, fears, and concerns.	Provides data and assist health-care team in helping family to cope.	Describe any feelings, fears, or concerns expressed by family members.
	Encourage family members to meet own basic needs, such as eating and resting appropriately. Reassure family members that infant will be well cared for in their absence.	Provides family members with the ability to better meet their own and infant's needs.	Document whether family members were able to meet basic needs.
TEACHING GOALS Family will be able to verbalize 4 signs/symptoms of ineffective family coping such as • inability to leave infant's bedside • inappropriate emotions (e.g., anger) toward members of the health-care team	Teach family about characteristics of ineffective family coping. Assess and record results.	Increased knowledge will assist the family in recognizing and reporting changes.	Document whether teaching was done and describe results.

(continued)

Nursing Diagnosis: Compromised Family Coping *(continued)*			
Expected Outcomes	**Possible Nursing Interventions**	**Rationale**	**Evaluation for Charting**
• inability to meet own basic needs • inability to ask for or accept outside help			
Family will be able to verbalize knowledge of care such as • assistance with seeking outside help (e.g., a visiting nurse agency the electric company, a medical supply company, financial resources) • identification of any signs/symptoms of ineffective family coping (such as those listed under Assessment) • when to contact health-care provider	Teach family about care (effective coping). Assess and record family's knowledge of and participation in care regarding assistance with seeking outside help, etc.	Education of family will allow for accurate care.	Document whether teaching was done and describe results.

Related Nursing Diagnoses

Impaired Level of Consciousness*	*related to* hypoxia secondary to apneic episodes
Decreased Cardiac Output	*related to* bradycardia
Fear: Parental	*related to* a. breathing pattern of infant b. responsibility for infant's survival when infant is discharged
Grieving: Family	*related to* the possibility of infant's death

*Non-NANDA diagnosis.

TWO

ASTHMA/REACTIVE AIRWAY DISEASE
MEDICAL DIAGNOSIS

PATHOPHYSIOLOGY Asthma, or reactive airway disease, is the most common chronic respiratory disease of childhood, responsible for the majority of school absenteeism, physical disability, and hospitalization of children. Asthma continues to increase in prevalence, morbidity, and mortality in the United States and other nations. In the United States, asthma severity is greater in the urban minority groups of African Americans and Hispanics. It is an airway disease that is characterized by airway narrowing and hyperresponsiveness due to inflammation, bronchospasm, and tenacious secretions.

Asthma is a complex disorder in which clinical pattern, severity, and natural history of the disease vary considerably. Many factors—including biochemical, immunological, infectious, metabolic, and psychological—can be involved. The impact of these factors varies from individual to individual. The predominant risk factor for persistent asthma in childhood is a personal or family history of allergy. Allergy also influences the severity, as well as the persistence, of asthma. In the airways, there is an initial acute allergic reaction to a trigger, but there is also a delayed bronchial response that can persist for hours, days, or weeks.

Asthma is a chronic inflammatory disorder of the airways that involves multiple cell types. Asthma's pathophysiology reflects a complex interplay between airway inflammation, structural airway changes, and airway responsiveness. Even the youngest child with the mildest asthma has airway inflammation. The underlying inflammation found in asthmatic airways results from a complex orchestration of inflammatory cells (such as mast cells, eosinophils, T lymphocytes, and neutrophils), chemical mediators (such as histamines, leukotrienes, etc.), and chemotactic factors (such as cytokines, etc.).

The inflammation in asthma contributes to several processes in the airways of the lungs. These processes are airway hyperresponsiveness to various stimuli, pathologic airway changes, and airflow obstruction. Airway hyperresponsiveness is characterized by the airways constricting in response to allergens, irritants, viral infections, and exercise. Pathologic airway changes secondary to the inflammation include not only the influx of inflammatory cells into the airways, but airway edema, increased mucus production, epithelial cell damage, and airway remodeling. Airway remodeling is the irreversible thickening of the subepithelial basement membrane and proliferation of smooth muscle cells which, over time, may lead to irreversible structural changes (e.g., decreased airway elasticity) and a progressive loss of pulmonary function for the child. Forms of airflow obstruction include bronchoconstriction (acute, due to smooth muscle contraction or delayed, due to inflammation), airway edema, mucus plug formation, and airway wall remodeling. All of these forms of airflow obstruction can lead to the symptoms of cough, wheeze, shortness of breath, and chest tightness.

During asthma exacerbations, the occurrence of bronchospasms, mucosal edema, and mucus plugging causes the airways to narrow significantly, resulting in decreased expiratory airflow and hyperinflation of the lungs. These factors, along with the increasing severity of bronchial obstruction, lead to reduced alveolar ventilation with carbon dioxide retention, hypoxemia, respiratory acidosis, and eventually respiratory failure.

The diagnosis of asthma is made after a thorough history, physical examination, and if possible, objective measurement of pulmonary function (spirometry). The degree of airway inflammation is reflected in the severity of the child's signs and symptoms. The National Heart, Lung, and Blood Institute of the National Institutes of Health (NIH) has established recommendations for the classification of asthma severity (intermittent, mild persistent, moderate persistent, and severe persistent) and management guidelines, which are published in *Guidelines for the Diagnosis and Management of Asthma*. The frequency of daytime and nighttime symptoms, the frequency and severity of exacerbations, and lung function were used to determine these classifications and stepwise pharmacologic management.

Optimal treatment goals for a child with asthma include pharmacologic therapy, family and child education (including self-management skills, and environmental control). Currently, medications used for the treatment of asthma are divided into two categories, those used for long-term control and the prevention of symptoms and those used for quick relief of acute symptoms and exacerbations. Long-acting bronchodilators, inhaled corticosteroids, and leukotriene receptor antagonist or modifiers are used for long-term control and the prevention of symptoms. Methylxanthines (theophylline) and Cromolyn sodium (a nonsteroidal antiinflammatory drug) continue to be used as alternative therapies. Short-acting bronchodilators, anticholinergics, and systemic corticosteroids are used for quick relief of acute symptoms. Bronchial thermoplasty, a bronchoscopic procedure used to reduce the mass of airway smooth muscle and reduce bronchoconstriction, has resulted in improvement for those children with moderate to severe asthma.

Treatment goals for asthma exacerbations include provision of prompt relief of airflow obstruction with inhaled bronchodilators, the suppression and reversal of airway inflammation with systemic corticosteroids, and relief of hypoxemia with oxygen. Monitoring the child's response to therapy with serial measurements of respiratory function is essential. Education for the child and family begins at diagnosis and must be integrated into every step of care. A written asthma management plan must be provided.

Primary Nursing Diagnosis   Impaired Gas Exchange

Definition
Alteration in the exchange of oxygen and carbon dioxide in the lungs and/or at the cellular level

Possibly Related to
- Airway inflammation
- Spasms of the smooth muscles of the bronchi and bronchioles
- Accumulation of tenacious secretions
- Edema of the mucous membranes of the airways
- Allergies
- Respiratory infection

Primary Nursing Diagnosis: Impaired gas exchange related to airway inflammation, spasms of the smooth muscles of the bronchi and bronchioles, accumulation of tenacious secretions, edema of the mucous membranes of the airways, allergies, respiratory infection.

Assessment/Defining Characteristics of Child and/or Family (Subjective & Objective Data):

- Wheezing (expiratory and/or inspiratory)
- Decreased breath sounds
- Tachypnea
- Retractions
- Use of accessory muscles
- Nasal flaring
- Dyspnea
- Prolonged expiratory time
- Cough
- Crackles, rhonchi
- Tight feeling in the chest
- Inability to take a deep breath

- Anxiety
- Fatigue
- Hypoxia
- Hypercarbia
- Acidosis
- Cyanosis
- Hyperinflation of the lungs revealed on chest X-ray
- Tachycardia
- Restlessness
- Irritability
- Lethargy

Primary Nursing Diagnosis: Impaired Gas Exchange (continued)

Expected Outcomes	Possible Nursing Interventions	Rationale	Evaluation for Charting

Child will have adequate gas exchange as evidenced by
 	
• clear and equal breath sounds bilaterally A & P
• respiratory rate within acceptable range (state specific range)
• absence of
  1. retractions
  2. use of accessory muscles
  3. nasal flaring
  4. cough
  5. tightness in chest
  6. inability to take a deep breath
  7. extreme anxiety
  8. extreme fatigue
  9. extreme restlessness
  10. extreme irritability
  11. extreme lethargy
  12. cyanosis
	Assess and record the following every 2 to 4 hours and PRN:
	
	• breath sounds
	• RR, HR
	• signs/symptoms of impaired gas exchange (such as those listed under Assessment)
		If child experiences impaired gas exchange the RR and HR will change, and the child will work harder to breathe.	Document range of RR and HR. Describe breath sounds and any signs/ symptoms of impaired gas exchange noted.

	When using a pulse oximeter, record reading every 1 to 2 hours and PRN.	Pulse oximetry detects the oxygen saturation in the bloodstream. It is important to detect small changes in oxygen saturation before the child starts displaying overt characteristics of impaired gas exchange.	Document range of oxygen saturation.
• clear chest X-ray with appropriate A-P diameter • oxygen saturation (via pulse oximeter) from 94 to 100% on room air • arterial pH of 7.35 to 7.45	Assess and record arterial blood gas values when indicated. Report any abnormalities to the physician.	Provides data on child's oxygenation status (hypoxemia, hypercapnia). Determines if treatment is adequate or if a change in treatment is needed.	Document range of blood gas results and determine the physiologic process (e.g., respiratory acidosis). Describe any therapeutic measures used to improve arterial blood gas values. Document their effectiveness.
• $PaCO_2$ from 35 to 45 mmHg • PaO_2 from 75 to 100 mmHg	Check and record results of chest X-ray when indicated.	Changes in chest X-ray results may indicate need for a change in therapy.	Document results of chest X-ray when indicated.
• arterial bicarbonate level of 22 to 28 mEq/L • heart rate within acceptable range (state specific range)	Administer humidified oxygen in correct amount and route of delivery. Record percent of oxygen and route of delivery. Assess and record effectiveness of therapy.	Humidified oxygen will dilate the pulmonary vasculature, which increases surface area available for gas exchange. Extra source oxygen will also allow for better oxygenation to body tissues and thus help improve gas exchange.	Document amount and route of oxygen delivery. Describe effectiveness.
• lack of signs/ symptoms of impaired gas exchange (such as those listed under Assessment)	Keep head of bed elevated at a 30° to 45° angle.	Elevating the head of the bed to a 30° or 45° angle causes a shift of the abdominal contents downward and this in turn will allow for increased lung expansion in order to help improve gas exchange.	Document whether head of bed was kept elevated.

(continued)

Primary Nursing Diagnosis: Impaired Gas Exchange *(continued)*			
Expected Outcomes	**Possible Nursing Interventions**	**Rationale**	**Evaluation for Charting**
	Administer bronchodilators on schedule. Assess and record effectiveness and any side effects (e.g., tachycardia, GI disturbance).	Bronchodilators are administered to reverse the bronchoconstriction present in airways due to the inflammation, spasms, and accumulation of secretions.	Document whether bronchodilators were administered on schedule. Describe effectiveness and any side effects noted.
	Administer steroids on schedule. Assess and record effectiveness and any side effects (e.g., GI disturbance, headache).	Steroids are administered to reduce the inflammation present in the airways.	Document whether steroids were administered on schedule. Describe effectiveness and any side effects noted.
TEACHING GOALS Child and/or family will be able to verbalize 4 signs/symptoms of impaired gas exchange such as • wheezing • rapid respirations • retractions • cough • tight feeling in the chest • anxiety • lethargy	Teach child/family about characteristics of impaired gas exchange. Assess and record results.	Increased knowledge will assist the child/family in recognizing and reporting changes in the child's condition.	Document whether teaching was done and describe results.
Child and/or family will be able to verbalize knowledge of care such as • medication administration (preventive, routine, and rescue) • effective coughing in order to expectorate mucus • remaining calm while child is experiencing breathing difficulty; way to regain control in crisis situation (e.g., assist child by positioning, breathe with child to calm child) • use of peak flow meter	Teach child/family about care. Assess and record child's/family's knowledge of and participation in care regarding medication administration, etc.	Education of child/family will allow for accurate care.	Document whether teaching was done and describe results.

Expected Outcomes	Possible Nursing Interventions	Rationale	Evaluation for Charting
Primary Nursing Diagnosis: Impaired Gas Exchange *(continued)*			
• use of games (e.g., blowing bubbles through a straw) to practice breathing exercise • head elevated positioning • identification of any signs/symptoms of impaired gas exchange (such as those listed under Assessment) • when to contact health-care provider			

Nursing Diagnosis

Deficient Knowledge: Child/Family

Definition

Lack of information concerning the child's disease and care

Possibly Related to

- Unfamiliarity with child's disease
- Limited understanding of home management
- Immediate and continuing management of breathing difficulty

Nursing Diagnosis: Deficient knowledge: child/family related to unfamiliarity with child's disease, limited understanding of home management, immediate and continuing management of breathing difficulty

Assessment/Defining Characteristics of Child and/or Family (Subjective & Objective Data):

- Verbalization by child/family indicating a lack of knowledge regarding asthma and the care needed
- Relation of incorrect information to members of the health-care team
- Inability to correctly repeat information previously explained
- Inability to correctly demonstrate skills previously taught (e.g., medication administration)

Expected Outcomes	Possible Nursing Interventions	Rationale	Evaluation for Charting
TEACHING GOALS Child/family will have an adequate knowledge base concerning the child's illness and care as evidenced by • ability to correctly state information previously taught regarding	Listen to child's/family's concerns and fears. Document findings.	Allows child/family to express feelings and concerns and provides them with a way to gain knowledge.	Describe child's/family's concerns and fears and any successful measures used to encourage family to express their feelings.

(continued)

Nursing Diagnosis: Deficient Knowledge: Child/Family *(continued)*

Expected Outcomes	Possible Nursing Interventions	Rationale	Evaluation for Charting
asthma and child's care (e.g., how to allergy-proof the home, correct use of hand-operated inhalers, appropriate exercise activities like swimming) • ability to correctly demonstrate skills previously taught (e.g., medication administration) • ability to relate appropriate information to the health-care team • ability to request additional information and/or clarification of information	Assess and record child's/family's knowledge of and understanding of child's illness. Encourage questions.	Generates a baseline of knowledge, which allows for teaching of accurate information and dispelling of incorrect knowledge.	Document whether teaching was done and describe results.
	Provide child/family with information about asthma, including • breathing exercises. • medication administration (preventive, routine, and rescue) • use of peak flow meter. • identification of precipitating factors (e.g., stress, allergens, exercise) • environmental control (avoidance of second hand smoke) and ways to allergy-proof the home • use of written action plans • overdependence of child and/or overprotectiveness of family • support organizations (such as American Lung Association) • identification of any signs/symptoms of asthma • when to contact health-care provider.	Education of child/family will allow for accurate care and increase coping ability of child/family.	Document whether teaching was done and describe results. Describe ability of child/family to repeat information correctly and perform skills adequately.

Related Nursing Diagnoses

Fear: Child   *related to*
    a. respiratory distress
    b. treatments and procedures
    c. unfamiliar surroundings
    d. hospitalization

Deficient Fluid Volume   *related to*
    a. respiratory distress
    b. increased insensible water loss from rapid respiratory rate

Activity Intolerance   *related to*
    a. dyspnea
    b. fatigue

Compromised Family Coping   *related to*
    a. repeated hospitalization of child
    b. respiratory distress of child

THREE

BRONCHIOLITIS
MEDICAL DIAGNOSIS

PATHOPHYSIOLOGY Bronchiolitis is one of the most serious lower respiratory tract infections that affects young children. Bronchiolitis is a widespread inflammation and obstruction of the bronchioles resulting from a viral infection of the lower airways. The respiratory syncytial virus (RSV) is the causative organism in approximately 50 to 90% of diagnosed cases. There are 2 strains of RSV, A and B, with numerous genotypes and serotypes. This virus spreads easily through respiratory secretions and can be shed for prolonged periods. The infection usually occurs from October through April and is uncommon in children older than 2 years of age. Environmental (daycare attendance, exposure to passive smoke, etc.) and genetics (family members with asthma) contribute to the development and severity of the disease. Other causative organisms include the parainfluenza virus, rhinovirus, and adenovirus.

In bronchiolitis, the viral organism infects the bronchiolar epithelium with subsequent inflammation and submucosal edema. These changes contribute to the formation of mucus filled with cellular debris. The inflammation, edema, and mucus plugs cause areas of the small, distal airways to become partially or completely obstructed. The infant is able to get air into the lungs but has difficulty expelling it. Hyperinflation occurs where air has been trapped secondary to partial occlusion. Atelectasis develops where complete obstruction exists. This airway plugging can interfere with gas exchange, and the infant may develop hypoxemia, hypercarbia, and apnea.

The infant with bronchiolitis presents with an acute illness characterized by rhinorrhea, cough, and low-grade fever. The infant may be restless and drinking less. Clinical findings include tachypnea, nasal flaring, retractions, wheezes or crackles, with poor air movement and a prolonged expiratory phase. Secondary to ventilation-perfusion mismatch, hypoxemia may be present. Infants with underlying conditions, such as prematurity, bronchopulmonary dysplasia, cystic fibrosis, asthma, congenital heart disease, or immunodeficiencies may exhibit the complications of apnea or respiratory failure. The infant may also have conjunctivitis or otitis media. Hyperinflation and patchy infiltrates can be seen on chest x-ray. Viral diagnostic testing can be useful in limiting the inappropriate use of antibiotics and to indicate the type of infection control measures to implement.

The primary treatment for a hospitalized infant with bronchiolitis is supportive, and includes supplemental oxygen and hydration. Oxygen saturation should be performed routinely (as it indicates severity of disease and cyanosis is difficult to detect). Specific medications for the treatment of bronchiolitis remain controversial. Included in this list are bronchodilators, racemic epinephrine, corticosteroids, antibiotics, and Ribavirin (the most controversial antiviral agent). Prophylaxis for RSV (palivizumab) is currently being administered to premature and high-risk infants.

Primary Nursing Diagnosis   Ineffective Breathing Pattern

Definition   A breathing pattern that results in inadequate oxygen consumption (failure to meet the cellular requirements of the body)

Possibly Related to   • Inflammation of the lower airways secondary to a viral invasion

Primary Nursing Diagnosis: Ineffective breathing pattern related to inflammation of the lower airways secondary to a viral invasion

Assessment/Defining Characteristics of Child and/or Family (Subjective & Objective Data):

- Tachypnea
- Retractions at test
- Nasal flaring
- Crackles
- Dry, hacking cough
- Wheezing
- Decreased breath sounds
- Cyanosis
- Evidence of air trapping revealed on chest X-ray
- Tachycardia
- Low-grade fever

Expected Outcomes	Possible Nursing Interventions	Rationale	Evaluation for Charting

Infant will have an effective breathing pattern as evidenced by
 	
• respiratory rate within acceptable range (state specific range)
• clear and equal breath sounds bilaterally A & P
• absence of
  1. cough
  2. nasal flaring
  3. retractions
  4. cyanosis
• clear chest X-ray with acceptable A-P diameter
• oxygen saturation (via pulse oximeter) from 94 to 100% on room air
• arterial pH of 7.35 to 7.45
• $PaCO_2$ from 35 to 45 mmHg
• PaO_2 from 75 to 100 mmHg
• arterial bicarbonate level of 22 to 28 mEq/L
• temperature within acceptable range of 36.5° to 37.2°
• heart rate within acceptable range (state specific range)
• lack of signs/symptoms of ineffective breathing pattern (such as those listed under Assessment)
	Assess and record the following every 4 hours and PRN
	
	• RR, HR, and T
	• breath sounds
	• signs/symptoms of ineffective breathing pattern (such as those listed under Assessment). Notify physician of any abnormalities.
		If the infant experiences an ineffective breathing pattern the RR, HR, and T will change, and the infant will work harder to breath.	Document range of RR, HR, and T. Describe breath sounds and any signs/symptoms of ineffective breathing pattern noted.

	When using a pulse oximeter, record reading every 1 to 2 hours and PRN.	Indirectly measures oxygen saturation and can be used to determine if treatment is effective or to indicate need for change in treatment.	Document range of oxygen saturation.
	Assess and record arterial blood gas values when indicated. Report any abnormalities to the physician.	Provides data on infant's oxygenation status (hypoxemia, hypercapnia). Determines if treatment is adequate or if a change in treatment is needed.	Document range of blood gas results and determine the physiological process (e.g., respiratory acidosis). Describe any therapeutic measures used to improve arterial blood gas values. Document their effectiveness.
	Administered humidified oxygen in correct amount and route of delivery. Record percent of oxygen and route of delivery. Assess and record effectiveness of therapy.	Humidified oxygen will dilate the pulmonary vasculature, which increases surface area available for gas exchange. Extra source oxygen will also allow for better oxygenation to body tissues and thus help improve gas exchange.	Document amount and route of oxygen delivery. Describe effectiveness.

(continued)

Primary Nursing Diagnosis: Ineffective Breathing Pattern *(continued)*

Expected Outcomes	Possible Nursing Interventions	Rationale	Evaluation for Charting
	Keep head of bed elevated at a 30° angle (may use infant seat if infant can support head in midline position).	Elevating the head of the bed to a 30° angle causes a shift of the abdominal contents downward and this in turn will allow for increased lung expansion in order to help improve breathing pattern.	Document whether infant was kept in a head elevated position.
	When indicated, administer aerosolized bronchodilators on schedule. Assess and record effectiveness and any side effects (e.g., tachycardia, GI disturbance).	Bronchodilators are administered to dilate the airways that are narrowed due to the inflammation and accumulation of secretions.	Document whether bronchodilators were administered on schedule. Describe effectiveness and any side effects noted.
	When indicated, administer steroids on schedule. Assess and record effectiveness and any side effects (e.g., GI disturbance, hypertension).	Steroids are administered to reduce the inflammation present in the airways.	Document whether steroids were administered on schedule. Describe effectiveness and any side effects noted.
	When, indicated, administer aerosolized racemic epinephrine on schedule. Assess and record effectiveness and any side effects (e.g., tachycardia, hypertension).	Reduces upper airway obstruction and relieves respiratory distress by promoting relaxation of bronchial smooth muscle and inhibiting the release of histamine.	Document whether racemic epinephrine was administered on schedule. Describe effectiveness and any side effects noted.
	Administer antibiotics (that may be given for a secondary bacterial infection) on schedule. Assess and record any side effects (e.g., rash, diarrhea).	Antibiotics are given to combat infection.	Document whether antibiotics were administered on schedule. Describe any side effects noted.
	Ensure that contact isolation is maintained.	Necessary to prevent spread of infection.	Document whether contact isolation was maintained.
	Check and record results of chest X-ray when indicated.	Changes in chest X-ray results may indicate need for a change in therapy.	Document results of chest X-ray when indicated.
	Suction PRN if infant is unable to clear airway. Record amount and characteristics of secretions.	Suctioning assists in removing excess secretions and this in turn helps to improve breathing pattern.	Document frequency and type of suctioning if indicated. Describe amount and characteristics of secretions.

Primary Nursing Diagnosis: Ineffective Breathing Pattern *(continued)*

Expected Outcomes	Possible Nursing Interventions	Rationale	Evaluation for Charting
	When indicated, administer antipyretics on schedule. Assess and record effectiveness.	Antipyretics are used to reduce fever.	Document whether an antipyretic was needed and describe effectiveness.
TEACHING GOALS Family will be able to verbalize 4 signs/symptoms of ineffective breathing pattern such as • rapid respirations • nasal flaring • dry, hacking cough • wheezing • color change from pink/tan to gray or blue	Teach family about characteristics of ineffective breathing pattern. Assess and record results.	Increased knowledge will assist the family in recognizing and reporting changes in the infant's condition.	Document whether teaching was done and describe results.
Family will be able to verbalize knowledge of care such as • medication administration • identification of any signs/symptoms of ineffective breathing pattern (such as those listed under Assessment) • when to contact health-care provider	Teach family about care. Assess and record family's knowledge of and participation in care regarding medication administration, etc.	Education of family will allow for accurate care.	Document whether teaching was done and describe results.

Nursing Diagnosis

Deficient Fluid Volume

Definition   Decrease in the amount of circulating fluid volume

Possibly Related to
- Respiratory distress
- Decreased fluid intake
- Increased insensible water loss from rapid respirations

Nursing Diagnosis: Deficient fluid volume related to respiratory distress, decreased fluid intake, increased insensible water loss from rapid respirations

Assessment/Defining Characteristics of Child and/or Family (Subjective & Objective Data):

- Inability to tolerate fluids by mouth
- Decreased urine output
- Increased urine specific gravity
- Tachypnea
- Tachycardia
- Hypotension
- Dry mucous membranes
- Decreased skin turgor (skin recoil greater than 2 to 3 seconds)
- Sunken fontanel

Expected Outcomes	Possible Nursing Interventions	Rationale	Evaluation for Charting
Infant will have an adequate fluid volume as evidenced by • adequate fluid intake, IV and/or oral (state specific amount of intake needed for each child) • adequate urine output (state specific range; 1 to 2 ml/kg/hr) • urine specific gravity from 1.008 to 1.020 • respiratory rate, heart rate, and blood pressure within acceptable range (state specific range for each) • moist mucous membranes • flat fontanel • rapid skin recoil (less than 2 to 3 seconds) • lack of signs/ symptoms of deficient fluid volume (such as those listed under Assessment)	Keep accurate record of intake and output. When indicated, encourage oral fluids.	Provides information on infant's hydration status. Decreased urine output can indicate dehydration.	Document intake and output.
	Assess and record • IV fluids and condition of IV site every hour • RR, HR, BP, and signs/ symptoms of deficient fluid volume (such as those listed under Assessment) every 4 hours and PRN	Provides information about fluid status of the infant. If patient has deficient fluid volume, the HR will increase at first, and eventually decrease. The RR will increase. The BP will eventually decrease. It is necessary to record the amount of IV fluids every hour to make sure the child is not being over or under hydrated. The IV site needs to be assessed every hour for signs of redness or swelling. If RR is increased, the child may have insensible water loss contributing to dehydration.	Document amount of IV fluids and describe condition of IV site along with any interventions needed. Document range of RR, HR, and BP. Describe any signs/ symptoms of deficient fluid volume noted.
	Check and record urine specific gravity with every void or as indicated.	Urine specific gravity provides information about hydration status.	Document range of urine specific gravity.
	Assess and record condition of fontanel, mucous membranes, and skin turgor every shift and PRN.	Provides information on hydration status.	Describe status of fontanel, mucous membranes, and skin turgor.

Nursing Diagnosis: Deficient Fluid Volume *(continued)*

Expected Outcomes	Possible Nursing Interventions	Rationale	Evaluation for Charting
TEACHING GOALS Family will be able to verbalize at least 4 characteristics of deficient fluid volume such as • inability to tolerate fluids by mouth • decreased urine output • dry mucous membranes • sunken fontanel	Teach family about characteristics of deficient fluid volume. Assess and record results.	Increased knowledge will assist the family in recognizing and reporting changes in the child's condition.	Document whether teaching was done and describe results.
Family will be able to verbalize knowledge of care such as • infant's need for appropriate fluids • monitoring intake and output • identification of any signs/symptoms of deficient fluid volume (such as those listed under Assessment) • when to contact health-care provider	Teach family about care. Assess and record family's knowledge of and participation in care regarding infant's need for appropriate fluids, monitoring intake and output, etc.	Education of family will allow for accurate care.	Document whether teaching was done and describe results.

Related Nursing Diagnoses

Imbalanced Nutrition: Less than Body Requirements

related to
a. respiratory distress
b. refusal of solid foods
c. lethargy

Fear: Parental

related to
a. hospitalization of infant/child
b. knowledge deficit about disease state
c. stress of seeing infant with respiratory distress

Risk for Further Infection*

related to
a. increased respiratory secretions
b. young age of child

*Non-NANDA diagnosis.

FOUR

BRONCHOPULMONARY DYSPLASIA
MEDICAL DIAGNOSIS

PATHOPHYSIOLOGY Bronchopulmonary dysplasia (BPD) is a chronic lung disease associated with premature birth and early lung injury. Classic BPD is believed to be caused by exposure to high oxygen concentrations and prolonged or extended use of positive-pressure ventilation via endotracheal intubation or continuous positive airway pressure (CPAP). These treatments are used to treat infants with respiratory distress syndrome (also known as hyaline membrane disease). Risk factors such as fluid overload and patent ductus arteriosus (PDA) contribute to the lung injury in BPD. The pulmonary changes in classic BPD result in thickening and necrosis of the alveolar wall and bronchiolar lining, which impairs the diffusion of oxygen from the alveoli to the capillaries. Use of an endotracheal tube for mechanical ventilation impairs ciliary action, preventing clearance of mucus and resulting in airway obstruction, atelectasis, and cystlike patterns that indicate developing emphysema. The thickening of the alveolar walls leads to respiratory acidosis and results in pulmonary hypertension, which can lead to right heart failure. Long-term problems for a child with this severe form of BPD can include airway hyperreactivity, hyperexpansion, airway obstruction, increased incidence of respiratory infections, and growth failure.

With the discovery and use of surfactant and improved respiratory care, and the more common use of antenatal steroids, the classic form of BPD is occurring less frequently. A new form of chronic lung disease is occurring in an increasing number of small preterm infants. These infants are usually extremely low birth weight and require ventilatory support for apnea and poor respiratory effort. They also have received antenatal steroids, postnatal surfactant therapy, and are not exposed to high oxygen concentrations or aggressive ventilation. However, deterioration in lung function develops over time possibly due to trauma to the airways, hyperoxia, pulmonary edema, and/or sepsis. It is thought that inflammation plays a major role in the pathogenesis of this form of BPD. The inflammation can be triggered by such factors as ante- or postnatal systemic or pulmonary infections, free oxygen radicals, increased blood flow to the lungs due to a PDA, or ventilation with excessive tidal volumes. The lungs of the infants with this form of BPD reveal more uniform inflation and less fibrosis than those infants with "classic" BPD. Smooth muscle hypertrophy and fibrosis, along with both small and large airway epithelial metaplasia are also absent in this "new" BPD. Prematurity, the presence of a symptomatic PDA, and systemic infections are associated with a significantly higher risk for developing BPD. These infants with BPD are often rehospitalized with pneumonia, asthma exacerbations, respiratory syncytial virus (RSV) infection, or worsening BPD. Prophylaxis against viral infections has decreased the rates of rehospitalization.

The infant with BPD will present with varying degrees of respiratory compromise, depending on their current situation. He or she may have tachypnea, retractions, changes in breath sounds (such as wheezing and/or crackles), nasal flaring, and grunting. Over time, the chest becomes barrel shaped. The infant's coloring can be dusky or cyanotic. The chest radiograph of an infant with BPD will often show abnormalities, such as hyperexpansion or atelectasis (some of the structural changes will persist into adolescence or adulthood). The infant can be agitated or irritable. Fine and gross motor skills may be impaired, and there can be cognitive and/or speech delays. Many of these infants have failure to thrive and may require a nasogastric or gastrostomy tube in an attempt to receive adequate calories.

Goals of treatment in these infants start with preventing the disease in susceptible infants and avoiding progression of the disease while maintaining adequate oxygenation and lung function. Promoting growth and development is also important and a challenge in these children who have great metabolic needs. To achieve these goals treatment may include: lowest peak inspiratory pressure possible to minimize injury to the lung, lowest oxygen concentration possible, aerosolized or systemic bronchodilators, inhaled corticosteroids, diuretics, anti-inflammatories, electrolyte supplements, and fluid maintenance or restriction. A diet that provides adequate nutrition is vital to optimize lung growth and repair. The PDA may be managed with drugs or surgery. Many of these infants can be discharged home when their oxygen need is low and they are gaining weight. Education and ongoing support for the parents can smooth the transition home for these infants and their families.

Primary Nursing Diagnosis   Impaired Gas Exchange

Definition   Alteration in the exchange of oxygen and carbon dioxide in the lungs and/or at the cellular level

Possibly Related to
- Long-term ventilator therapy
- Barotrauma from mechanical ventilation
- Prolonged high oxygen concentrations
- Respiratory infection
- Systemic infection
- Increased blood flow going to the lungs through the patent ductus arteriosus
- Inflammatory response of airways

Primary Nursing Diagnosis: Impaired gas exchange related to long-term ventilator therapy, barotrauma from mechanical ventilation, prolonged high oxygen concentrations, respiratory infection, systemic infection, increased blood flow going to the lungs through the patent ductus arteriosus, inflammatory response of airways

Assessment/Defining Characteristics of Child and/or Family (Subjective & Objective Data):

- Tachypnea
- Retractions
- Crackles
- Diminished or unequal breath sounds
- Wheezing
- Barrel-chest appearance
- Cyanosis
- Tachycardia
- Resolving diffuse opacifications, atelectasis, and air cysts revealed on X-ray and indicating developing emphysema, flattened diaphragms, and hyperexpansion

Expected Outcomes	Possible Nursing Interventions	Rationale	Evaluation for Charting

Infant will maintain adequate gas exchange as evidenced by
 	
• respiratory rate within acceptable range (state specific range)
• clear and equal breath sounds bilaterally A & P
• absence of
  1. retractions
  2. cyanosis
• oxygen saturation (via pulse oximeter) from 94 to 100% on room air
• heart rate within acceptable range (state specific range)
• lack of signs/ symptoms of impaired gas exchange (such as those listed under Assessment)
	Assess and record the following every 2 to 4 hours and PRN:
	
	• breath sounds
	• RR and HR
	• signs/symptoms of impaired gas exchange (such as those listed under Assessment)
		If infant experiences impaired gas exchange the RR and HR will change and the infant will work harder to breathe.	Document range of RR and HR. Describe breath sounds and any signs/ symptoms of impaired gas exchange noted.

	Administer humidified oxygen in correct amount and route of delivery. Record percent of oxygen and route of delivery. Assess and record effectiveness of therapy.	Humidified oxygen will dilate the pulmonary vasculature, which increases surface area available for gas exchange. Extra source oxygen will also allow for better oxygenation to body tissues and thus help combat impaired gas exchange.	Document amount and route of oxygen delivery. Describe effectiveness.

(continued)

Primary Nursing Diagnosis: Impaired Gas Exchange *(continued)*

Expected Outcomes	Possible Nursing Interventions	Rationale	Evaluation for Charting
	Ensure that chest physiotherapy is done on schedule. Record effectiveness and infant's response to treatment.	Chest percussion loosens secretions and positioning can help to assist the flow of secretions out of the lungs by gravity. This will aid in improving gas exchange.	Document whether chest physiotherapy was done on schedule. Describe effectiveness and infant's response to treatment.
	Administer aerosolized or systemic bronchodilators on schedule. Assess and record effectiveness and any side effects (e.g., tachycardia, GI disturbance).	Aerosolized or systemic bronchodilators are administered to dilate the airways in order to improve gas exchange.	Document whether bronchodilators were administered on schedule. Describe effectiveness and any side effects noted.
	When using a pulse oximeter, record reading every 1 to 2 hours and PRN.	Pulse oximetry detects the oxygen saturation in the bloodstream. It is important to detect small changes in oxygen saturation before the infant starts displaying overt characteristics of impaired gas exchange.	Document range of oxygen saturation.
	Suction PRN if infant is unable to clear airway. Record amount and characteristics of secretions.	Suctioning assists in removing excess secretions and this in turn helps to improve gas exchange.	Document frequency and type of suctioning if indicated. Describe amount and characteristics of secretions.
	When indicated, administer inhaled steroids on schedule. Assess and record effectiveness and any side effects (e.g., GI disturbance, headache).	Inhaled steroids are administered to reduce the inflammation present in the airways.	Document whether inhaled steroids were administered on schedule. Describe effectiveness and any side effects noted.
	Administer diuretics on schedule. Assess and record effectiveness and any side effects noted (e.g., hypokalemia or dehydration).	Diuretics are given in order to decrease excess intravascular fluid through increased urine output, which will decrease the workload on the heart, thereby improving gas exchange.	Document whether diuretics were administered on schedule. Describe effectiveness and any side effects noted.

Primary Nursing Diagnosis: Impaired Gas Exchange *(continued)*

Expected Outcomes	Possible Nursing Interventions	Rationale	Evaluation for Charting
	Check and record results of chest X-ray when indicated.	Changes in chest X-ray results may indicate need for a change in therapy.	Document results of chest X-ray when indicated.
TEACHING GOALS Family will be able to verbalize 4 signs/symptoms of impaired gas exchange such as • rapid respirations • wheezing • retractions • color change from pink/tan to gray or blue	Teach family about characteristics of impaired gas exchange. Assess and record results.	Increased knowledge will assist the family in recognizing and reporting changes in the infant's condition.	Document whether teaching was done and describe results.
Family will be able to verbalize knowledge of care such as • medication administration • chest physiotherapy • setup, connection, and maintenance of oxygen therapy • suctioning of infant • infant CPR • identification of any signs/symptoms of impaired gas exchange (such as those listed under Assessment) • when to contact health-care provider	Teach family about care. Assess and record family's knowledge of and participation in care regarding medication administration, etc.	Education of family will allow for accurate care.	Document whether teaching was done and describe results.

Nursing Diagnosis   Excess Fluid Volume

Definition

Increase in the amount of circulating fluid volume (which can eventually lead to interstitial or intracellular fluid overload)

Possibly Related to

• Increased pulmonary vascular resistance
• Right heart failure

Nursing Diagnosis: Excess fluid volume related to increased pulmonary vascular resistance, right heart failure

Assessment/Defining Characteristics of Child and/or Family (Subjective & Objective Data):
- Sudden weight gain
- Edema
- Tachypnea
- Crackles
- Deceased urine output
- Increased urine specific gravity (greater than 1.020)
- Hepatosplenomegaly

Expected Outcomes	Possible Nursing Interventions	Rationale	Evaluation for Charting
Infant will resume appropriate fluid balance as evidenced by • adequate urine output (state specific range; 1 to 2 ml/kg/hr) • respiratory rate within acceptable range (state specific range) • clear and equal breath sounds bilaterally A & P • urine specific gravity from 1.008 to 1.020 • lack of 1. sudden weight gain 2. edema 3. hepatosplenomegaly • lack of signs/ symptoms of excess fluid volume (such as those listed under Assessment)	Keep accurate record of intake and output. Be sure infant does not exceed maximal intake ordered.	Fluids may need to be restricted in order to decrease extravascular fluid volume and pulmonary congestion.	Document intake and output.
	Assess and record • amount and location of edema at least once/ shift and PRN • RR and breath sounds every 4 hours and PRN • signs/symptoms of excess fluid volume (such as those listed under Assessment) every 4 hours and PRN	Edema is due to fluid retention. RR will change with fluid retention and breath sounds will become abnormal (crackles) if pulmonary congestion is present.	Describe amount and location of edema. Document range of RR. Describe breath sounds. Describe any signs/symptoms of excess fluid volume (such as those listed under Assessment).
	Check and record urine specific gravity every 4 hours or as indicated.	Urine specific gravity provides information about hydration status.	Document range of urine specific gravity.
	Weigh infant daily on same scale at same time of day. Document results and compare to previous weight.	Provides information about the infant's fluid status. An increase in the weight can indicate fluid retention. A decrease in the weight can indicate dehydration.	Document weight and determine if it was an increase or decrease from the previous weight.
	Administer diuretics on schedule. Assess and record effectiveness and any side effects noted (e.g., hypokalemia or dehydration).	Diuretics are given in order to decrease excess intravascular fluid through increased urine output, which will decrease the workload on the heart.	Document whether diuretics were administered on schedule. Describe effectiveness and any side effects noted.

Nursing Diagnosis: Excess Fluid Volume *(continued)*

Expected Outcomes	Possible Nursing Interventions	Rationale	Evaluation for Charting
TEACHING GOALS Family will be able to verbalize 4 signs/symptoms of excess fluid volume such as • sudden weight gain • edema • rapid respirations • decreased urine output	Teach family about characteristics of excess fluid volume. Assess and record results.	Increased knowledge will assist the family in recognizing and reporting changes in the infant's condition.	Document whether teaching was done and describe results.
Family will be able to verbalize knowledge of care such as • monitoring intake and output • medication administration • monitoring weight • identification of any signs/symptoms of excess fluid volume (such as those listed under Assessment) • when to contact health-care provider	Teach family about care. Assess and record family's knowledge of and participation in care regarding monitoring intake and output, medication administration, etc.	Education of family will allow for accurate care.	Document whether teaching was done and describe results.

Related Nursing Diagnoses

Decreased Cardiac Output	*related to* a. pulmonary hypertension b. right heart failure
Imbalanced Nutrition: Less than Body Requirements	*related to* a. maximal respiratory effort requiring increased caloric consumption secondary to respiratory distress b. difficulty sucking and breathing simultaneously c. fatigue
Compromised Family Coping	*related to* a. need for repeated hospitalizations b. difficulty in obtaining competent babysitters c. financial burden d. delayed infant growth and development e. guilt (unfounded) when infant becomes ill and has to be admitted to the hospital
Risk for Infection	*related to* increased pulmonary secretions

FIVE

CYSTIC FIBROSIS
MEDICAL DIAGNOSIS

PATHOPHYSIOLOGY Cystic fibrosis (CF) is one of the most common fatal genetic disorders in the United States. It is an autosomal recessive disease, meaning that both parents must be carriers and contribute one defective gene for a child to be born with CF. Each child born in these families has a 25% chance of having the disease, a 50% chance of being a carrier, and a 25% chance of neither having the disease nor being a carrier. More than 95% of all documented cases affect white persons. Although it is rare, CF does also occur in the African American, Hispanic, and Asian populations. Gender is not a factor in incidence. Prenatal diagnosis is now possible, and some states provide newborn screening for CF. Although genotyping is currently available, clinical criteria, family history, and the sweat test remain important in making a diagnosis of CF. A sweat test with a chloride concentration of 60 mEq/L or greater is considered diagnostic. The sweat of individuals with CF has abnormally high sodium and chloride concentrations; parents frequently complain of their infants tasting "salty" when kissed.

Cystic fibrosis is caused by a defect in a single gene isolated on the long arm of chromosome 7. This mutation results in abnormalities in the production or function of a protein product of the gene. This protein product is known as the cystic fibrosis transmembrane conductance regulator (CFTR). It resides on the apical membrane lining the airways, biliary tree, intestines, vas deferens, sweat ducts, and pancreatic ducts. In the absence of functional CFTR, there is decreased chloride secretion and increased sodium absorption due to a defective chloride-ion transport across the exocrine and epithelial cells. Secretions of the respiratory, gastrointestinal, and reproductive systems become more viscous or precipitate and obstruct the ducts. This in turn leads to plugging, dysfunction, and damage at the organ level, reduction in fluid volume, an exaggerated inflammatory response, decreased bacterial killing, and increased sodium reabsorption. All body organs with mucus ducts become affected.

The child with CF usually exhibits symptoms of a classic diagnostic triad that includes chronic pulmonary disease, pancreatic insufficiency, and elevated sweat chloride concentrations. The hepatic and reproductive systems are also affected. The progression and severity of the clinical manifestations in children with CF vary greatly.

All parts of the respiratory tract (nasal epithelium, sinuses, airways, and lungs) can be affected in a child with CF. Cough is the predominant symptom in the early stages of CF. The cough becomes classic as the lungs are filled with thick mucus, which the respiratory cilia cannot clear. Hyperinflation and atelectasis result as air becomes trapped in the small airways. Opacification of the sinuses is very common, nasal polyps are less common. Clubbing of the distal phalanges of the fingers and toes may be present due to chronic fibrotic changes within the lungs. Involvement of the lung by the CF disease process accounts for most of the morbidity and mortality from CF.

Frequent pulmonary exacerbations are the usual course of CF lung disease. *Haemophilus influenzae*, *Staphylococcus aureus*, and *P. aeruginosa* are the most prevalent early pathogens. Bacterial infection and its subsequent intense inflammatory response cause hypertrophy and hyperplasia of the mucus-secreting apparatus and progressive damage to the airway wall. Throughout his or her life the person with CF experiences the vicious cycle of infection, inflammation, and airway damage. Chronic lung infections, host response, and airway damage contribute to progressive obstructive lung disease, followed by respiratory insufficiency. Pulmonary complications include hemoptysis and pneumothorax.

In a child with CF, gastrointestinal symptoms result when abnormal secretions obstruct the pancreatic ducts, preventing essential pancreatic enzymes from reaching the duodenum. This results in malabsorption of fats and proteins, and a deficiency of fat-soluble vitamins. Many children experience failure to thrive due to the poor digestion and malabsorption. Steatorrhea (fatty stools) and azotorrhea (nitrogen loss in the stool) are common. Rectal prolapse is a common gastrointestinal complication of children with CF, especially during infancy or early childhood, when the child experiences frequent loosely formed foul-smelling stools. Some infants may present in the newborn period with meconium ileus. Eventually constipation becomes a common problem partially due to blockage of the bowel by the thick secretions. In older children, intestinal obstruction may occur.

The reproductive system of both males and females are affected by cystic fibrosis. In males, the blockage or absence of the vas deferens causes sterility. Females have difficulty conceiving because of the thickened mucous secretions in the reproductive tract that interfere with the passage of sperm, or because of chronic illness.

The goals in the management of a child with CF include: to delay and prevent the development of lung disease, to prevent and minimize pulmonary complications, to promote adequate nutrition for normal growth, to treat any other complications of the disease, and to support the child and family in adapting to a chronic disease. Therapies for managing pulmonary problems in a child with CF are directed at preventing and treating infections by improving aeration; thinning, loosening, and removing mucopurulent secretions; and administering antibiotics (orally, intravenously, or aerosolized). The course of treatment may also include the administration of bronchodilators, recombinant human deoxyribonuclease (DNase), corticosteroids, and/or other anti-inflammatory medications and oxygen. Chest physiotherapy (CPT) remains essential to maintain pulmonary hygiene. Lung or heart-lung transplantations remain options for those with end-stage CF. Good nutrition and growth are promoted by pancreatic enzyme replacement, fat-soluble vitamin replacement, and a high-protein, high-calorie diet. Double-lung transplantation is considered for those in the end sages of CF.

For those with CF, the mean age of survival has been increasing steadily during the past 3 decades, currently hovering around 30 years of age, but there are also long-term survivors. The focus of research for new technologies and treatment modalities has changed from treatment of the end results of CF to determining how to lessen the effects of the CFTR mutation and deal more directly with the defect. For the children with CF and their families, these changes increase the probability that they will survive into adulthood.

Primary Nursing Diagnosis   Ineffective Airway Clearance

Definition Condition in which secretions cannot adequately be cleared from the airways

Possibly Related to
- Excessive mucus
- Bacterial infection

Primary Nursing Diagnosis: Ineffective airway clearance related to excessive mucus, bacterial infection

Assessment/Defining Characteristics of Child and/or Family (Subjective & Objective Data):
- Decreased breath sounds
- Cough
- Tachypnea
- Dyspnea
- Wheezes, diffuse crackles, and rhonchi
- Use of accessory muscles for breathing
- Frequent respiratory infections
- Barrel-chest
- Cyanosis
- Digital clubbing
- Tachycardia

Expected Outcomes	Possible Nursing Interventions	Rationale	Evaluation for Charting
Child will have adequate airway clearance as evidenced by • clear and equal breath sounds bilaterally A & P • respiratory rate within acceptable range (state specific range) • heart rate within acceptable range (state specific range)	Assess and record the following every 4 hours and PRN • RR and HR • breath sounds • amount and characteristics of secretions • signs/symptoms of ineffective airway clearance (such as those listed under Assessment)	If child experiences ineffective airway clearance the RR and HR will increase and the breath sounds may be abnormal. It is important to record the amount and characteristics of secretions in order to detect changes (such as increase in the amount and color change of secretions).	Document range of RR and HR. Describe breath sounds, amount and characteristics of secretions, and any signs/symptoms of ineffective airway clearance noted.

(continued)

Primary Nursing Diagnosis: Ineffective Airway Clearance *(continued)*

Expected Outcomes	Possible Nursing Interventions	Rationale	Evaluation for Charting

• oxygen saturation (via pulse oximeter) from 94 to 100% on room air
• absence of
  1. constant cough
  2. dyspnea
  3. cyanosis
• lack of signs/ symptoms of ineffective airway clearance (such as those listed under Assessment)
	Ensure chest physiotherapy is performed on schedule. Encourage child to cough during and after treatment. Assess and record effectiveness of treatments.	Chest percussion loosens secretions and positioning can help to assist the flow of secretions out of the lungs by gravity. This will aid in improving airway clearance.	Document whether chest physiotherapy was done on schedule. Describe effectiveness and child's response to treatment.

	Administer aerosolized bronchodilators on schedule. Assess and record effectiveness and any side effects (e.g., tachycardia, dizziness).	Bronchodilators are administered to dilate the airways that are narrowed by the accumulation of thick secretions and inflammation.	Document whether bronchodilators were administered on schedule. Describe effectiveness and any side effects noted.
	Administer antibiotics (orally, intravenous, and/ or aerosolized) on schedule. Assess and record any side effects (e.g., rash, diarrhea).	Antibiotics are administered to combat respiratory infection.	Document whether antibiotics were administered on schedule. Describe any side effects noted.
	Administer corticosteroids on schedule. Assess and record effectiveness and any side effects (e.g., GI disturbance, headache).	Steroids are administered to reduce the inflammation present in the airways.	Document whether steroids were administered on schedule. Describe effectiveness and any side effects noted.
	Administer aerosolized recombinant human deoxyribonuclease (e.g., Pulmozyme) on schedule. Assess and record effectiveness and any side effects (e.g., sore throat, rash).	Decreases the viscosity of mucus in the airways.	Document whether recombinant human deoxyribonuclease medications were administered on schedule. Describe effectiveness and any side effects noted.
	When indicated, administer humidified oxygen in correct amount and route of delivery. Record percent of oxygen and route of delivery. Assess and record effectiveness of therapy.	Humidified oxygen will dilate the pulmonary vasculature, which increases surface area available for gas exchange.	Document amount and route of oxygen delivery. Describe effectiveness.
	Check and record results of chest X-ray when indicated.	Changes in chest X-ray results may indicate need for a change in therapy.	Document results of chest X-ray when indicated.
	Encourage fluid intake (240 ml 8 times/24 hours).	Helps to thin secretions.	Document intake.

Primary Nursing Diagnosis: Ineffective Airway Clearance (*continued*)

Expected Outcomes	Possible Nursing Interventions	Rationale	Evaluation for Charting
	Instruct child to spit out secretions in a tissue and dispose of tissue in waste container.	Helps to decrease spread of infection.	Document whether child was compliant with secretion disposal.
	When using a pulse oximeter, record reading every 1 to 2 hours and PRN.	Pulse oximetry detects the oxygen saturation in the bloodstream. It is important to detect small changes in oxygen saturation before the child starts displaying overt characteristics of ineffective airway clearance.	Document range of oxygen saturation.
TEACHING GOALS Child and/or family will be able to verbalize 4 signs/symptoms of ineffective airway clearance such as • rapid respirations • increased coughing • use of accessory muscles for breathing • color change from pink/tan to gray or blue	Teach child/family about characteristics of ineffective airway clearance. Assess and record results.	Increased knowledge will assist the child/family in recognizing and reporting changes in the child's condition.	Document whether teaching was done and describe results.
Child and/or family will be able to verbalize knowledge of care such as • medication administration • chest physiotherapy • central line (portacath) care • identification of any signs/symptoms of ineffective airway clearance (such as those listed under Assessment) • when to contact health-care provider	Teach child/family about care. Assess and record child's/family's knowledge of and participation in care regarding medication administration, chest physiotherapy, etc.	Education of child/family will allow for accurate care.	Document whether teaching was done and describe results.

Nursing Diagnosis Imbalanced Nutrition: Less Than Body Requirements

Definition Insufficient nutrients to meet body requirements

Possibly Related to
- Malabsorption secondary to absence of pancreatic enzymes
- Infection

Nursing Diagnosis: Imbalanced nutrition: less than body requirements related to malabsorption secondary to absence of pancreatic enzymes, infection			
Assessment/Defining Characteristics of Child and/or Family (Subjective & Objective Data): • Failure to gain weight • Voracious appetite (together with a failure to gain weight due to malabsorption) • Malabsorption of fat-soluble vitamins		• Frequent foul-smelling, loosely formed, bulky stools • Steatorrhea (fatty stools) • Azotorrhea (nitrogen loss in the stool)	
Expected Outcomes	**Possible Nursing Interventions**	**Rationale**	**Evaluation for Charting**
Child will be adequately nourished as evidenced by • absorption of adequate amount of calories, parenterally and/or orally (state specific amount for each child, usually 1½ to 2 times RDA for age for children with CF) • steady weight gain or lack of weight loss • lack of signs/symptoms of imbalanced nutrition (such as those listed under Assessment)	Keep accurate record of intake and output.	Provides information on child's hydration status.	Document intake and output.
	Assess and record any signs/symptoms of imbalanced nutrition (such as those listed under Assessment) every 8 hours and PRN.	Provides information on nutritional status of child.	Describe any signs/symptoms of imbalanced nutrition noted.
	Weigh child daily on same scale at same time of day. Document results and compare to previous weight.	Provides information on child's hydration and nutritional status. Decrease in weight may be due to malabsorption.	Document weight and determine if it was an increase or decrease from the previous weight.
	If indicated, maintain and record daily calorie counts.	Provides information on actual caloric intake.	Document calorie count if indicated.
	Assess child's food likes/dislikes and, when possible, provide foods that child likes to eat.	Encourages child to eat.	Describe any therapeutic measures used to maintain adequate nutrition. Document their effectiveness.
	Offer between-meal snacks and high caloric supplements. When indicated, administer gastrostomy tube feedings on schedule.	Increases caloric intake.	Describe any therapeutic measures used to maintain adequate nutrition. Document their effectiveness.

Nursing Diagnosis: Imbalanced Nutrition: Less than Body Requirements *(continued)*

Expected Outcomes	Possible Nursing Interventions	Rationale	Evaluation for Charting
	Organize care to conserve energy.	Conserving energy will help to maintain adequate nutrition.	Describe any therapeutic measures used to maintain adequate nutrition. Document their effectiveness.
	Administer oral pancreatic enzymes on schedule (before meals and snacks). It may be necessary to disguise the taste of the enzymes in foods such as applesauce. Assess and record effectiveness.	Needed for replacement. Aids in digestion.	Document weather pancreatic enzymes were administered on schedule. Describe effectiveness.
	Administer multivitamins and fat-soluble vitamins (in a water-miscible preparation) on schedule.	Multivitamins are needed to prevent vitamin deficiency and fat-soluble vitamins are needed for replacement.	Document if vitamins were administered on schedule.
	Initiate consultation with dietician, when indicated.	Provides nutritional support for child and/or family regarding adequate nutrition.	Document if dietician was consulted.
TEACHING GOALS Child and/or family will be able to verbalize at least 3 characteristics of imbalanced nutrition such as • failure to gain weight • frequent foul-smelling, loosely formed, bulky stools • decreased appetite	Teach child/family about characteristics of imbalanced nutrition. Assess and record results.	Increased knowledge will assist the child/family in recognizing and reporting changes in the child's condition.	Document whether teaching was done and describe results.
Child and/or family will be able to verbalize knowledge of care such as • medication administration • monitoring intake and output • care of gastrostomy tube, when indicated	Teach child/family about care. Assess and record child's/family's knowledge of and participation in care regarding medication administration, monitoring intake and output, etc.	Education of child/family will allow for accurate care.	Document whether teaching was done and describe results.

(continued)

Nursing Diagnosis: Imbalanced Nutrition: Less than Body Requirements *(continued)*			
Expected Outcomes	**Possible Nursing Interventions**	**Rationale**	**Evaluation for Charting**
• consultation with dietician when indicated • identification of any signs/symptoms of imbalanced nutrition (such as those listed under Assessment) • when to contact health-care provider			

Related Nursing Diagnoses

Compromised Family Coping *related to*
    a. child's long-term illness
    b. fatal disease
    c. financial considerations
    d. guilt secondary to the genetic nature of the disease

Deficient Knowledge: Child/Family *related to*
    a. disease state and prognosis
    b. treatments and procedures
    c. home care maintenance

Disturbed Body Image *related to*
    a. child's chronic long-term illness
    b. delayed development of secondary sex characteristics
    c. copious amounts of viscid, purulent sputum
    d. inability to maintain average weight

Risk for Infection *related to* invasion of the respiratory tract by bacterial organisms

Grieving *related to* presence of chronic and fatal illness

SIX

FOREIGN BODY ASPIRATION
MEDICAL DIAGNOSIS

PATHOPHYSIOLOGY Foreign body aspiration is a common occurrence in children. A child can potentially aspirate any object put into the mouth, which can then lead to serious illness or death. Children 6 months to 4 years are most commonly affected. Food items are most frequently aspirated, with nuts, popcorn, uncut hot dogs, and grapes being common hazards. Older children and preteens tend to aspirate nonfood items such as buttons, coins, paperclips, and small toy parts. Balloon aspiration can be fatal.

Any section of the airway, from the larynx to the bronchi, may be the site of a foreign body aspiration (FBA). Normally the airways expand on inspiration and contract on expiration. This helps explain the different degrees of obstruction possible. If a particle is very small, air could flow in and out around the object. Usually a wheeze is audible in this situation. When an aspirated object is a little larger, it may allow air to enter the airways, but the air distal to the obstruction is trapped during expiration due to narrowing of the airways on expiration. Some aspirated objects can be large enough to obstruct airflow in and out of the airways. The air distal to the obstruction is absorbed, and atelectasis results. The right main stem bronchus is the most common site because it is shorter and wider than the left main stem bronchus and comes off the trachea in a straighter angle.

The clinical manifestations and degree of severity of FBA depend on the child's age, what has been aspirated and its location, and the time lapsed since the aspiration. Initially, the child may exhibit coughing, choking, gasping, and respiratory distress because of airway obstruction. A phase where the child may not have any symptoms follows. Next, symptoms of complications such as infection may develop. Whenever a child is afebrile and has a sudden onset of respiratory distress, FBA should be considered.

Imaging studies can often assist with the diagnosis for foreign body aspiration, but they have limitations. Between 50 and 70% of children with FBA will have a normal chest film. Radiographs initially are the most useful, but computed tomography (CT) scans and fluoroscopy may be needed in children who have persistent symptoms. At times, the diagnosis of FBA is delayed. The reasons for this can be either physician- or parent-related. Parental delay in seeking medical care for the child is usually because the aspiration episode was unwitnessed or symptoms were mild or absent. Physician-related factors contributing to a delay in diagnosis include the child having a normal chest film or symptoms leading to misdiagnosis.

Removal of the foreign body by rigid bronchoscopy or laryngoscopy should be done as soon as possible. Having a foreign object in the airways triggers a progressive inflammatory process, or a chemical pneumonia may develop. The food matter can soften making removal difficult. After the foreign object is removed, the child may require high humidity, pulmonary toilet, antibiotics, and bronchodilators.

Primary Nursing Diagnosis   Ineffective Airway Clearance

Definition   Condition in which secretions cannot adequately be cleared from the airways

Possibly Related to   • Airway obstruction by a small object (specify if object can be identified)

Primary Nursing Diagnosis: Ineffective airway clearance related to airway obstruction by a small object (specify if object can be identified)

Assessment/Defining Characteristics of Child and/or Family (Subjective & Objective Data):

INITIAL CHARACTERISTICS

- Choking
- Rhonchi
- Wheezing
- Gagging

- Sudden, periodic coughing
- Periods during which child is asymptomatic for days or weeks after initial onset of symptoms

SECONDARY CHARACTERISTICS

- Fever
- Tachypnea
- Tachycardia
- Dyspnea
- Asymmetrical chest expansion

- Decreased breath sounds over affected area
- Recurrent pneumonia
- Diaphragm low and fixed on the obstructed side as revealed on expiration chest X-ray (sometimes)

LOCATIONAL CHARACTERISTICS

- **Larynx:**
  1. hoarseness
  2. croupy cough
  3. inspiratory stridor
  4. inability to vocalize
- **Trachea:**
  1. cough

  2. dyspnea
  3. hoarseness
  4. cyanosis
- **Bronchus:**
  1. cough
  2. blood-tinged sputum
  3. dyspnea

Expected Outcomes	Possible Nursing Interventions	Rationale	Evaluation for Charting
Child will have adequate airway clearance as evidenced by • respiratory rate within acceptable range (state specific range) • heart rate within acceptable range (state specific range) • clear and equal breath sounds bilaterally A & P • symmetrical chest expansion • thin, clear secretions • ability to vocalize • oxygen saturation (via pulse oximeter) from 94 to 100% on room air • temperature within acceptable range of 36.5° to 37.2°	Assess and record the following every 4 hours and PRN: • RR, HR, and T • breath sounds • amount and characteristics of secretions • signs/symptoms of ineffective airway clearance (such as those listed under Assessment)	If child experiences ineffective airway clearance the RR and HR will increase, and the breath sounds may be abnormal. It is important to record the amount and characteristics of secretions in order to detect changes (such as increase in the amount and color change of secretions). If a respiratory infection is present the T will increase.	Document range of RR, HR, and T. Describe breath sounds, amount and characteristics of secretions, and any signs/symptoms of ineffective airway clearance noted.

Primary Nursing Diagnosis: Ineffective Airway Clearance (*continued*)

Expected Outcomes	Possible Nursing Interventions	Rationale	Evaluation for Charting
• lack of signs/symptoms of ineffective airway clearance (such as those listed under Assessment)	When using a pulse oximeter, record reading every 1 to 2 hours and PRN.	Pulse oximetry detects the oxygen saturation in the bloodstream. It is important to detect small changes in oxygen saturation before the child starts displaying overt characteristics of ineffective airway clearance.	Document range of oxygen saturation.
	When indicated, administer humidified oxygen in correct amount and route of delivery. Record percent of oxygen and route of delivery. Assess and record effectiveness of therapy.	Humidified oxygen will dilate the pulmonary vasculature, which increases surface area available for gas exchange.	Document amount and route of oxygen delivery. Describe effectiveness.
	When indicated, administer antipyretics on schedule. Assess and record effectiveness.	Antipyretics are used to reduce fever.	Document whether an antipyretic was needed and describe effectiveness.
	Administer aerosolized bronchodilators on schedule. Assess and record effectiveness and any side effects (e.g., tachycardia, GI disturbance).	Bronchodilators are administered to dilate the airways that are narrowed by the accumulation of secretions and inflammation secondary to the foreign body.	Document whether bronchodilators were administered on schedule. Describe effectiveness and any side effects noted.
	Administer antibiotics on schedule. Assess and record any side effects (e.g., rash, diarrhea).	Antibiotics are administered to combat respiratory infection.	Document whether antibiotics were administered on schedule. Describe any side effects noted.
	Explain to child/family any indicated treatments or procedures and their rationale.	Provides knowledge and rationale for treatments or procedures.	Document if teaching was done and describe child's/family's response to explanation.
	Prepare child for surgical treatments such as bronchoscopy.	Surgical treatments may be necessary to remove foreign body.	Describe child's level of tolerance for any procedures that might have been done, such as bronchoscopy.

(*continued*)

Primary Nursing Diagnosis: Ineffective Airway Clearance *(continued)*			
Expected Outcomes	**Possible Nursing Interventions**	**Rationale**	**Evaluation for Charting**
	Keep child NPO following bronchoscopy until gag reflex has fully returned. Ensure that a high humidity atmosphere is maintained following procedure.	If the gag reflex has not fully returned, the child could aspirate if fluids or food are given. A high humidity atmosphere is needed to prevent drying and irritation of the airways and facilitate removal of secretions.	If bronchoscopy is done, document whether high-humidity mist is maintained and whether the child's gag reflex returns.
	If indicated, ensure chest physiotherapy is performed on schedule. Assess and record effectiveness of treatments.	Chest percussion loosens secretions and positioning can help to assist the flow of secretions out of the lungs by gravity. This will aid in improving airway clearance.	Document whether chest physiotherapy was done on schedule. Describe effectiveness and child's response to treatment.
	Check and record results of chest X-ray, CT scans, and/or fluoroscopy when indicated.	Changes in chest X-ray, CT scans, or fluoroscopy results may indicate need for a change in therapy.	Document results of chest X-ray, CT scan, and/or fluoroscopy when indicated.
TEACHING GOALS Child and/or family will be able to verbalize 4 signs/symptoms of ineffective airway clearance such as • choking • gagging • sudden, periodic coughing • hoarseness • color change from pink/tan to gray or blue	Teach child/family about characteristics of ineffective airway clearance. Assess and record results.	Increased knowledge will assist the child/family in recognizing and reporting changes in the child's condition.	Document whether teaching was done and describe results.
Child and/or family will be able to verbalize knowledge of care such as • back blows or abdominal thrust to loosen or expel aspirated items (Heimlich maneuver) • hazards of aspiration in relation to developmental age of child	Teach child/family about care. Assess and record child's/family's knowledge of and participation in care regarding safety and age related aspiration hazards, medication administration, etc.	Education of child/family will allow for accurate care.	Document whether teaching was done and describe results.

Primary Nursing Diagnosis: Ineffective Airway Clearance (continued)			
Expected Outcomes	**Possible Nursing Interventions**	**Rationale**	**Evaluation for Charting**
• medication administration • chest physiotherapy • identification of any signs/symptoms of ineffective airway clearance (such as those listed under Assessment) • when to contact health-care provider			

Nursing Diagnosis   Fear: Child

Definition   Feeling of apprehension resulting from a known cause

Possibly Related to
- Respiratory distress
- Unfamiliar surroundings
- Forced contact with strangers
- Treatments and procedures
- Hospitalization

Nursing Diagnosis: Fear: child related to respiratory distress, unfamiliar surroundings, forced contact with strangers, treatments and procedures, hospitalization

Assessment/Defining Characteristics of Child and/or Family (Subjective & Objective Data):
- Uncooperativeness
- Regressed behavior
- Hostile behavior
- Decreased communication
- Decreased attention span
- Verbal expression of fear to the health-care team
- Restlessness
- Constant crying
- Tachypnea
- Tachycardia
- Diaphoresis

Expected Outcomes	**Possible Nursing Interventions**	**Rationale**	**Evaluation for Charting**
Child will exhibit only a minimal amount of fear as evidenced by • ability to relate appropriately to family members • ability to rest and sleep between treatments and procedures	Assess and record any physiological signs/symptoms of fear manifested by the child (e.g., increased respiratory rate, increased heart rate, diaphoresis), level of child's fear, and the source of the fear every 4 hours and PRN.	Provides information about the level of fear and possibly the source of the fear. If child is experiencing fear, the RR and HR will increase.	Document RR, HR, level of child's fear, and any identified sources of the fear.

(continued)

	Nursing Diagnosis: Fear: Child *(continued)*		
Expected Outcomes	**Possible Nursing Interventions**	**Rationale**	**Evaluation for Charting**
• lack of constant crying • respiratory rate within acceptable range (state specific range) • heart rate within acceptable range (state specific range) • lack of diaphoresis • lack of signs/ symptoms of fear (such as those listed under Assessment)	Decrease child's fears when possible by • encouraging family members to stay with child • encouraging child/family members to participate in care • assigning same staff members to provide care for child • spending extra time with child when family members are unable to be present • encouraging family members to bring in familiar articles and toys from home	These measures will help to make the child more comfortable and can help to decrease fear.	Document any measures used to help alleviate fear. Document effectiveness of measures.
	Initiate age-appropriate therapeutic play when indicated. Document effectiveness.	Play can be a useful distraction or outlet to help decrease fears.	Document whether therapeutic play was used and its effectiveness.
	Encourage child to express fears to members of the health-care team.	Expression and identification of fears can help the child find ways to manage these fears.	Document any identified fears.
TEACHING GOALS Child and/or family will be able to verbalize at least 4 characteristics of fear such as • uncooperativeness • regressed behavior • hostile behavior • decreased communication • verbal communication of fear	Teach child/family about characteristics of fear. Assess and record results.	Increased knowledge will assist the child/ family in recognizing and reporting changes in the child's condition.	Document whether teaching was done and describe results.

Nursing Diagnosis: Fear: Child *(continued)*			
Expected Outcomes	**Possible Nursing Interventions**	**Rationale**	**Evaluation for Charting**
Child and/or family will be able to verbalize knowledge of care such as • appropriate diversional activities • identification of any signs/symptoms of fear (such as those listed under Assessment) • when to contact health-care provider	Teach child/family about care. Assess and record child's/family's knowledge of and participation in care regarding appropriate diversional activities, etc.	Education of child/family will allow for accurate care.	Document whether teaching was done and describe results.

Related Nursing Diagnosis

Deficient Fluid Volume   *related to*
 a. dyspnea
 b. choking

Risk for Infection   *related to*
 a. aspiration
 b. invasive procedures

Deficient Knowledge: Parental   *related to* care and safety of a young child

SEVEN

LARYNGOTRACHEOBRONCHITIS/ VIRAL CROUP
MEDICAL DIAGNOSIS

PATHOPHYSIOLOGY Laryngotracheobronchitis (LTB), the most common form of the croup syndromes, is a viral infection that affects the larynx, trachea, and bronchi, thus involving both the upper and lower airways. The viral organism invades the mucosa lining of the airways, resulting in inflammation and edema. The inflammation and edema narrow the airways, sometimes obstructing them. This obstruction is greatest in the subglottic area, usually the narrowest part of the airways. The hallmark sound of children with LTB is inspiratory stridor, a shrill, harsh, "crowing" respiratory sound. This sound is the result of increased velocity and turbulence of airflow through a narrowed (extrathoracic) airway. When air passes through the constricted airway, the negative pressure tends to further narrow the already comprised airway, producing the stridor sound.

Laryngotracheobronchitis is more common in boys than in girls and typically occurs in children between 6 months and 6 years of age, with the peak incidence at 18 months of age. The most common viral agents causing LTB are parainfluenza viruses (types 1 and 3)

(65% of cases), influenza viruses, rhinoviruses, and the respiratory syncytial virus (RSV). Most cases of laryngotracheobronchitis occur during the late fall and early winter, which corresponds to the seasonal prevalence of the pathogens.

The child with LTB usually presents with a history of upper airway congestion, low-grade or no fever, and the classic clinical findings of a hoarse voice, inspiratory stridor, and a barking cough, which tends to be worse at night. In severe cases of croup, the inspiratory stridor is audible when the child is at rest and other signs of respiratory distress, such as nasal flaring and intercostal retractions, are present. Neck radiographs may be used to confirm the diagnosis. The classical "steeple sign" in the subglottal area will usually be visible on the anteroposterior radiograph.

The main goals of treatment for the child with laryngotracheobronchitis are airway maintenance and provision for adequate airway exchange. This is usually accomplished with a combination of humidified air or oxygen, nebulized epinephrine (racemic epinephrine), and corticosteroids.

Primary Nursing Diagnosis   Ineffective Breathing Pattern

Definition   Breathing pattern that results in inadequate oxygen consumption (failure to meet the cellular requirements of the body)

Possibly Related to   • Viral infection of the larynx, trachea, and bronchi

---

Primary Nursing Diagnosis: Ineffective breathing pattern related to viral infection of the larynx, trachea, bronchi

Assessment/Defining Characteristics of Child and/or Family (Subjective & Objective Data):

- Tachypnea
- Inspiratory stridor
- Hoarseness
- "Barky" cough
- Dyspnea
- Diminished breath sounds bilaterally
- Crackles and rhonchi
- Substernal, intercostal and/or suprasternal retractions
- Nasal flaring
- Fever
- Tachycardia
- Irritability and restlessness
- Cyanosis (late sign)

Primary Nursing Diagnosis: Ineffective Breathing Pattern (continued)

Expected Outcomes	Possible Nursing Interventions	Rationale	Evaluation for Charting

Child will have an effective breathing pattern as evidenced by
 	
• respiratory rate within acceptable range (state specific range)
• clear and equal breath sounds bilaterally A & P
• heart rate within acceptable range (state specific range)
• oxygen saturation (via pulse oximeter) from 94 to 100% on room air
• temperature within acceptable range of 36.5° to 37.2°
• **Absence of**
  1. hoarseness
  2. "barky" cough
  3. extreme irritability
  4. retractions
• **Absence of signs/symptoms or increasing respiratory obstruction**
  1. inspiratory stridor at rest
  2. tachypnea at rest
  3. tachycardia
  4. circumoral or orbital cyanosis
  5. restlessness
• **Absence of signs/symptoms of respiratory failure**
  1. listlessness
  2. decrease in stridor and retractions without clinical improvement
  3. diminished breath sounds
• lack of signs/symptoms of ineffective breathing pattern (such as those listed under Assessment)
	Assess and record the following every 4 hours and PRN:
	
	• RR, HR, and T
	• breath sounds
	• signs/symptoms of ineffective breathing pattern (such as those listed under Assessment). Notify physician of any abnormalities.
		If the child experiences an ineffective breathing pattern the RR, HR, and T will change, and the child will work harder to breathe.	Document range of RR, HR, and T. Describe breath sounds and any signs/symptoms of ineffective breathing pattern noted.

	When using a pulse oximeter, record reading every 1 to 2 hours and PRN.	Indirectly measures oxygen saturation and can be used to determine if treatment is effective or to indicate need for change in treatment.	Document range of oxygen saturation.
	If indicated, ensure that cool mist is administered by ordered route of delivery.	Cool mist is believed to soothe the inflammation of the larynx and may help to thin airway secretions.	Document whether cool mist was administered and the route of delivery. Describe effectiveness.
	Administer aerosolized bronchodilators (such as racemic epinephrine) on schedule. Assess and record effectiveness and any side effects (e.g., tachycardia, GI disturbance).	Bronchodilators are administered to dilate the airways that are narrowed due to the inflammation and accumulation of secretions.	Document whether bronchodilators were administered on schedule. Describe effectiveness and any side effects noted.
	When indicated, administer antipyretics on schedule. Assess and record effectiveness.	Antipyretics are used to reduce fever.	Document whether an antipyretic was needed and describe effectiveness.
	If indicated, administer antibiotics on schedule. Assess and record any side effects (e.g., rash, diarrhea).	Antibiotics may be given to combat a secondary infection that may be present.	Document whether antibiotics were administered on schedule. Describe any side effects noted.

(continued)

Primary Nursing Diagnosis: Ineffective Breathing Pattern *(continued)*

Expected Outcomes	Possible Nursing Interventions	Rationale	Evaluation for Charting
	If indicated, administer steroids (such as dexamethasone) on schedule. Assess and record effectiveness and any side effects (e.g., GI disturbance, hypertension).	Steroids are administered to reduce the inflammation present in the upper and lower airways.	Document whether steroids were administered on schedule. Describe effectiveness and any side effects noted.
	When indicated, administer humidified oxygen in correct amount and route of delivery. Record percent of oxygen and route of delivery. Assess and record effectiveness of therapy. Be aware that more than 40% oxygen may mask symptoms of increasing respiratory distress.	Humidified oxygen will dilate the pulmonary vasculature, which increases surface area available for gas exchange.	Document amount and route of oxygen delivery. Describe effectiveness.
	Assess and record arterial blood gas values when indicated. Report any abnormalities to the physician.	Provides data on infant's oxygenation status (hypoxemia, hypercapnia). Determines if treatment is adequate or if a change in treatment is needed.	Document range of blood gas results and determine the physiological process (e.g., respiratory acidosis). Describe any therapeutic measures used to improve arterial blood gas values. Document their effectiveness.
	Deep suction only if specifically ordered. Record amount and characteristics of secretions.	Suctioning assists in removing excess secretions and this in turn helps to improve breathing pattern.	Document frequency and type of suctioning if indicated. Describe amount and characteristics of secretions.
	Provide rest and a quiet atmosphere.	Helps to decrease work of breathing.	Document whether a restful and quiet atmosphere was provided. Describe effectiveness.
TEACHING GOALS Family will be able to verbalize 4 signs/symptoms of ineffective breathing pattern such as • inspiratory stridor • hoarseness • "barky" cough • color change from pink/tan to gray or blue	Teach family about characteristics of ineffective breathing pattern. Assess and record results.	Increased knowledge will assist the family in recognizing and reporting changes in the child's condition.	Document whether teaching was done and describe results.

Primary Nursing Diagnosis: Ineffective Breathing Pattern *(continued)*

Expected Outcomes	Possible Nursing Interventions	Rationale	Evaluation for Charting
Family will be able to verbalize knowledge of care such as • delivery of cool mist via humidifier at home • maintenance of home humidifier (cleaning of unit) • mist provided by steaming up bathroom (constant and careful supervision will be needed) • medication administration • identification of any signs/symptoms of ineffective breathing pattern (such as those listed under Assessment) • when to contact health-care provider	Teach family about care. Assess and record family's knowledge of and participation in care regarding delivery of cool mist via humidifier, medication administration, etc.	Education of family will allow for accurate care.	Document whether teaching was done and describe results.

Nursing Diagnosis   Deficient Fluid Volume

Definition   Decrease in the amount of circulating fluid volume

Possibly Related to

- Respiratory difficulty
- Sore throat resulting in decreased intake by mouth
- Increased insensible water loss from rapid respirations
- Fever

Nursing Diagnosis: Deficient fluid volume related to respiratory difficulty, sore throat resulting in decreased intake by mouth, increased insensible water loss from rapid respirations, fever

Assessment/Defining Characteristics of Child and/or Family (Subjective & Objective Data):

- Anorexia
- Inability to tolerate fluids by mouth
- Decreased urine output
- Vomiting
- Tachypnea
- Tachycardia
- Hypotension

- Fever
- Malaise
- Dry mucous membranes
- Decreased skin turgor (skin recoil greater than 2 to 3 seconds)
- Increased urine specific gravity

Expected Outcomes	Possible Nursing Interventions	Rationale	Evaluation for Charting
Child will have an adequate fluid volume as evidenced by • adequate fluid intake, IV and/or oral (state specific amount of intake needed for each child) • adequate urine output (state specific range; 1 to 2 ml/kg/hr) • urine specific gravity from 1.008 to 1.020 • moist mucous membranes • rapid skin recoil (less than 2 to 3 seconds) • respiratory rate, heart rate, and blood pressure within acceptable range (state specific range for each) • temperature within acceptable range of 36.5° to 37.2° • absence of anorexia, vomiting, and malaise • lack of signs/symptoms of deficient fluid volume (such as those listed under Assessment)	Keep accurate record of intake and output. When indicated, encourage oral fluids.	Provides information on child's hydration status. Decreased urine output can indicate dehydration.	Document intake and output.
	Assess and record • IV fluids and condition of IV site every hour • RR, HR, and T every 4 hrs and PRN • signs/symptoms of deficient fluid volume (such as those listed under Assessment) every 4 hours and PRN	Provides information about fluid status of patient. It is necessary to record the amount of IV fluids every hour to make sure the child is not being over or under hydrated. The IV site needs to be assessed every hour for signs of redness or swelling. If patient has deficient fluid volume, the HR will increase at first, and eventually decrease. The BP will eventually decrease. If RR and T are increased, the child may have insensible water loss contributing to dehydration.	Document amount of IV fluids and describe condition of IV site along with any interventions needed. State range of RR, HR, BP, and T. Describe any signs/symptoms of deficient fluid volume noted.
	Check and record urine specific gravity with every void or as indicated.	Urine specific gravity provides information about hydration status.	Document range of urine specific gravity.
	Provide mouth care every 4 hours and PRN.	Mouth care is necessary to counteract the dry mucous membranes.	Document whether mouth care was done and describe effectiveness.
TEACHING GOALS Family will be able to verbalize at least 4 characteristics of	Teach family about characteristics of deficient fluid volume. Assess and record results.	Increased knowledge will assist the family in recognizing and reporting changes in the child's condition.	Document whether teaching was done and describe results.

	Possible Nursing		Evaluation for
Expected Outcomes	**Interventions**	**Rationale**	**Charting**
deficient fluid volume such as • anorexia • inability to tolerate fluids by mouth • vomiting • decreased urine output • fever			
Family will be able to verbalize knowledge of care such as • child's need for appropriate fluids • monitoring intake and output • identification of any signs/symptoms of deficient fluid volume (such as those listed under Assessment) • when to contact health-care provider	Teach family about care. Assess and record family's knowledge of and participation in care regarding child's need for appropriate fluids, monitoring intake and output, etc.	Education of family will allow for accurate care.	Document whether teaching was done and describe results.

Nursing Diagnosis: Deficient Fluid Volume *(continued)*

Related Nursing Diagnoses

Fear: Child

related to
a. respiratory distress
b. unfamiliar surroundings
c. forced contact with strangers
d. treatments and procedures
e. confinement to mist area

Activity Intolerance

related to
a. respiratory difficulty
b. fatigue
c. confinement to mist area

Acute Pain

related to sore throat

Compromised Family Coping

related to
a. respiratory distress of child
b. hospitalization of child
c. guilt secondary to delay in seeking health care
d. knowledge deficit regarding home care

EIGHT

PERTUSSIS (WHOOPING COUGH)
MEDICAL DIAGNOSIS

PATHOPHYSIOLOGY Pertussis, or whooping cough, is an acute bacterial respiratory infection caused by *Bordetella pertussis*, a highly communicable gram-negative coccobacillus. This organism multiplies only in association with the respiratory epithelial cells, causing necrosis and desquamation of the superficial epithelium. When this process occurs in the small bronchi, bronchopneumonia develops. The accumulation of mucus secretions can also result in bronchiolar obstruction and atelectasis.

Transmission of *B. pertussis* occurs with exposure to the aerosol droplets from the respiratory tract of infected individuals or from direct contact with their nasopharyngeal secretions. The incubation period is usually 7 to 10 days. Although pertussis can occur at any age, severe illness is most common in infants and young children. Infants and young children are frequently infected by older siblings and adults who have a mild or atypical illness. Approximately 80% of susceptible persons become infected with pertussis after close contact with an infected household member. Immunization has reduced the incidence and mortality rate of pertussis, but it does not provide permanent or complete immunity. Two new booster vaccines for adolescents and adults, Boostrix and Adacel, produce antibodies that may decline at the same rate following natural *B. pertussis* infection. These vaccines help prevent the spread of the disease from adolescents and adults to infants and children.

Pertussis progresses through three stages. During the catarrhal stage, which lasts 1 to 2 weeks, the symptoms of a mild upper respiratory tract infection, such as runny nose, sneezing, and cough, are present. The paroxysmal stage, lasting 2 to 4 weeks, is characterized by a paroxysmal or spasmodic cough, accompanied by a characteristic inspiratory whoop. Coughing spasms are often followed by vomiting. During the convalescent stage, which usually lasts 1 to 2 weeks, the severity and frequency of the symptoms gradually decrease, although the cough may persist for several months. Paroxysmal cough and post-tussive vomiting are the most common presenting symptoms. Complications of pertussis include apneic episodes, pneumonia, dehydration, weight loss, seizures, and, rarely, encephalopathy or death. Nasopharyngeal cultures confirm the diagnosis of a pertussis infection.

The treatment of pertussis is supportive and may include hydration, nutrition, oxygen, and cardiorespiratory monitoring for complications. The American Academy of Pediatrics (AAP) recommends erythromycin as treatment to prevent transmission of pertussis. Gastrointestinal side effects (such as nausea, emesis, and diarrhea) and increased risk of pyloric stenosis in infants younger than 2 months can occur with erythromycin. Newer generation macrolides (e.g., azithromycin [Zithromax] and clarithromycin [Biaxin]) have less risk of side effects and similar bacterial eradication rates as erythromycin. Corticosteroids, bronchodilators, antihistamines, and pertussis-specific immunoglobulin are sometimes used as adjunct therapies. If children are not treated during the catarrhal stage, they are considered contagious until 3 weeks after the paroxysmal stage ends or until 5 days after starting antibiotics. Antibiotic prophylaxis is recommended in those who are in close contact with the infected individual, especially incompletely immunized persons who are also in close contact with high-risk children. The hospital infection control team and local public health officials should be notified of all suspected and confirmed cases of pertussis.

Primary Nursing Diagnosis   Ineffective Airway Clearance

Definition   Condition in which secretions cannot adequately be cleared from the airways

Possibly Related to
- Accumulation of mucus secretions, including mucus plugs
- Bacterial infection of the lungs
- Spasmodic coughing episodes

Primary Nursing Diagnosis: Ineffective airway clearance related to accumulation of mucus secretion, including mucus plugs; bacterial infection of the lungs; spasmodic coughing episodes

Assessment/Defining Characteristics of Child and/or Family (Subjective & Objective Data):

- Severe paroxysms of cough with an inspiratory whoop, often followed by vomiting
- Possible facial redness, cyanosis, bulging eyes, protrusion of the tongue, tearing, salivation, and distension of neck veins accompanying coughing episodes
- Diminished breath sounds
- Diffuse rhonchi and crackles
- Perihilar infiltrates, atelectasis, or emphysema revealed on chest X-ray
- Tachypnea
- Fever
- Tachycardia
- Apneic episodes
- Lethargy

Expected Outcomes	Possible Nursing Interventions	Rationale	Evaluation for Charting
Child will have adequate airway clearance as evidenced by • clear and equal breath sounds bilaterally A & P • respiratory rate within acceptable range (state specific range) • oxygen saturation (via pulse oximeter) from 94 to 100% on room air • clear chest X-ray with appropriate A-P diameter • lack of spasmodic coughing episodes • lack of lethargy • lack of apneic episodes • temperature within acceptable range of 36.5° to 37.2° • heart rate within acceptable range (state specific range) • lack of signs/symptoms of ineffective airway clearance (such as those listed under Assessment)	Assess and record the following every 4 hours and PRN: • breath sounds, RR, HR, and T • coughing episodes and any accompanying signs • amount and characteristics of secretions • signs/symptoms of ineffective airway clearance or respiratory distress (such as those listed under Assessment)	If child experiences ineffective airway clearance the RR, HR, T, and breath sounds may be abnormal. If coughing episodes increase this may diminish airway clearance. It is important to record the amount and characteristics of secretions in order to detect changes (such as increase in the amount and color change of secretions).	Document range of RR, HR, and T. Describe breath sounds, coughing episodes, amount and characteristics of secretions, and any signs/symptoms of ineffective airway clearance noted.
	When using a pulse oximeter, record reading every 1 to 2 hours and PRN.	Pulse oximetry detects the oxygen saturation in the blood stream. It is important to detect small changes in oxygen saturation before the child starts displaying overt characteristics of ineffective airway clearance.	Document range of oxygen saturation.
	Administer antibiotics on schedule. Assess and record any side effects (e.g., rash, diarrhea).	Antibiotics are administered to combat respiratory infection.	Document whether antibiotics were administered on schedule. Describe any side effects noted.
	When indicated, administer corticosteroids on schedule. Assess and record effectiveness and any side effects (e.g., GI disturbance, hypertension).	Steroids are administered to reduce the inflammation present in the airways.	Document whether steroids were administered on schedule. Describe effectiveness and any side effects noted.

(continued)

Primary Nursing Diagnosis: Ineffective Airway Clearance *(continued)*

Expected Outcomes	Possible Nursing Interventions	Rationale	Evaluation for Charting
	When indicated, administer aerosolized bronchodilators on schedule. Assess and record effectiveness and any side effects (e.g., tachycardia, GI disturbance).	Bronchodilators are administered to dilate the airways that are narrowed by the accumulation of thick secretions and inflammation.	Document whether bronchodilators were administered on schedule. Describe effectiveness and any side effects noted.
	When indicated, administer pertussis-specific immunoglobulin. Assess and record effectiveness and any side effects noted (e.g., rash, mild headache).	Immunoglobulins are administered to enhance respiratory and systemic immune response.	Document whether immunoglobulins were administered on schedule. Describe effectiveness and any side effects noted.
	When indicated, administer humidified oxygen in correct amount and route of delivery. Record percent of oxygen and route of delivery. Assess and record effectiveness of therapy.	Humidified oxygen will dilate the pulmonary vasculature, which increases surface area available for gas exchange.	Document amount and route of oxygen delivery. Describe effectiveness.
	Encourage fluid intake (e.g., 240 ml 8 times/ 24 hours).	Helps to thin secretions.	Document intake.
	Ensure chest physiotherapy is performed on schedule. Assess and record effectiveness of treatments.	Chest percussion loosens secretions and positioning can help to assist the flow of secretions out of the lungs by gravity. This will aid in improving airway clearance.	Document whether chest physiotherapy was done on schedule. Describe effectiveness and child's response to treatment.
	Suction gently PRN if infant or child is unable to clear airway. Record amount and characteristics of secretions.	Suctioning assists in removing excess secretions and this in turn in helps to improve breathing pattern.	Document frequency and type of suctioning if indicated. Describe amount and characteristics of secretions.
	Ensure that respiratory isolation is maintained.	Necessary to prevent spread of infection.	Document whether respiratory isolation was maintained.
	Check and record results of chest X-ray when indicated.	Changes in chest X-ray results may indicate need for a change in therapy.	Document results of chest X-ray when indicated.

Primary Nursing Diagnosis: Ineffective Airway Clearance *(continued)*

Expected Outcomes	Possible Nursing Interventions	Rationale	Evaluation for Charting
	Keep head of bed elevated at a 30° angle (may use infant seat if infant can support head in midline position).	Elevating the head of the bed to a 30° angle causes a shift of the abdominal contents downward and this in turn will allow for increased lung expansion in order to help improve breathing pattern.	Document whether head of bed was kept elevated.
TEACHING GOALS Family will be able to verbalize 4 signs/symptoms of ineffective airway clearance such as • severe paroxysms of cough with an inspiratory whoop, often followed by vomiting • facial redness, bulging eyes, protrusion of the tongue • lethargy • color change from pink/tan to gray or blue	Teach family about characteristics of ineffective airway clearance. Assess and record results.	Increased knowledge will assist the family in recognizing and reporting changes in the child's condition.	Document whether teaching was done and describe results.
Family will be able to verbalize knowledge of care such as • identification and avoiding triggers of the coughing episodes (e.g., lying flat in bed). • medication administration • chest physiotherapy • prophylaxis treatment for family members • identification of any signs/symptoms of ineffective airway clearance (such as those listed under Assessment) • when to contact health-care provider	Teach family about care. Assess and record family's knowledge of and participation in care regarding medication administration, etc.	Education of family will allow for accurate care.	Document whether teaching was done and describe results.

Nursing Diagnosis   Fear: Parental

Definition   Feeling of apprehension resulting from a known cause

Possibly Related to
- Child's spasmodic coughing episodes
- Child's acute illness
- Hospitalization of infant or young child
- Communicability of child's illness to siblings
- Guilt if child has not been immunized
- Feelings of dread regarding child's outcome
- Apprehension surrounding child's coughing episodes

Nursing Diagnosis: Fear: parental related to child's spasmodic coughing episodes, child's acute illness, hospitalization of infant or young child, communicability of child's illness to siblings, guilt if child has not been immunized, feelings of dread regarding child's outcome, apprehension surrounding child's coughing episodes

Assessment/Defining Characteristics of Child and/or Family (Subjective & Objective Data):
- Avoidance of child or inability to leave child's side
- Decreased attention span
- Decreased communication
- Inability to participate in child's care
- Reports of somatic discomfort

Expected Outcomes	Possible Nursing Interventions	Rationale	Evaluation for Charting
Parents will exhibit only a minimal amount of fear as evidenced by • decreased reports of somatic discomfort • ability to leave child's bedside for short periods, especially to care for own basic needs such as eating meals and getting rest • ability to express fears to members of the health-care team or supportive family and friends • participation in child's care • ability to verbalize understanding of explanations regarding child's illness, treatments, and procedures	Assess and record level of parental fear and the source of the fear.	Provides information about the level of fear and possibly the source of the fear.	Document level of fear and any identified sources of the fear.
	Decrease parents' fears when possible by • encouraging family members to stay with child. • encouraging family members to participate in care. • assigning same staff members to provide care for child. • spending extra time with child when family members are unable to be present. • encouraging family members to bring in familiar articles and toys from home. • explaining to family what to expect during this recovery phase.	These measures will help to make the parents be more comfortable and can help to decrease fear.	Document any measures used to help alleviate fear. Describe effectiveness of measures.

Nursing Diagnosis: Fear: Parental *(continued)*			
Expected Outcomes	**Possible Nursing Interventions**	**Rationale**	**Evaluation for Charting**
	Encourage parents to express fears to members of the health-care team.	Expression and identification of fears can help the parents to find ways to manage these fears.	Document any identified fears.
	Encourage parents to meet basic needs, such as eating and resting appropriately. Assist them as needed.	Assist parents in decreasing stress, which can help to identify and alleviate fears.	Document whether parents were able to separate for short periods so that they could meet their own basic needs.
	Listen as parents express fears. If possible, encourage mastery of the situation (e.g., identifying and avoiding triggers of child's cough, responding appropriately to a coughing episode).	Expression and identification of fears can help the parents to find ways to manage these fears.	Document any identified fears and describe any measures used to help decrease parental fears.
TEACHING GOALS Parents will be able to verbalize at least 4 characteristics of fear such as • avoidance of child or inability to leave child's side • decreased attention span • decreased communication • inability to participate in child's care	Teach parents about characteristics of fear. Assess and record results.	Increased knowledge will assist the parents in recognizing and reporting changes in the child's condition.	Document whether teaching was done and describe results.
Parents will be able to verbalize knowledge of care such as • identifying and avoiding trigger of child's cough • responding appropriately to a coughing episode • identification of any signs/symptoms of fear (such as those listed under Assessment) • when to contact health-care provider	Teach parents about care. Assess and record parents' knowledge of and participation in care regarding responding appropriately to a coughing episode, etc.	Education of parents will allow for accurate care.	Document whether teaching was done and describe results.

Related Nursing Diagnoses

Ineffective Breathing Pattern	*related to* a. spasmodic coughing episodes b. infection of the lungs
Deficient Fluid Volume	*related to* a. vomiting after spasmodic coughing episodes b. decreased fluid intake c. drinking triggering spasmodic cough d. fever
Imbalanced Nutrition: Less than Body Requirements	*related to* a. vomiting after spasmodic coughing episodes b. decreased food intake c. eating triggering spasmodic cough d. increased caloric need related to increased energy expenditure secondary to fever or work of breathing
Impaired Home Maintenance	*related to* a. communicable disease b. lack of knowledge

NINE

PNEUMONIA
MEDICAL DIAGNOSIS

PATHOPHYSIOLOGY Pneumonia is an inflammation of the lungs characterized by consolidation due to exudate filling the alveoli and bronchioles. Once the lower respiratory tract has been infected, the normal inflammatory response occurs, along with the accompanying airway obstruction. Blood is shunted around these nonfunctioning areas, resulting in hypoxemia. Pneumonia usually occurs as a primary disease or less commonly, after hematogenous spread. It can be localized to one specific area (lobular pneumonia) or disseminated throughout the lungs (bronchopneumonia). The causative organism can be bacterial, viral, or mycoplasmal. Bacterial pneumonia is commonly caused by pneumococcus, streptococcus, or staphylococcus. The respiratory syncytial virus (RSV) is the causative organism in the majority of viral pneumonias. Other causative organisms include influenza viruses, adenoviruses, rhinovirus, rubeola, and varicella. Mycoplasmal pneumonia generally occurs in older children and young adults. Children with cystic fibrosis, aspiration syndromes, immunodeficiencies, neurologic impairments, or congenital or acquired pulmonary malformations are at a higher risk for pneumonia.

The clinical manifestations of pneumonia will vary depending on the child's age, the child's systemic response to the infection, the etiologic agent, the extent of lung involvement, and airway obstruction. Tachypnea, fever, and cough are frequently present in children with pneumonia, as well as use of accessory muscles and abnormal breath sounds. Radiographic examination and a variety of laboratory studies (such as culture of sputum, white blood cell count, etc.) will assist with diagnosis.

Treatment for pneumonia is generally symptomatic and supportive. It can include some or all of the following: oxygen administration, chest physiotherapy, suctioning, pharmacotherapy (such as antibiotics, antipyretics, and bronchodilators), hydration, and rest.

Primary Nursing Diagnosis   Ineffective Breathing Pattern

Definition   Breathing pattern that results in inadequate oxygen consumption (failure to meet the cellular requirements of the body)

Possibly Related to   • Infection of the lungs (state whether bacterial, viral, or mycoplasmal)

Primary Nursing Diagnosis: Ineffective breathing pattern related to infection of the lungs (state whether bacterial, viral, or mycoplasmal)

Assessment/Defining Characteristics of Child and/or Family (Subjective & Objective Data):

- Cough, unproductive in early stages but later becoming productive
- Nasal discharge
- Dyspnea
- Tachypnea
- Diminished breath sounds
- Grunting respirations
- Retractions
- Fever
- Tachycardia
- Diaphoresis
- Crackles
- Cyanosis
- Leukocytosis
- Evidence of infiltration revealed on chest X-ray

(continued)

Primary Nursing Diagnosis: Ineffective Breathing Pattern (*continued*)

Expected Outcomes	Possible Nursing Interventions	Rationale	Evaluation for Charting

Child will have an effective breathing pattern as evidenced by
 	
• respiratory rate within acceptable range (state specific range)
• clear and equal breath sounds bilaterally A & P
• absence of
  1. cough
  2. nasal discharge
  3. retractions
  4. cyanosis
  5. diaphoresis
• clear chest X-ray with acceptable A-P diameter
• oxygen saturation (via pulse oximeter) from 94 to 100% on room air
• temperature within acceptable range of 36.5° to 37.2°
• heart rate within acceptable range (state specific range)
• WBC count within acceptable range (state specific range)
• lack of signs/ symptoms of ineffective breathing pattern (such as those listed under Assessment)
	Assess and record the following every 4 hours and PRN:
	
	• RR, HR, and T
	• breath sounds
	• signs/symptoms of ineffective breathing pattern (such as those listed under Assessment). Notify physician of any abnormalities.
		If the child experiences ineffective breathing pattern the RR, HR, and T will change, and the child will work harder to breathe.	Document range of RR, HR, and T. Describe breath sounds and any signs/symptoms of ineffective breathing pattern noted.

	When using a pulse oximeter, record reading every 1 to 2 hours and PRN.	Indirectly measures oxygen saturation and can be used to determine if treatment is effective or to indicate need for change in treatment.	Document range of oxygen saturation.
	Administered humidified oxygen in correct amount and route of delivery. Record percent of oxygen and route of delivery. Assess and record effectiveness of therapy.	Humidified oxygen will dilate the pulmonary vasculature, which increases surface area available for gas exchange. Extra source oxygen will also allow for better oxygenation to body tissues and thus help improve gas exchange.	Document amount and route of oxygen delivery. Describe effectiveness.
	When indicated, administer antibiotics on schedule. Assess and record any side effects (e.g., rash, diarrhea).	Antibiotics are given to combat infection.	Document whether antibiotics were administered on schedule. Describe any side effects noted.
	Ensure chest physiotherapy is performed on schedule. Encourage child to cough during and after treatment. Assess and record effectiveness of treatments.	Chest percussion loosens secretions and positioning can help to assist the flow of secretions out of the lungs by gravity. This will aid in improving airway clearance and breathing pattern.	Document whether chest physiotherapy was done on schedule. Describe effectiveness and child's response to treatment.
	When indicated, administer antipyretics on schedule. Assess and record effectiveness.	Antipyretics are used to reduce fever.	Document whether an antipyretic was needed and describe effectiveness.

Primary Nursing Diagnosis: Ineffective Breathing Pattern *(continued)*

Expected Outcomes	Possible Nursing Interventions	Rationale	Evaluation for Charting
	Suction child PRN if unable to clear airway. Record amount and characteristics of secretions.	Suctioning assists in removing excess secretions and this in turn in helps to improve breathing pattern.	Document frequency and type of suctioning if indicated. Describe amount and characteristics of secretions.
	Check and record results of chest X-ray when indicated.	Changes in chest X-ray results may indicate need for a change in therapy.	Document results of chest X-ray when indicated.
	Check and record results of WBC. Notify physician if results are out of the normal range.	Abnormal WBC results may indicate an infection.	Document CBC results if available.
TEACHING GOALS Child and/or family will be able to verbalize 4 signs/symptoms of ineffective breathing pattern such as • cough • rapid respirations • nasal discharge • color change from pink/tan to gray or blue • fever	Teach child/family about characteristics of ineffective breathing pattern. Assess and record results.	Increased knowledge will assist the child/family in recognizing and reporting changes in the child's condition.	Document whether teaching was done and describe results.
Child and/or family will be able to verbalize knowledge of care such as • chest physiotherapy • medication administration • identification of any signs/symptoms of ineffective breathing pattern (such as those listed under Assessment) • when to contact health-care provider	Teach child/family about care. Assess and record child's/family's knowledge of and participation in care regarding chest physiotherapy, medication administration, etc.	Education of child/family will allow for accurate care.	Document whether teaching was done and describe results.

Nursing Diagnosis   Deficient Fluid Volume

Definition   Decrease in the amount of circulating fluid volume

Possibly Related to
- Respiratory distress
- Decreased fluid intake
- Increased insensible water loss from rapid respirations
- Fever

Nursing Diagnosis: Deficient fluid volume related to respiratory distress, decreased fluid intake, increased insensible water loss from rapid respirations, fever

Assessment/Defining Characteristics of Child and/or Family (Subjective & Objective Data):

- Loss of desire for food or liquids
- Listlessness
- Lethargy
- Fever
- Tachypnea
- Tachycardia
- Hypotension

- Vomiting
- Diarrhea
- Dry mucous membranes
- Decreased skin turgor (skin recoil greater than 2 to 3 seconds)
- Decreased urine output

Expected Outcomes	Possible Nursing Interventions	Rationale	Evaluation for Charting
Child will have an adequate fluid volume as evidenced by • adequate fluid intake, IV and/or oral (state specific amount of intake needed for each child) • temperature within acceptable range of 36.5° to 37.2° • respiratory rate, heart rate, and blood pressure within acceptable range (state specific range for each) • adequate urine output (state specific range; 1 to 2 ml/kg/hr) • urine specific gravity from 1.008 to 1.020 • moist mucous membranes • rapid skin recoil (less than 2 to 3 seconds)	Keep accurate record of intake and output. When indicated, encourage oral fluids.	Provides information on child's hydration status. Decreased urine output can indicate dehydration.	Document intake and output.
	Assess and record • IV fluids and condition of IV site every hour • RR, HR, BP and T every 4 hrs and PRN • signs/symptoms of deficient fluid volume (such as those listed under Assessment) every 4 hours and PRN	Provides information about fluid status of patient. It is necessary to record the amount of IV fluids every hour to make sure the child is not being over or under hydrated. The IV site needs to be assessed every hour for signs of redness or swelling. If patient has deficient fluid volume, the HR will increase at first, and eventually decrease. The BP will eventually decrease. If RR and T are increased, the child may have insensible water loss contributing to dehydration.	Document amount of IV fluids and describe condition of IV site along with any interventions needed. Document range of RR, HR, BP, and T. Describe any signs/symptoms of deficient fluid volume noted.

Nursing Diagnosis: Deficient Fluid Volume *(continued)*

Expected Outcomes	Possible Nursing Interventions	Rationale	Evaluation for Charting
• absence of 1. lethargy 2. listlessness 3. vomiting, diarrhea • lack of signs/ symptoms of deficient fluid volume (such as those listed under Assessment)	Check and record urine specific gravity with every void or as indicated.	Urine specific gravity provides information about hydration status.	Document range of urine specific gravity.
	Assess and record condition of mucous membranes and skin turgor every shift and PRN.	Provides information on hydration status.	Describe status of mucous membranes, and skin turgor.
	Provide mouth care every 4 hours and PRN.	Mouth care is necessary to counteract the dry mucous membranes.	Document whether mouth care was done and describe effectiveness.
TEACHING GOALS Child and/or family will be able to verbalize at least 4 characteristics of deficient fluid volume such as • loss of desire for food or liquids • lethargy • vomiting • decreased urine output • fever	Teach child/family about characteristics of deficient fluid volume. Assess and record results.	Increased knowledge will assist the child/ family in recognizing and reporting changes in the child's condition.	Document whether teaching was done and describe results.
Child and/or family will be able to verbalize knowledge of care such as • child's need for appropriate fluids • monitoring intake and output • identification of any signs/symptoms of deficient fluid volume (such as those listed under Assessment) • when to contact health-care provider	Teach child/family about care. Assess and record child's/family's knowledge of and participation in care regarding child's need for appropriate fluids, monitoring intake and output, etc.	Education of child/ family will allow for accurate care.	Document whether teaching was done and describe results.

Related Nursing Diagnoses

Imbalanced Nutrition: Less than Body Requirements	*related to* a. respiratory distress b. anorexia c. vomiting d. increased caloric needs secondary to infection
Acute Pain	*related to* a. headache b. chest pain
Activity Intolerance	*related to* a. respiratory distress b. lethargy c. listlessness d. decreased fluid and food intake e. fever
Anxiety: Child	*related to* a. hospitalization b. respiratory distress

TUBERCULOSIS
MEDICAL DIAGNOSIS

PATHOPHYSIOLOGY Tuberculosis is a bacterial infection caused by tubercle bacillus, a member of the Mycobacteriaceae family. In the United States, disease caused by *Mycobacterium tuberculosis* is most common. In parts of the world that do not control tuberculosis in cattle or pasteurize milk, disease caused by *M. bovis* also exists.

Infection with *M. tuberculosis* occurs when micro-droplets contaminated with infectious tuberculosis are inhaled and reach the terminal bronchioles and alveoli. Therefore, most primary lesions are in the lungs. At the focal site, an inflammatory reaction occurs, followed by a localized acute bronchopneumonia. The typical tubercle forms when the proliferating epithelial cells surround and encapsulate the multiplying bacilli in an attempt to wall off the invading organisms. The disease can also spread via intracellular multiplication of tubercle bacilli or via the bloodstream from the focal site to the lymph system, the reticuloendothelial system, and other organ systems. The lymph nodes, meninges, and bones are frequently affected. The tuberculosis bacilli have the ability to remain dormant for many years. Reactivation of the disease may occur at a later date if the child's resistance decreases. Childhood tuberculosis can be classified as intrathoracic (most pediatric cases) or extrathoracic.

Children are usually infected with tuberculosis by adults with progressive cavitary lesions who discharge infected droplets into the air. Prolonged contact (such as through repeated exposure to coughing, kissing, and environmental dust) is necessary before a child will develop the active disease. Several factors increase the communicability of tuberculosis. Poverty and over-crowding can foster poor hygiene, and malnutrition and fatigue can lower one's resistance to the disease. Currently, the highest rates of infection are among minority groups. Patients with AIDS also have an increased incidence of tuberculosis.

Children with tuberculosis may be asymptomatic or develop a broad range of symptoms. The infection often resolves spontaneously without progressing to a clinical disease. Hospitalization is usually needed only for children with the more serious forms of the disease or to perform diagnostic tests. Isolation is rarely needed, as most children with active primary pulmonary tuberculosis are noninfectious. Children are often considered noninfectious as their lesions are limited, output of bacilli is small, and cough is minimal or nonexistent. The diagnosis of tuberculosis in otherwise healthy children is usually made if the child has been exposed to an infectious case, has a positive tuberculin test, and an abnormal chest X-ray. New diagnostic methods are being investigated to confirm tuberculosis in children.

Antituberculosis drugs are used to treat tuberculosis on a long-term basis (minimum of 6 months). Pyridoxine and/or corticosteroids may be used as adjunctive therapy. Directly observed therapy (DOT) may be necessary when compliance is a concern. Directly observed therapy entails treatment provided directly to the child by a health-care worker or trained third party (not a relative or friend) to assure that the child takes each dose of medication.

Primary Nursing Diagnosis   Ineffective Airway Clearance

Definition   Condition in which secretions cannot adequately be cleared from the airways

Possibly Related to   • Bacterial infection of the lungs

Primary Nursing Diagnosis: Ineffective airway clearance related to bacterial infection of the lungs

Assessment/Defining Characteristics of Child and/or Family (Subjective & Objective Data):

- Persistent cough (slowly progressing over weeks to months)
- Aching pain and tightness in the chest
- Fever
- Tachycardia
- Diminished breath sounds
- Crackles
- Rhonchi
- Tachypnea
- Wheezing
- Stridor
- Lobar infiltration, segmental atelectasis, lobar emphysema, or pleural effusion revealed on chest X-ray

Expected Outcomes	Possible Nursing Interventions	Rationale	Evaluation for Charting

Child will have adequate airway clearance as evidenced by
 	
• clear and equal breath sounds bilaterally A & P
• improved chest X-ray with absence of atelectasis and pleural effusion
• oxygen saturation (via pulse oximeter) from 94 to 100% on room air
• respiratory rate within acceptable range (state specific range)
• temperature within acceptable range of 36.5° to 37.2°
• absence of
  1. persistent cough
  2. aching pain or tightness in the chest
  3. stridor
• heart rate within acceptable range (state specific range)
• lack of signs/symptoms of ineffective airway clearance (such as those listed under Assessment)
	Assess and record the following every 4 hours and PRN:
	
	• RR, HR, and T
	• breath sounds
	• amount and characteristics of secretions
	• signs/symptoms of ineffective airway clearance or respiratory distress (such as those listed under Assessment)
		If child experiences ineffective airway clearance the RR, HR, T, and breath sounds may be abnormal. If coughing episodes increase this may diminish airway clearance. It is important to record the amount and characteristics of secretions in order to detect changes (such as increase in the amount and color change of secretions).	Document range of RR, HR, and T. Describe breath sounds, coughing episodes, amount and characteristics of secretions, and any signs/symptoms of ineffective airway clearance noted.

	When using a pulse oximeter, record reading every 1 to 2 hours and PRN.	Pulse oximetry detects the oxygen saturation in the bloodstream. It is important to detect small changes in oxygen saturation before the child starts displaying overt characteristics of ineffective airway clearance.	Document range of oxygen saturation.
	Administer bacteriocidal antituberculosis agents (e.g., isoniazid, rifampin, pyrazinamide) on schedule. Assess and record any side effects (e.g., GI distress, hypersensitivity reactions, neurologic complications).	Bacteriocidal antituberculosis agents are administered to combat the bacterial infection.	Document whether bacteriocidal antituberculosis agents were administered on schedule. Describe any side effects noted.
	When indicated, administer antipyretics on schedule. Assess and record effectiveness.	Antipyretics are used to reduce fever.	Document whether an antipyretic was needed and describe effectiveness.

Primary Nursing Diagnosis: Ineffective Airway Clearance *(continued)*

Expected Outcomes	Possible Nursing Interventions	Rationale	Evaluation for Charting
	When indicated, administer pyridoxine (vitamin B₆) on schedule. Assess and record effectiveness any side effects (e.g., GI distress, headache, sleepiness).	Pyridoxine is administered in order to combat the toxic effects of isoniazid.	Document whether pyridoxine was administered on schedule. Describe effectiveness and any side effects noted.
	When indicated, administer corticosteroids on schedule. Assess and record effectiveness and any side effects (e.g., GI disturbance, hypertension).	Steroids are administered to reduce the inflammation present in the airways.	Document whether steroids were administered on schedule. Describe effectiveness and any side effects noted.
	When indicated, administer humidified oxygen in correct amount and route of delivery. Record percent of oxygen and route of delivery. Assess and record effectiveness of therapy.	Humidified oxygen will dilate the pulmonary vasculature, which increases surface area available for gas exchange.	Document amount and route of oxygen delivery. Describe effectiveness.
	Ensure chest physiotherapy is performed on schedule. Encourage child to cough during and after treatment. Assess and record effectiveness of treatments.	Chest percussion loosens secretions and positioning can help to assist the flow of secretions out of the lungs by gravity. This will aid in improving airway clearance and breathing pattern.	Document whether chest physiotherapy was done on schedule. Describe effectiveness and child's response to treatment.
	Suction gently PRN if infant or child is unable to clear airway. Record amount and characteristics of secretions.	Suctioning assists in removing excess secretions and this in turn helps to improve breathing pattern.	Document frequency and type of suctioning if indicated. Describe amount and characteristics of secretions.
	Encourage fluid intake (e.g., 240 ml 8 times/ 24 hours).	Helps to thin secretions.	Document intake.
	Check and record results of chest X-ray when indicated.	Changes in chest X-ray results may indicate need for a change in therapy.	Document results of chest X-ray when indicated.
	Keep head of bed elevated at a 30° angle (may use infant seat if infant can support head in midline position).	Elevating the head of the bed to a 30° angle causes a shift of the abdominal contents downward and this in turn will allow for increased lung expansion in order to help improve breathing pattern.	Document whether head of bed was kept elevated.

(continued)

Primary Nursing Diagnosis: Ineffective Airway Clearance *(continued)*			
Expected Outcomes	**Possible Nursing Interventions**	**Rationale**	**Evaluation for Charting**
	If child produces sputum, instruct child to spit out secretions in a tissue and dispose of tissue in waste container. Adhere to Centers for Disease Control (CDC) guidelines and/or institutional policy for current precautions/isolation techniques.	Prevents spread of infection. The CDC guidelines provide the latest information on the standard of care.	Document maintenance of isolation/precaution techniques.
TEACHING GOALS Child and/or family will be able to verbalize 4 signs/symptoms of ineffective airway clearance such as • persistent cough • wheezing • aching pain and tightness in the chest • fever	Teach child/family about characteristics of ineffective airway clearance. Assess and record results.	Increased knowledge will assist the child/family in recognizing and reporting changes in the child's condition.	Document whether teaching was done and describe results.
Child and/or family will be able to verbalize knowledge of care such as • medication administration and long-term compliance • chest physiotherapy • disposal of child's soiled tissues • identification of any signs/symptoms of ineffective airway clearance (such as those listed under Assessment) • when to contact health-care provider	Teach child/family about care. Assess and record child's/family's knowledge of and participation in care regarding medication administration and long-term compliance, etc.	Education of child/family will allow for accurate care.	Document whether teaching was done and describe results.

Nursing Diagnosis Deficient Knowledge: Parental

Definition Lack of information concerning the child's disease and care

Possibly Related to
- Unfamiliarity with child's disease and its communicability
- Cognitive or cultural-language limitations
- Guilt secondary to child's acquiring disease

Nursing Diagnosis: Deficient knowledge: parental related to unfamiliarity with child's disease and its communicability, cognitive or cultural-language limitations, guilt secondary to child's acquiring disease

Assessment/Defining Characteristics of Child and/or Family (Subjective & Objective Data):
- Verbalization by parents indicating a lack of knowledge regarding tuberculosis and the care needed
- Relation of incorrect information to members of the health-care team
- Inability to correctly repeat information previously explained
- Inability to correctly demonstrate skills previously taught (e.g., medication administration)

Expected Outcomes	Possible Nursing Interventions	Rationale	Evaluation for Charting
TEACHING GOALS Parents will have an adequate knowledge base concerning the child's illness and care as evidenced by • ability to correctly state information previously taught regarding tuberculosis and child's care (e.g., communicability, need to identify the person from whom the child contracted the illness, testing for other family members, home care, medication administration, compliance with treatment, future test of child) • ability to correctly demonstrate skills previously taught (e.g., medication administration, hygiene) • ability to relate appropriate information to the health-care team	Listen to parents' concerns and fears. Document findings.	Allows parents to express fears, feelings, and concerns. This provides them with a way to accept new information.	Describe parents' concerns and fears and any successful measures used to encourage family to increase parental knowledge.
	Assess and record parents' knowledge of and understanding of child's illness. Encourage questions.	Generates a baseline of knowledge, which allows for teaching of accurate information and dispelling of incorrect knowledge.	Document whether teaching was done and describe results.
	Provide parents with information about tuberculosis, including • hygiene • medication administration and long-term compliance • nutrition • activity level • isolation from others who are susceptible • overdependence of child and/or overprotectiveness of family	Education of parents will allow for accurate care and increase coping ability of parents.	Document whether teaching was done and describe results. Describe ability of parents to repeat information correctly and perform skills adequately.

(continued)

Expected Outcomes	Possible Nursing Interventions	Rationale	Evaluation for Charting
Nursing Diagnosis: Deficient Knowledge: Parental *(continued)*			
• ability to request additional information and/or clarification of information	• identification of any signs/symptoms of ineffective airway clearance such as those listed under Assessment		
	When indicated, obtain an interpreter.	Necessary in order to make sure parents understand teaching.	Document whether an interpreter was needed and effectiveness of teaching.

Related Nursing Diagnoses

Activity Intolerance

related to
a. fever
b. anorexia
c. increased respiratory effort

Imbalanced Nutrition: Less than Body Requirements

related to
a. increased metabolic state
b. decreased food intake

Noncompliance

related to
a. long duration of treatment
b. cognitive or cultural-language limitations

Impaired Home Maintenance

related to
a. communicable disease
b. lack of knowledge
c. lack of resources and support systems

CARE OF
CHILDREN WITH
UROGENITAL
DYSFUNCTION

11

| ONE |

ACUTE POSTINFECTIOUS GLOMERULONEPHRITIS
MEDICAL DIAGNOSIS

PATHOPHYSIOLOGY Inflammation of the glomeruli is known as glomerulonephritis. Poststreptococcal glomerulonephritis is the most common type in children. Other bacteria (such as *Staphylococcus* or *Pneumococcus*), viruses (such as coxsackievirus), pharmacological and toxic agents, and autoimmune diseases may also be underlying causes of glomerulonephritis. Acute post-streptococcal glomerulonephritis can follow pharyngitis or skin infections with a beta-hemolytic nephritogenic strain of streptococcus. It usually occurs 1 to 12 weeks after the initial infection. The incidence of acute glomerulonephritis is highest in children ages 2 to 12 and it is more common in boys than girls. Acute glomerulonephritis is an important cause of acute and chronic renal failure in children.

Postinfectious glomerulonephritis occurs as a result of damage to the glomerular capillary wall due to immune-mediated (both cellular and humoral) responses to a stimulus (the streptococcal antigen). This is followed by inflammation, which may progress to fibrosis and irreversible scarring. Antigen-antibody complexes affix themselves in the glomeruli, resulting in a proliferative and exudative process (immune complex disease). The antigen-antibody complexes become entrapped in the glomerular membrane, causing obstruction, inflammation, and edema in the kidney. The affected area of the kidney is infiltrated by white blood cells, and the glomerular endothelial and epithelial cells proliferate, become edematous, and occlude the glomeruli. Renal capillary permeability increases, and there is renal vascular spasm. These processes lead to decreased glomerular filtration. Water and sodium are retained; causing increased intravascular and interstitial fluid volume (edema). The edema is usually confined to the face, except in cases of severe disease when it may be more generalized. Proteinuria occurs when the nonoccluded glomeruli malfunction and allow protein to leak into the glomerular filtrate. If the membranes rupture, red cells may pass into the urine (hematuria) as well. If the inflammatory process does not resolve, glomerular sclerosing and chronic interstitial damage will occur.

Half of all children with acute glomerulonephritis will be asymptomatic, with the glomerulonephritis self-resolving. The most severely affected children will present with the classic presentation of puffy eyelids, facial edema, hypertension, and scant, dark urine with microscopic hematuria and proteinuria. Other clinical manifestations can include flank or midabdominal pain, irritability, malaise, fever, headache, nausea, vomiting, oliguria, dysuria, or costovertebral tenderness.

Treatment goals for the child with acute postinfectious glomerulonephritis include preserving renal function and preventing complications. This is done by relieving symptoms, such as hypertension, reestablishing fluid and electrolyte balance, and preventing infection and skin breakdown. The child's nutritional and emotional needs also must be addressed. In severe cases of acute postinfectious glomerulonephritis, control of the hypertension and treatment with dialysis can be life saving for the child. Prognosis is usually good.

Primary Nursing Diagnosis   Excess Fluid Volume

Definition	Increase in the amount of circulating fluid volume, which can eventually lead to interstitial or intracellular fluid overload
Possibly Related to	• Poststreptococcal infection • Antigen antibody reaction • Pathological changes in the glomeruli

Primary Nursing Diagnosis: Excess fluid volume related to poststreptococcal infection, antigen antibody reaction, pathological changes in the glomeruli

Assessment/Defining Characteristics of Child and/or Family (Subjective & Objective Data):

- Oliguria
- Microscopic or gross hematuria (coke- or tea-colored urine)
- Proteinuria
- Increased urine specific gravity (greater than 1.030)
- Edema (usually facial, especially periorbital)
- Hypertension
- Headache
- Sudden weight gain
- Increased blood urea nitrogen (BUN)

Expected Outcomes	Possible Nursing Interventions	Rationale	Evaluation for Charting
Child will resume appropriate fluid balance as evidenced by - adequate urine output (state specific range; 1 to 2 ml/kg/hr) - clear, pale yellow urine - blood pressure within acceptable range (state specific range) - lack of 1. proteinuria 2. hematuria 3. edema 4. headache 5. sudden weight gain - urine specific gravity from 1.008 to 1.020 - BUN from 5 to 18 mg/dl - lack of signs/symptoms of excess fluid volume (such as those listed under Assessment)	Keep accurate record of intake and output. Be sure child does not exceed maximal intake ordered. Record characteristics of urine output, including presence of proteinuria and hematuria.	Provides information on child's hydration status. Fluids may need to be restricted in order to decrease extravascular fluid volume and blood pressure.	Document intake and outputs. Describe characteristics of urine output.
	Check and record urine specific gravity, protein, and blood every 4 hours or as indicated.	Urine specific gravity provides information about hydration status. The presence of protein and blood can indicate the amount of glomerular damage.	Document range of urine specific gravity, protein, and blood.
	Assess and record - amount and location of edema at least once/shift and PRN - BP every 4 hours and PRN - IV fluids and condition of IV site every hour - laboratory values as indicated. Report abnormalities to the physician. - signs/symptoms of excess fluid volume (such as those listed under Assessment) every 4 hours and PRN	Provides information about fluid status of the child. It is necessary to record the amount of IV fluids every hour to make sure the child is not being over or under hydrated. The IV site needs to be assessed every hour for signs of redness or swelling. Edema is due to fluid retention. BP will change with fluid retention.	Describe amount and location of edema. Document range of BP. Document amount of IV fluids and describe condition of IV site along with any interventions needed. Document results of laboratory values when indicated and determine if the values are an increase or decrease from the previous values. Describe any signs/symptoms of excess fluid volume.
	Weigh child daily on same scale at same time of day. Document results and compare to previous weight.	Provides information on child's hydration and nutritional status.	Document weight and determine if it was an increase or decrease from the previous weight.

(continued)

Primary Nursing Diagnosis: Excess Fluid Volume *(continued)*

Expected Outcomes	Possible Nursing Interventions	Rationale	Evaluation for Charting
	Administer antihypertensive medications on schedule. Assess and record effectiveness and any side effects (e.g., dizziness, hypotension, GI disturbance).	Antihypertensive drugs work in various ways to lower BP in order to reach the ultimate goal of decreasing workload on the heart.	Document whether antihypertensive drugs were administered on schedule. Describe effectiveness and any side effects noted.
	Administer diuretics (e.g., furosemide) on schedule. Assess and record effectiveness and any side effects (e.g., dizziness, dehydration, hypokalemia).	Diuretics are administered to decrease excess intravascular fluid through increased urine output, which will decrease the workload on the heart.	Document whether diuretics were administered on schedule. Describe effectiveness and any side effects noted.
	When indicated, restrict dietary sodium and/or potassium.	Sodium may need to be restricted in order to reduce fluid overload. Potassium may need to be restricted due to the body's inability to excrete potassium.	Describe any dietary restrictions used to improve fluid balance. Document their effectiveness.
TEACHING GOALS Child and/or family will be able to verbalize 4 signs/symptoms of excess fluid volume such as • sudden weight gain • edema • headache • decreased urine output	Teach child/family about characteristics of excess fluid volume. Assess and record results.	Increased knowledge will assist the child/family in recognizing and reporting changes in the child's condition.	Document whether teaching was done and describe results.
Child and/or family will be able to verbalize knowledge of care such as • medication administration • monitoring intake and output • fluid and/or diet restriction • identification of any signs/symptoms of excess fluid volume (such as those listed under Assessment) • when to contact health-care provider	Teach child/family about care. Assess and record child's/family's knowledge of and participation in care regarding medication administration, monitoring intake and output, etc.	Education of child/family will allow for accurate care.	Document whether teaching was done and describe results.

Nursing Diagnosis   Disturbed Body Image

Definition   Condition in which the child has a negative self-view

Possibly Related to   • Facial/periorbital edema
                            • Sudden weight gain

Nursing Diagnosis: Disturbed body image related to facial/periorbital edema, sudden weight gain

Assessment/Defining Characteristics of Child and/or Family (Subjective & Objective Data):

• Verbalization of displeasure in body
• Refusal to look in a mirror

• Refusal to participate in care or play and social activities
• Decreased interest in appearance

Expected Outcomes	Possible Nursing Interventions	Rationale	Evaluation for Charting
Child will indicate acceptance of body image as evidenced by • ability to verbally describe self positively • ability to look in mirror • willingness to participate in care • willingness to participate in play and social activities • developmentally appropriate interest in appearance	Assess and record child's/family's ability to accept body image.	Provides a baseline, which can be used to describe increased or decreased acceptance of body image.	Describe child's/family's ability to accept body image.
	Encourage child to express feelings, fears, or concerns regarding illness and appearance.	Provides information about child's feelings, fears, and concerns related to their appearance.	Describe any feelings, fears, or concerns that child expressed.
	Clarify any misconceptions child may express regarding illness and appearance.	Provides an opportunity for health-care team to correct any misinformation.	Document any misinformation stated by child and measures used to dispel misinformation.
	Provide child with opportunities for age-appropriate therapeutic play.	Provides an outlet for child to express their feelings.	Describe any therapeutic play measures used to help child express their feelings.
	Encourage child to maintain usual state of grooming and appearance.	Helps to increase child's body image.	Describe any therapeutic measures used to help child improve their body image.
	Encourage child/family to participate in care when possible.	This may increase the comfort level of the child and thus help child to have an improved body image.	Document whether child/family participated in care and if this was successful in helping child to have an improved body image.
	Encourage child/family to focus on nonphysical qualities.	This may increase the comfort level of the child and thus help child to have an improved body image.	Describe any therapeutic measures used to improve body image. Document their effectiveness.

(continued)

Nursing Diagnosis: Disturbed Body Image *(continued)*			
Expected Outcomes	**Possible Nursing Interventions**	**Rationale**	**Evaluation for Charting**
TEACHING GOALS Child and/or family will be able to verbalize at least 4 characteristics of disturbed body image such as • verbalization about displeasure with body • refusal to look in mirror • refusal to participate in care or play and social activities • decreased interest in appearance	Teach child/family about characteristics of disturbed body image. Assess and record results.	Increased knowledge will assist the child/family in recognizing and reporting changes in the child's condition.	Document whether teaching was done and describe results.
Child and/or family will be able to verbalize knowledge of care such as • participating in care regarding promoting a positive body image • identification of any signs/symptoms of impaired mobility (such as those listed under Assessment) • when to contact health-care provider	Teach child's/family about care. Assess and record child/family's knowledge of and participation in care regarding ways to promote a positive body image.	Education of child/family will allow for accurate care.	Document whether teaching was done and describe results.

Related Nursing Diagnoses

Activity Intolerance	*related to* fatigue
Impaired Skin Integrity	*related to* a. immobility b. edema
Deficient Knowledge: Child/Parental	*related to* home care secondary to diet restrictions and medication administration
Imbalanced Nutrition: Less than Body Requirements	*related to* anorexia

TWO

CHRONIC RENAL FAILURE
MEDICAL DIAGNOSIS

PATHOPHYSIOLOGY In chronic renal failure (CRF), kidney function deteriorates over time as the nephrons suffer irreversible damage. Congenital abnormalities and infections of the kidneys and urinary tract are the most common causes of CRF. Other causes include glomerulonephritis, acute tubular necrosis, diabetes mellitus, immune system disorders, metabolic disorders, and obstructions. CRF occurs in approximately 18 out of 1 million children.

Insult to the kidneys results in tissue scarring and structural and functional damage to the nephrons, especially to the glomeruli. Initially undamaged nephrons compensate, but eventually nephron function deterioration becomes secondary to injury from hyperfiltration (the increased filtration load) and renal insufficiency. The glomerular filtration rate (GFR) continues to decrease, impairing the body's ability to excrete nitrogenous wastes, causing metabolic, biochemical, and clinical disturbances.

There are five stages of CRF. In Stage 1, the child has decreased renal reserve but is asymptomatic, has normal or increased GFR, and has normal blood urea nitrogen (BUN) and serum creatinine levels. In Stage 2, the GFR is mildly reduced, and BUN and serum creatinine levels are rising. In Stage 3, there is moderate reduction of the GFR, and in Stage 4, there is severe reduction of the GFR. In Stage 5, end stage renal disease (ESRD), 90% of the nephrons have been destroyed, the GFR is 10% of normal, BUN and serum creatinine levels rise sharply, and all of the body's systems are adversely affected. Hypertension, anemia, and bone disease are long-term complications of ESRD and CRF.

Azotemia and/or uremia, an elevation in BUN and creatinine levels, occurs as renal function decreases and nitrogenous wastes are retained. Metabolic acidosis occurs for several reasons: the blood levels of acids increase because of their decreased excretion, the kidney is unable to excrete hydrogen ions, the distal tubules' ability to produce ammonia is decreased, and urinary bicarbonate wasting related to impaired tubular function occurs. Decreased GFR and abnormal reabsorptive function in damaged tubules result in fluid alterations and electrolyte imbalances as well.

Sodium and fluid excretion may initially increase as the undamaged nephrons try to compensate by filtering an increased solute load, causing diuresis with possible dehydration. As renal failure progresses, the very low GFR and the continued alterations in the kidneys' dilutional ability cause sodium and fluid retention. An activated renin-angiotensin system leads to hyperaldosteronism, further compounding sodium and water retention. Hypoproteinemia, caused by the excessive loss of serum proteins through the damaged glomeruli (proteinuria), can compound the already existing edema.

As long as fluid and acid-base balance are maintained, hyperkalemia is not a problem in children with CRF. Hyperkalemia can occur, though, from the ingestion of a large potassium load, from hemolysis, as metabolic acidosis ensues, or from a catabolic state associated with fever.

Impaired renal absorption of calcium and decreased tubular excretion of phosphorus result in hypocalcemia and hyperphosphatemia, which in turn causes a rebound effect of increased parathyroid hormone production. Calcium absorption from the gastrointestinal tract is reduced as the increased phosphorus level impairs the kidney's ability to produce usable vitamin D. Hypocalcemia causes bone resorption and bone abnormalities collectively known as renal osteodystrophy. Osteodystrophy increases the child's risk for spontaneous fractures, rickets, and valgus deformity of the legs.

Impaired red cell production and a shortened red blood cell life span due to uremia result in anemia. Impaired release of stored iron, inadequate iron intake, and the detrimental effects of nitrogenous wastes on platelet function lead to bleeding tendencies and also contribute to the anemia. The severity of the anemia is proportional to the decline in renal function.

The child with CRF can develop growth retardation, affected by such factors as the etiology of the primary disease, the age of onset, acidosis, and the presence of renal osteodystrophy. Disturbances in the metabolism of calcium, phosphorus, and vitamin D, as well as a decreased caloric intake, also contribute to the child's growth retardation. CRF and its treatment also present many social and developmental issues for the child.

The onset of CRF is insidious; with the symptoms often presenting only after severe kidney damage has occurred. The child with CRF may present with edema, symptomatic hypertension, gross hematuria, or a urinary tract infection. Persistent proteinuria is an important marker of kidney damage. The child with ESRD develops uremic symptoms. These include nausea, vomiting, anorexia, uremic breath odor, progressive anemia, uremic frost (urea crystals deposited on the skin), pruritis, malaise, headache, progressive confusion, tremors, pulmonary edema, dyspnea, and congestive heart failure. The degree of the child's chronic renal disease is determined by the glomerular filtration rate, which is the best measurement of overall kidney function. Other blood and urine laboratory evaluations, as well as imaging studies are used to monitor the child's disease process.

Most children with chronic renal failure are treated conservatively with pharmacologic, dietetic, and supportive therapy to preserve the remaining kidney function, maintain fluid and electrolyte balance, prevent complications, and promote growth and development. Dialysis is initiated when, despite the conservative treatment, the child progresses to ESRD. Kidney transplantation is considered the only alternative to long-term dialysis for children. Transplants performed before the child needs dialysis, have better long-term outcomes, as do living donor transplants as opposed to cadaver transplants.

Primary Nursing Diagnosis   Impaired Metabolic Function*

Definition

Imbalance or altered utilization of specific body biochemicals

Possibly Related to

- Accumulation of nitrogenous waste products, decreased ammonia excretion, decreased acid excretion, and fluid and electrolyte imbalances secondary to irreversibly damaged nephrons

*Non-NANDA diagnosis.

Primary Nursing Diagnosis: Impaired metabolic function related to accumulation of nitrogenous waste products, decreased ammonia excretion, decreased acid excretion, and fluid and electrolyte imbalances secondary to irreversibly damaged nephrons

Assessment/Defining Characteristics of Child and/or Family (Subjective & Objective Data):

- Elevated BUN (greater than 20 mg/dL)
- Elevated serum creatinine level (greater than 1.5 mg/dL)
- Decreased serum bicarbonate (less than 2.0 mEq/L)
- Skin dryness
- Pruritis (uremic frost)
- Uremic breath
- Nausea
- Vomiting
- Anorexia
- Uremic neuropathy (muscle cramps, tetany, weakness, muscle wasting)
- Uremic encephalopathy (irritability, lethargy, seizures)

Expected Outcomes	Possible Nursing Interventions	Rationale	Evaluation for Charting
Child will have improved metabolic function as evidenced by • BUN from 5 to 18 mg/dL • serum creatinine from 0.3 to 1.0 mg/dL • serum bicarbonate 22 to 29 mEq/L	Assess and record • IV fluids and condition of IV site every hour • laboratory values as indicated. Report abnormalities to the physician.	If child experiences impaired metabolic function the lab values will be out of the normal range and the child may exhibit the signs/symptoms listed under Assessment. It is necessary to record the amount of IV fluids	Document current ranges of laboratory values and any signs/symptoms of metabolic dysfunction noted. Document amount of IV fluids and describe condition of IV site along with any interventions needed.

Primary Nursing Diagnosis: Impaired Metabolic Function *(continued)*

Expected Outcomes	Possible Nursing Interventions	Rationale	Evaluation for Charting
• lack of 　1. skin dryness 　2. pruritis 　3. uremic breath 　4. nausea 　5. vomiting 　6. anorexia 　7. muscle cramps 　8. tetany 　9. weakness 　10. muscle wasting 　11. irritability 　12. lethargy 　13. seizures • lack of signs/symptoms of impaired metabolic function (such as those listed under Assessment)	• signs/symptoms of impaired metabolic function (such as those listed under Assessment) every 4 hours and PRN	every hour to keep make sure the child is not being over or under hydrated. The IV site needs to be assessed every hour for signs of redness or swelling.	
	When indicated, ensure that peritoneal dialysis is done according to institutional policy, including • maintaining a closed sterile system • using aseptic technique whenever the system is opened • warming the dialysate. • obtaining daily cultures (e.g., site, fluid) • changing the tubing and catheter site dressing using sterile technique	Dialysis is used to rid the body of waste products and accumulated electrolytes.	Document whether dialysis was used. Describe effectiveness of procedure and child's response.
	When indicated, ensure child keeps scheduled hemodialysis appointments. Assess and record condition of access site. Record child's response to dialysis.	Dialysis is used to rid the body of waste products and accumulated electrolytes.	Document whether dialysis was used. Describe effectiveness of procedure and child's response.
	When indicated, restrict dietary protein, sodium, phosphorus, and potassium intake.	These restrictions may be necessary to prevent build up of electrolytes and waste products in the body.	Document whether dietary restrictions were necessary and describe effectiveness of measures.
	Administer dietary supplements (e.g., water-soluble vitamins) on schedule. Assess and record effectiveness.	Dietary supplements are necessary to promote growth and development.	Document whether dietary supplements were administered on schedule. Describe effectiveness.
	When indicated, administer alkalizing agents (e.g., sodium bicarbonate). Assess and record effectiveness and any side effects (e.g., stomach cramps, severe headaches).	Alkalizing agents can be administered to treat metabolic acidosis.	Document whether alkalizing agents were administered on schedule. Describe effectiveness and any side effects noted.

(continued)

Primary Nursing Diagnosis: Impaired Metabolic Function *(continued)*			
Expected Outcomes	**Possible Nursing Interventions**	**Rationale**	**Evaluation for Charting**
	Initiate and maintain consultation with dietitian.	Provides information and support for child and family on dietary matters.	Document whether consultation with dietitian was needed and describe effectiveness.
	Initiate and maintain consultation with visiting nurses and/or other home-care providers.	Provides support for care of child in the home setting.	Document whether any other support services were consulted. Describe their effectiveness.
	Consult social services to assist the family in identifying and using available resources (e.g., financial, transportation).	Provides support for care of child.	Document whether social services were consulted. Describe their effectiveness.
TEACHING GOALS Child and/or family will be able to verbalize at least 4 characteristics of impaired metabolic function such as • nausea • vomiting • anorexia • easy bruising • skin dryness	Teach child/family about characteristics of impaired metabolic function. Assess and record results.	Increased knowledge will assist the child/family in recognizing and reporting changes in the child's condition.	Document whether teaching was done and describe results.
Child and/or family will be able to verbalize knowledge of care such as • dietary restrictions • medication administration • compliance with dialysis schedule and techniques • identification of any signs/symptoms of impaired metabolic function (such as those listed under Assessment) and the correct action for each • when to contact health-care provider	Teach child/family about care. Assess and record child's/family's knowledge of and participation in care regarding dietary restriction, medication administration, etc.	Education of child/family will allow for accurate care.	Document whether teaching was done and describe results.

Nursing Diagnosis Deficient Fluid Volume: Intravascular and/or Excess Fluid Volume: Extravascular or Intravascular

Definition Decrease in the amount of circulating fluid volume *and/or* interstitial fluid overload *or* increased intravascular volume (which can eventually lead to interstitial or intracellular fluid overload)

Possibly Related to
- Reduced renal function due to irreversible nephron damage secondary to glomerular diseases
- Congenital abnormalities of the kidneys or urinary tract (e.g., renal hypoplasia, severe bilateral vesicoureteral reflux)
- Pyelonephritis with reflux
- Hereditary renal diseases
- Miscellaneous disorders

Nursing Diagnosis: Deficient fluid volume: intravascular *and/or* excess fluid volume: extravascular or intravascular related to

- Reduced renal function due to irreversible nephron damage secondary to
  1. glomerular diseases
  2. congenital abnormalities of the kidneys or urinary tract (e.g., renal hypoplasia, severe bilateral vesicoureteral reflux)
  3. pyelonephritis with reflux
  4. hereditary renal diseases
  5. miscellaneous disorders

Assessment/Defining Characteristics of Child and/or Family (Subjective & Objective Data):
- Initial polydipsia
- Diuresis
- Nocturia or polyuria (in renal insufficiency where more than 75% of the nephrons are destroyed and GFR is 25% of normal)
- Oliguria
- Edema
- Hypertension
- Either dehydration or circulatory overload with tachycardia, tachypnea, and crackles
- Unconcentrated urine

Expected Outcomes	Possible Nursing Interventions	Rationale	Evaluation for Charting
Child will have improved fluid balance as evidenced by • adequate urine output (state specific range; 1 to 2 ml/kg/hr) • heart rate, respiratory rate, and blood pressure within acceptable range (state specific range for each)	Keep accurate record of intake and output. If Foley catheter is in place, note hourly output. Maintain aseptic technique when emptying urine and caring for catheter.	Provides information on child's hydration status. Decreased urine output can indicate reduced renal function. Aseptic technique is necessary when caring for the Foley catheter in order to prevent infection.	Document intake and output. Document whether aseptic technique was used when providing Foley care.

(continued)

Nursing Diagnosis: Deficient Fluid Volume: Intravascular and/or Excess Fluid Volume: Extravascular or Intravascular *(continued)*

Expected Outcomes	Possible Nursing Interventions	Rationale	Evaluation for Charting

• lack of
  1. edema
  2. dehydration
  3. circulatory over-
     load, accompanied
     by tachycardia,
     tachypnea, and/or
     crackles
  4. polydipsia
• clear and equal breath
  sounds bilaterally
  A & P
• urine specific gravity
  from 1.008 to 1.020
• lack of signs/symptoms
  of fluid imbalance
  (such as those listed
  under Assessment)
	Restrict or replace fluids as indicated. Assess and record child's response.	Promotes improved fluid balance.	Describe any therapeutic measures used to improve fluid balance. Document their effectiveness and child's response.

	Assess and record • HR, RR, BP, and breath sounds every 4 hours and PRN • IV fluids and condition of IV site every hour • urine specific gravity every 4 hours or as indicated • signs/symptoms of fluid imbalance (such as those listed under Assessment) every 4 hours and PRN	If patient has fluid imbalance, the HR, RR, BP, and breath sounds will change. Specific gravity provides information about fluid status of patient. It is necessary to record the amount of IV fluids every hour to make sure the child is not being over or under hydrated. The IV site needs to be assessed every hour for signs of redness or swelling.	Document range of HR, RR, BP, and urine specific gravity. Describe breath sounds. Document amount of IV fluids and describe condition of IV site along with any interventions needed. Describe any signs/symptoms of fluid imbalance noted.
	Administer diuretics on schedule (ensure that dose has been adjusted to avoid toxicity from inadequate renal clearance). Assess and record effectiveness and any side effects (e.g., hypokalemia, dehydration).	Diuretics are administered to decrease excess intravascular fluid through increased urine output, which will decrease the workload on the heart.	Document whether diuretics were administered on schedule. Describe effectiveness and any side effects noted.
	Administer antihypertensives on schedule (ensure that dose has been adjusted to avoid toxicity from inadequate renal clearance). Assess and record effectiveness and any side effects noted (e.g., dizziness, hypotension, GI disturbance).	Antihypertensive drugs work in various ways to lower BP in order to reach the ultimate goal of decreasing workload on the heart.	Document whether antihypertensive drugs were administered on schedule. Describe effectiveness and any side effects noted.
	Weigh child daily on same scale at same time each day. Record results and compare to previous weight.	Sudden increase in weight gain may indicate extravascular fluid overload and may result in decreased cardiac output.	Document weight and determine if it was an increase or decrease from the previous weight.

Nursing Diagnosis: Deficient Fluid Volume: Intravascular and/or Excess Fluid Volume: Extravascular or Intravascular *(continued)*

Expected Outcomes	Possible Nursing Interventions	Rationale	Evaluation for Charting
	When prescribed, restrict dietary sodium intake.	Restriction may be necessary to help maintain fluid balance.	Document whether dietary restrictions were necessary and describe effectiveness of measure.
	When indicated, ensure that peritoneal dialysis is done on according to institutional policy, including • maintaining a closed sterile system • using aseptic technique whenever the system is opened • warming the dialysate • obtaining daily cultures (e.g., site, fluid) • changing the tubing and catheter site dressing using sterile technique	Dialysis is used to rid the body of waste products and accumulated electrolytes.	Document whether dialysis was used. Describe effectiveness of procedure and child's response.
	When indicated, ensure child keeps scheduled hemodialysis appointments. Assess and record condition of access site. Record child's response to dialysis.	Dialysis is used to rid the body of waste products and accumulated electrolytes.	Document whether dialysis was used. Describe effectiveness of procedure and child's response.
	Initiate and maintain consultation with dietitian.	Provides information and support for child and family on dietary matters.	Document whether consultation with dietitian was needed and describe effectiveness.
	Initiate and maintain consultation with visiting nurses and/or other home-care providers.	Provides support for care of child in the home setting.	Document whether any other support services were consulted. Describe their effectiveness.
	Consult social services to assist the family in identifying and using available resources (e.g., financial, transportation).	Provides support for care of child.	Document whether social services were consulted. Describe their effectiveness.

(continued)

Nursing Diagnosis: Deficient Fluid Volume: Intravascular and/or Excess Fluid Volume: Extravascular or Intravascular *(continued)*

Expected Outcomes	Possible Nursing Interventions	Rationale	Evaluation for Charting
TEACHING GOALS Child and/or family will be able to verbalize at least 4 characteristics of fluid imbalance such as • increased thirst • increased urine output • increased weight • edema	Teach child/family about characteristics of fluid imbalance. Assess and record results.	Increased knowledge will assist the child/family in recognizing and reporting changes in the child's condition.	Document whether teaching was done and describe results.
Child and/or family will be able to verbalize knowledge of care such as • monitoring of intake and output • medication administration • dietary changes • identification of any signs/symptoms of fluid imbalance (such as those listed under Assessment) and the correct action for each • when to contact health-care provider	Teach child/family about care. Assess and record child's/family's knowledge of and participation in care regarding monitoring intake and output, medication administration, etc.	Education of child/family will allow for accurate care.	Document whether teaching was done and describe results.

Related Nursing Diagnoses

Electrolyte Imbalance: Sodium Excess, Potassium Excess, Calcium Losses, Phosphate Losses*	*related to* irreversibly damaged nephrons
Imbalanced Nutrition: Less than Body Requirements	*related to* a. anorexia b. nausea c. vomiting d. inadequate intake e. catabolic state
Delayed Growth and Development	*related to* a. frequent biochemical and metabolic disturbances secondary to irreversible dysfunction b. noncompliance with treatment plan
Disturbed Body Image	*related to* a. altered growth and development b. dependency upon a dialysis machine c. edema

*Non-NANDA diagnosis.

THREE

NEPHROTIC SYNDROME
MEDICAL DIAGNOSIS

PATHOPHYSIOLOGY Nephrotic syndrome, a condition that results in alteration of renal function, is characterized by hypoalbuminemia, hyperlipidemia, massive proteinuria, edema, and altered immunity. It is classified as congenital, primary (idiopathic), or secondary. Congenital nephrotic syndrome, caused by a recessive gene on an autosome, is rare and responds poorly to usual therapy. Infants generally succumb to this form of the disease in the first or second year of life unless dialysis is initiated or the infant undergoes renal transplantation. Primary nephrotic syndrome involves only the kidney. Idiopathic (primary) nephrotic syndrome can be divided into 3 patterns. Minimal change nephrotic syndrome (MCNS), is the most common form of idiopathic nephrotic syndrome (approximately 80%), usually affects preschool children, and is twice as common in boys as in girls. The glomeruli, in a child with MCNS, appear normal or show minimal changes. The cause of MCNS is unknown. The other 2 types of idiopathic nephrotic syndrome are focal segmental glomerulosclerosis (FSGS) (10%) and mesangioproliferative glomerulonephritis (MesPGN) (5%). The secondary form of nephrotic syndrome develops during the course of other illnesses, such as acute or chronic glomerulonephritis, systemic lupus erythematous, diabetes mellitus, and acquired immunodeficiency syndrome (AIDS), or it may occur as the result of drug toxicity. The prognosis of nephrotic syndrome is dependent on the histologic type and early clinical course.

The pathogenesis of nephrotic syndrome is not clearly understood, but immune dysregulation, mainly cell-mediated immunity, is strongly suspected. An upper respiratory infection usually precedes the edema by approximately 2 to 3 days. A disturbance in the basement membrane of the glomeruli leads to increased permeability, which allows protein (especially albumin) to leak into the urine (proteinuria). This shift of protein out of the vascular system causes fluid from the plasma to seep into the interstitial spaces and body cavities, particularly the abdomen (ascites). Edema and hypovolemia result. The reduced vascular volume stimulates the renin-angiotensin system, which in turn leads to the secretion of aldosterone and antidiuretic hormone (ADH). Aldosterone increases the distal tubular reabsorption of sodium and water, adding to the edema already present. The liver's response to these events is to increase synthesis of lipoprotein. The hyperlipidemia is thought to occur because the lipoproteins are of higher molecular weight than albumin and therefore are not lost in the urine. Hyperlipidemia may cause an increase in platelet count. Urinary loss of antithrombin III and reduced levels of several clotting factors (IX, XI, and XII) may lead to hypercoagulability. The child is therefore at risk for thrombosis. Other complications include infections, hypertension, and renal failure. Relapses may occur especially after respiratory infections or live virus immunizations.

The clinical manifestations of nephrotic syndrome may include periorbital edema, generalized edema, ascites, dark and frothy urine, weight gain, irritability, abdominal pain, decreased appetite, nausea, vomiting, diarrhea, hypertension, and tachycardia. Diagnosis of nephrotic syndrome is based on the child's history, physical examination, and laboratory findings. The urinalysis reveals massive proteinuria. A complete blood count, coagulation studies, electrolytes (serum sodium will be decreased), serum creatinine, blood urea nitrogen (BUN), cholesterol, and albumin are also usually evaluated. A renal ultrasonography or single needle biopsy of the kidney may be performed in some cases.

Restoration of the intravascular fluid volume and maintenance of protein-free urine are the primary treatment goals of nephrotic syndrome. Corticosteroids are the mainstay of treatment. Additional therapies include diuretics, antihypertensives, alkylating agents (especially for those children with steroid resistant MCNS), and dietary salt restriction. Albumin may be indicated for those children with severe edema who are resistant to diuretics. Preventing infection, establishing good nutrition, and addressing the child's emotional needs are also important.

Primary Nursing Diagnosis

Deficient Fluid Volume: Intravascular and Excess Fluid Volume: Extravascular

Definition

Disturbance in the amount of circulating fluid volume with a decrease in intravascular fluid volume and an interstitial fluid overload

Possibly Related to

- Protein loss in the urine secondary to increased permeability of the glomeruli
- Increased water and sodium reabsorption from renal tubules secondary to increased secretion of aldosterone

Primary Nursing Diagnosis: Deficient fluid volume: intravascular and excess fluid volume: extravascular related to protein loss in the urine secondary to increased permeability of the glomeruli, increased water and sodium reabsorption from renal tubules secondary to increased secretion of aldosterone

Assessment/Defining Characteristics of Child and/or Family (Subjective & Objective Data):

- Marked generalized edema
- Ascites
- Possible diarrhea secondary to edema of the intestinal mucosa
- Dramatic weight gain
- Hypoproteinemia
- Hyperlipidemia
- Proteinuria
- Decreased urine output
- Frothy, dark-colored urine
- Blood pressure within acceptable limits or slightly decreased (usually)
- Increased urine specific gravity
- Tachycardia
- Tachypnea
- Nausea
- Vomiting
- Irritability
- Abdominal pain

Expected Outcomes	Possible Nursing Interventions	Rationale	Evaluation for Charting
Child will have an adequate intracellular and extracellular fluid volume as evidenced by	Keep accurate record of intake and output. Record characteristics of urine output.	Provides information on child's hydration status.	Document intake and output. Describe characteristics of urine output.

• adequate urine output (state specific range; 1 to 2 ml/kg/hr)
• clear, pale yellow urine
• return to usual weight
• blood pressure within acceptable range (state specific range)
• heart rate and respiratory rate within acceptable range (state specific range for each)
• lack of
  1. edema
  2. ascites
  3. hypoproteinemia
	Assess and record every 4 hours and PRN
	• BP, HR, and RR
	• abdominal girth
	• strip-test for presence of protein in the urine
	• urine specific gravity
	• laboratory values, as indicated. Report any abnormalities to the physician.
	• signs/symptoms of fluid imbalance (such as those listed under Assessment)
		Provides information about fluid status of patient. If patient has fluid imbalance, the BP, HR, RR, abdominal girth, and laboratory values will change.	Document range of BP, HR, and RR. Document current abdominal girth and indicate whether it has increased or decreased since previous measurement. Document range of urine protein and urine specific gravity. Document results of laboratory values when indicated and determine if the values are an increase or decrease from the previous values. Describe any signs/symptoms of fluid imbalance noted.

Primary Nursing Diagnosis: Deficient Fluid Volume: Intravascular and Excess Fluid Volume: Extravascular *(continued)*

Expected Outcomes	Possible Nursing Interventions	Rationale	Evaluation for Charting
4. hyperlipidemia 5. proteinuria 6. diarrhea 7. nausea 8. vomiting 9. irritability 10. abdominal pain • urine specific gravity from 1.008 to 1.020 • lack of signs/ symptoms of fluid imbalance (such as those listed under Assessment)	Weigh child daily on same scale at same time each day. Record results and compare to previous weight.	Sudden increase in weight gain may indicate extravascular fluid overload and may result in decreased cardiac output.	Document weight and determine if it was an increase or decrease from the previous weight.
	Handle edematous areas gently. Males may need to wear a scrotal support if scrotal edema is present.	Promotes comfort.	Document whether edematous areas were handled gently and describe effectiveness.
	Administer steroids on schedule. Assess and record effectiveness and any side effects (e.g., GI disturbance, headache).	Steroids indirectly help to decrease the loss of protein in the urine.	Document whether steroids were administered on schedule. Describe effectiveness and any side effects noted.
	If indicated, administer antacids on schedule. Assess and record effectiveness and any side effects (e.g., constipation, diarrhea, stomach cramps).	Antacids are administered to help prevent complication of GI bleeding from steroid therapy.	Document whether antacids were administered on schedule. Describe effectiveness and any side effects noted.
	Administer diuretics on schedule (ensure that dose has been adjusted to avoid toxicity from inadequate renal clearance). Assess and record effectiveness and any side effects (e.g., hypokalemia, dehydration).	Diuretics are administered to decrease excess intravascular fluid through increased urine output, which will decrease the workload on the heart.	Document whether diuretics were administered on schedule. Describe effectiveness and any side effects noted.
TEACHING GOALS Child and/or family will be able to verbalize at least 4 characteristics of fluid imbalance such as • marked generalized edema • increase abdominal girth • dramatic weight gain • decreased urine output	Teach child/family about characteristics of fluid imbalance. Assess and record results.	Increased knowledge will assist the child/family in recognizing and reporting changes in the child's condition.	Document whether teaching was done and describe results.

(continued)

Primary Nursing Diagnosis: Deficient Fluid Volume: Intravascular and Excess Fluid Volume: Extravascular *(continued)*

Expected Outcomes	Possible Nursing Interventions	Rationale	Evaluation for Charting
Child and/or family will be able to verbalize knowledge of care such as • monitoring of intake and output • test for protein in urine • medication administration • recognition of subtle signs/symptoms of infection (side effects of steroids may mast signs of infection) • identification of any signs/symptoms of fluid imbalance (such as those listed under Assessment) and the correct action for each • when to contact health-care provider	Teach child/family about care. Assess and record child's/family's knowledge of and participation in care regarding monitoring intake and output, etc.	Education of child/family will allow for accurate care.	Document whether teaching was done and describe results.

Nursing Diagnosis   Imbalanced Nutrition: Less Than Body Requirements

Definition   Insufficient nutrients to meet body requirements

Possibly Related to
- Malnutrition secondary to protein loss and decreased appetite
- Poor intestinal absorption secondary to edema of the intestinal mucosa

Nursing Diagnosis: Imbalanced nutrition: less than body requirements related to malnutrition secondary to protein loss and decreased appetite, poor intestinal absorption secondary to edema of the intestinal mucosa

Assessment/Defining Characteristics of Child and/or Family (Subjective & Objective Data):
- Anorexia
- Lethargy
- Hypoproteinemia
- Diarrhea

Expected Outcomes	Possible Nursing Interventions	Rationale	Evaluation for Charting
Child will be adequately nourished as evidenced by • absorption of adequate amount of calories (state specific amount for each child) • return of appetite • lack of hypoproteinemia • lack of signs/symptoms of imbalanced nutrition (such as those listed under Assessment)	Keep accurate record of intake and output.	Provides information on child's hydration status.	Document intake and output.
	Assess and record any signs/symptoms of imbalanced nutrition (such as those listed under Assessment) every 4 hours and PRN.	Provides information on nutritional status of child.	Describe any signs/symptoms of imbalanced nutrition noted.
	Weigh child daily on same scale at same time of day. Document results and compare to previous weight.	Provides information on child's hydration and nutritional status.	Document weight and determine if it was an increase or decrease from the previous weight.
	Assess child's food likes/dislikes and, when possible, provide foods that child likes to eat.	Encourages child to eat.	Describe any therapeutic measures used to maintain adequate nutrition. Document their effectiveness.
	Organize care to conserve energy. Encourage small frequent meals and snacks.	Conserving energy will help to maintain adequate nutrition.	Describe any therapeutic measures used to maintain adequate nutrition. Document their effectiveness.
	Ensure that child get prescribed diet. May need dietary salt restriction. If indicated, maintain calorie count.	Sodium restriction may be necessary due to the edema. Adequate calories are needed for the healing process.	Document whether dietary restrictions were necessary and describe effectiveness of measures. Document calorie count if indicated.
TEACHING GOALS Child and/or family will be able to verbalize at least 3 characteristics of imbalanced nutrition such as • anorexia • lethargy • diarrhea	Teach child/family about characteristics of imbalanced nutrition. Assess and record results.	Increased knowledge will assist the child/family in recognizing and reporting changes in the child's condition.	Document whether teaching was done and describe results.

(continued)

	Possible Nursing		Evaluation for
Expected Outcomes	**Interventions**	**Rationale**	**Charting**
Child and/or family will be able to verbalize knowledge of care such as • prescribed diet • organization of care and activity of child in order to conserve energy • identification of any signs/symptoms of imbalanced nutrition (such as those listed under Assessment) • when to contact health-care provider	Teach child/family about care. Assess and record child's/family's knowledge of and participation in care regarding prescribed diet, etc.	Education of child/family will allow for accurate care.	Document whether teaching was done and describe results.

Nursing Diagnosis: Imbalanced Nutrition: Less than Body Requirements *(continued)*

Related Nursing Diagnoses

Risk for Infection	*related to* a. edema fluid being excellent culture medium b. thin and stretched skin secondary to edema c. lowered resistance secondary to steroid therapy
Deficient Knowledge: Child/Family	*related to* disease state and home care
Impaired Skin Integrity	*related to* edema
Disturbed Body Image	*related to* edema

FOUR

VESICOURETERAL REFLUX
MEDICAL DIAGNOSIS

PATHOPHYSIOLOGY Vesicoureteral reflux (VUR) is the abnormal backflow of urine from the bladder into the ureters and possibly into the kidneys. VUR is the most common urologic abnormality in children, seen in 1% of healthy children, but in 30 to 50% of children who have a history of one or more urinary tract infections (UTIs). Siblings and offspring of affected individuals have an increased rate of VUR, suggesting a genetic component to its etiology. Higher rates of VUR are seen in whites, females, and children from birth to age 2. VUR is associated with an increased likelihood of pyelonephritis during UTIs. This may contribute to the development of renal scarring, hypertension, or renal failure.

Normally urine flows downward from the kidneys through the ureters into the bladder. The ureters are positioned at the posterior, lower aspect of the bladder at an oblique angle and tunnel through the bladder mucosa for a short distance before opening into the bladder. When the bladder becomes full of urine and voiding begins, the pressure in the bladder is increased and the bladder musculature contracts, compressing the tunneled portion of the ureters (similar to a valve) and preventing backflow of urine into the ureters. When voiding is complete, the bladder relaxes and the ureteral openings may drain once again.

Reflux occurs when the mechanism for compressing the tunneled portion of the ureters malfunctions. Primary reflux occurs with a congenital malformation in which the ureters enter the bladder at an abnormal acute angle and the tunneling of the ureters in the bladder mucosa is shortened, resulting in decreased compression. When pressure builds in the bladder, urine refluxes up into the ureters. If pressure is high enough, the urine can reflux into the kidneys and eventually cause hydronephrosis and renal damage. When voiding is complete, the bladder wall relaxes and the urine that was refluxed into the ureters returns to the bladder. Primary VUR may resolve spontaneously. Secondary reflux occurs as a result of increased bladder pressure secondary to bladder outlet obstruction (e.g., posterior urethral valves), abnormal attachment of the ureter (e.g., ectopic ureter), or associated urinary tract abnormalities that affect the insertion of the ureter (e.g., prune belly syndrome).

Vesicoureteral reflux ranges from mild to severe, with grading system from I to V used to describe the degree. In Grade I, urine is refluxed into the distal ureters only; Grade II reflux extends into the proximal ureter without dilatation, in Grade III urine is refluxed into the kidney with mild dilatation of the ureters and pelvis, Grade IV urine is refluxed into the kidney with moderate dilatation of the ureters and pelvis, Grade V indicates gross reflux of urine and severe dilatation of the ureters and renal pelvis.

During the evaluation for a UTI is when VUR is usually diagnosed. Renal sonography, and either voiding cystourethography (VCUG) or radionuclide cystography (RNC) provide imaging of the upper and lower urinary tracts. VUR is being diagnosed more often following the identification of hydronephrosis by fetal ultrasonography.

Most cases of VUR can be treated with conservative (nonsurgical) medical management, which includes continuous low-dose antibacterial therapy with frequent urine cultures. The goal of therapy is to prevent urinary tract infections in the hopes of preventing pyelonephritis and renal scarring. If reflux is mild (Grades I and II), it usually resolves spontaneously. Surgical correction is employed when (1) there is a significant anatomic abnormality, (2) the reflux is severe enough (Grade V) to cause ureteral dilatation and upper urinary tract dysfunction, and renal scarring, or (3) there is noncompliance with medical therapy or intolerance to antibiotics. Surgical correction is also considered for reflux that is persistent, bilateral, and diagnosed at a later age. When surgery is indicated, surgical options include ureteral reimplantation or endoscopic repair.

Postoperative Nursing Care Plan for Ureteral Implantation

Primary Nursing Diagnosis   Risk for Infection

Definition   Condition in which the body is at risk for being invaded by microorganisms

Possibly Related to   • Surgical wound

                        • Invasive urinary devices

Primary Nursing Diagnosis: Risk for infection related to surgical wound, invasive urinary devices			
Assessment/Defining Characteristics of Child and/or Family (Subjective & Objective Data):			
• Fever • Tachycardia • Tachypnea • Hypotension • Redness • Swelling • Purulent wound drainage		• Foul-smelling urine • Cloudy, hazy, or thick urine • Lower abdominal pain • Lethargy • Anorexia • Chills • Leukocytosis	
Expected Outcomes	**Possible Nursing Interventions**	**Rationale**	**Evaluation for Charting**
Child will be free of infection as evidenced by • body temperature within acceptable range of 36.5°C to 37.2°C • heart rate within acceptable range (state specific range) • respiratory rate within acceptable range (state specific range) • blood pressure within acceptable range (state specific range) • clear, pale yellow urine • return of appetite • WBC within acceptable range (state specific range) • lack of signs/symptoms of infection (such as those listed under Assessment)	Assess and record • T, HR, RR, and BP every 4 hours and PRN • IV fluids and condition of IV site every hour • laboratory values as indicated. Report abnormalities to the physician. • signs/symptoms of infection (such as those listed under Assessment) every 4 hours and PRN	If infection is present, the T, HR, RR, BP, and lab values will change. The signs/symptoms of infection (such as those listed under Assessment) may be present. Provides information about fluid status of the child. It is necessary to record the amount of IV fluids every hour to make sure the child is not being over or under hydrated. The IV site needs to be assessed every hour for signs or redness or swelling.	Document range of T, HR, RR, and BP. Document amount of IV fluids and describe condition of IV site along with any interventions needed. Document results of laboratory values when indicated and determine if the values are in increase or decrease from the previous values. Describe any signs/symptoms of infection.
	Maintain good hand-washing technique.	Good hand washing is the single most important measure in decreasing infection.	Document whether good hand-washing technique was used.

Primary Nursing Diagnosis: Risk for Infection *(continued)*

Expected Outcomes	Possible Nursing Interventions	Rationale	Evaluation for Charting
	Keep accurate record of intake and output. Use aseptic technique when emptying urine collection bags. Check and record urine output every hour for the first 24 hours and then at least every 4 hours. Record characteristics of urine.	Provides information on child's hydration status. Decreased urine output can indicate obstruction. Aseptic technique is necessary when caring for and emptying urine collection bags in order to prevent infection.	Document intake and output. Document whether aseptic technique was used when emptying urine collection bags. Describe characteristic of urine output.
	Secure tubing attached to urinary devices with tape. Include a stress loop for additional protection.	Necessary to prevent displacement.	Document whether tubing was secured and the effectiveness of the measure.
	Use aseptic technique when dressing changes are indicated. Assess and record location and characteristics of wound.	Helps prevent infection.	Document whether aseptic technique was used during dressing changes. Describe location and characteristics of wound.
	Administer antibiotics on schedule. Assess and record any side effects (e.g., rash, diarrhea).	Antibiotics are given to combat infection.	Document whether antibiotics were administered on schedule. Describe any side effects noted.
	When indicated, administer antipyretics on schedule and PRN. Assess and record effectiveness.	Antipyretics are used to reduce fever.	Document whether an antipyretic was needed and describe effectiveness.
	Check and record results of WBC. Notify physician if WBC is out of the stated range.	If infection is present, WBC results will change.	Document results of WBC if available.
	Ensure that proper collection of urine specimens for culture are obtained as indicated. Make sure that specimens are sent to the laboratory immediately after collection. Record results when available.	Necessary to prevent contamination of the specimen.	Document results of urine culture if available.

(continued)

Primary Nursing Diagnosis: Risk for Infection *(continued)*

Expected Outcomes	Possible Nursing Interventions	Rationale	Evaluation for Charting
TEACHING GOALS Child and/or family will be able to verbalize at least 4 characteristics of infection such as • fever • purulent wound drainage • foul-smelling urine • cloudy, hazy, or thick urine • lethargy • anorexia	Teach child/family about characteristics of risk for infection. Assess and record results.	Increased knowledge will assist the child/family in recognizing and reporting changes in the child's condition.	Document whether teaching was done and describe results.
Child and/or family will be able to verbalize knowledge of care such as • good hand-washing technique • fever control • medication administration • need for reminding child to empty bladder frequently • proper collection or urine specimen when indicated • need for reminding child to wear clean cotton underwear • good hygienic habits, including teaching females to wipe the perineal area from front to back • avoidance of harsh detergents and bubble baths • reminding child to drink liquids frequently • avoidance of tight-fitting clothing • identification of any signs/symptoms of further infection (such as those listed under Assessment) • when to contact health-care provider	Teach child/family about care. Assess and record child's/family's knowledge of and participation in care regarding good hand-washing technique, fever control, etc.	Education of child/family will allow for accurate care.	Document whether teaching was done and describe results.

Nursing Diagnosis Acute Pain

Definition Condition in which an individual experiences acute mild to severe pain

Possibly Related to
- Surgical incisions
- Bladder spasms

Nursing Diagnosis: Acute pain related to surgical incisions, bladder spasms

Assessment/Defining Characteristics of Child and/or Family (Subjective & Objective Data):
- Verbal communication of pain
- Facial grimacing
- Crying unrelieved by usual comfort measures
- Decreased activity, self-imposed
- Restlessness
- Rating of pain on pain-assessment tool
- Physical signs/symptoms (tachycardia, tachypnea, increased blood pressure, diaphoresis)

Expected Outcomes	Possible Nursing Interventions	Rationale	Evaluation for Charting

Child will have decreased pain or be free of severe and/or constant pain as evidenced by
 	
• verbal communication of comfort
• lack of
  1. constant crying
  2. facial grimacing
  3. restlessness
• heart rate within acceptable range (state specific range)
• respiratory rate within acceptable range (state specific range)
• blood pressure within acceptable range (state specific range)
• rating of decreased pain or no pain on pain-assessment tool
• lack of signs/symptoms of acute pain (such as those listed under Assessment)
	Assess and record HR, RR, BP, and any signs/symptoms of pain (such as those listed under Assessment) every 2 to 4 hours and PRN. Use age-appropriate pain-assessment tool.	Provides data regarding the level of pain child is experiencing.	Document range of HR, RR, BP, and degree of pain child was experiencing. Describe any successful measures used to decrease pain.

	Administer analgesics on schedule. Assess and record effectiveness and any side effects (e.g., constipation, nausea).	Analgesics are administered to decrease pain.	Document whether analgesics were administered on schedule. Describe effectiveness and any side effects noted.
	Administer antispasmodics on schedule. Assess and record effectiveness and any side effects (e.g., nausea, vomiting).	Helps relieve bladder and ureter spasms.	Document whether antispasmodics were administered on schedule. Describe effectiveness and any side effects noted.
	Handle child gently.	Helps to increase comfort.	Document if child was handled gently. Describe effectiveness.
	Encourage family members to stay and comfort child when possible.	Helps to comfort and support the child.	Document whether family was able to remain with child and describe effectiveness of their presence.
	Allow family members to participate in care of child when possible.	This may increase the comfort level of the child and thus help child in managing pain.	Document whether family participated in care and if this was successful in helping child with pain management.

(continued)

Nursing Diagnosis: Acute Pain (*continued*)

Expected Outcomes	Possible Nursing Interventions	Rationale	Evaluation for Charting
	Use diversional activities (e.g., music, television, playing games, relaxation) when appropriate.	Diversional activities can distract child and may help to decrease pain.	Document whether diversional activities were successful in helping to manage pain.
	If age appropriate, explain all procedures beforehand.	Allowing child some control can assist child with pain management.	Describe if this measure was effective in helping child to manage pain.
	If age appropriate, allow the child to participate in planning his or her care. Encourage the child to practice self-care (e.g., bathing, dressing).	Allowing child some control can assist child with pain management.	Describe if this measure was effective in helping child to manage pain.
	When indicated, institute additional pain relief measures, such as hypnosis and guided imagery. Assess and record effectiveness.	These nonpharmacologic measures may help decrease pain.	Document whether these measures were successful in helping to manage pain.
TEACHING GOALS Child and/or family will be able to verbalize at least 4 characteristics of pain such as • verbal communication of pain • crying unrelieved by usual comfort measures • decreased activity, self-imposed • rapid heart rate	Teach child/family about characteristics of pain. Assess and record results.	Increased knowledge will assist the child/family in recognizing and reporting changes in the child's condition.	Document whether teaching was done and describe results.
Child and/or family will be able to verbalize knowledge of care such as • medication administration • gentle handling of child • identification of any signs/symptoms of pain (such as those listed under Assessment) • when to contact health-care provider	Teach child/family about care. Assess and record child's/family's knowledge of and participation in care regarding medication administration, etc.	Education of child/family will allow for accurate care.	Document whether teaching was done and describe results.

Related Nursing Diagnoses

Deficient Knowledge: Child/Family	*related to* a. postoperative care of child b. prevention of further urinary tract infections
Compromised Family Coping	*related to* a. hospitalization of child b. guilt (if parents/family were noncompliant with medical management in past)
Fear: Child	*related to* a. hospitalization b. forced contact with strangers

FIVE

URINARY TRACT INFECTION/ PYELONEPHRITIS
MEDICAL DIAGNOSIS

PATHOPHYSIOLOGY Urinary tract infections (UTI) are caused by bacterial invasion of a normally sterile area in the urinary tract. Cystitis occurs when the infection is limited to the bladder or lower urinary tract; involvement of the upper urinary tract or kidneys is called pyelonephritis. In the pediatric population, the frequency of urinary tract infections is second only to that of respiratory tract infections. Age and sex are the two most important factors influencing the prevalence of UTIs. Urinary tract infections are more frequent in females except during the newborn period. The higher incidence of UTIs in males during that period is thought to be due to the increased incidence of anatomic abnormalities and there is also a slight increase in the incidence of urinary tract infections in uncircumcised males. UTI is more common in preschool-age children than in school-age children. There is an increased risk for developing UTIs during adolescence in sexually active girls and in homosexual boys. Vesicoureteral reflux (VUR) is the most important risk factor for the development of pyelonephritis.

Organisms can enter the urinary tract through the bloodstream (bloodborne), but more often they enter from the genital area, ascending through the urethra into the bladder. Except during the newborn period, pyelonephritis usually develops after fecal flora colonize in the urethra and then ascend into the bladder and kidneys. Facilitating entry of bacteria into the urinary system are structural factors (e.g., the short urethra and its close proximity to the anus in females), anatomical anomalies (e.g., obstruction, which may lead to reflux of urine from the bladder through the ureters to the kidneys because of the high voiding pressure needed to overcome the obstruction), urinary stasis (e.g., inadequate bladder innervation or neurogenic bladder), and introduction of urinary catheters. The bacterial organisms usually responsible are *Escherichia coli* (75 to 90% of the time), *Klebsiella*, enteric *Streptococci*, *Proteus*, *Pseudomonas*, *Enterobacter*, and *Staphylococcus* species.

The inflammation resulting from the bacterial invasion causes irritability and spasms of the bladder wall. The inflammation may also lead to hematuria. Changes in the bladder wall can occur after repeated infections, which may damage the vesicoureteral valves (where ureters enter the bladder) and result in reflux of urine into the ureters, especially during voiding. The ureters can become dilated and allow access of urine and bacteria into the upper urinary tract. Bacteria that reach the kidneys can cause inflammation, edema, necrosis of the renal cortex, scarring, and loss of renal tissue. The normal concentrating and filtering mechanisms of the kidneys may also be impaired. Long-term complications of pyelonephritis include recurrence, renal scarring, and hypertension.

Clinical manifestations vary with age and the area involved along the urinary tract. Infants with pyelonephritis may present with fever and irritability, as well as poor feeding and lethargy. Toddlers may complain of abdominal pain. Children can present with pyelonephritis without the typical symptoms of a lower tract infection. Older children with pyelonephritis may exhibit the typical signs of a UTI such as dysuria, urgency, and increased urinary frequency along with fever, chills, nausea, and flank pain. The diagnosis of UTI is confirmed by a properly obtained urine specimen, which will indicate a significant number of bacteria. Infrequently, imaging studies are needed to confirm a diagnosis of pyelonephritis. Computed tomography (CT) scans with contrast are more sensitive than ultrasonography in detecting changes consistent with pyelonephritis. A voiding cystourethrogram (VCUG) or radionuclide cystography (RNC) may be done to diagnose vesicoureteral reflux. Renal scintography can also confirm pyelonephritis as well as detect renal scarring.

Treatment goals for UTIs and pyelonephritis include eliminating the current infection, preventing systemic spread of the infection, preserving renal function, preventing renal scarring, and reducing the risk of recurrence. Various antimicrobial agents are useful for the treatment of UTIs and pyelonephritis.

Primary Nursing Diagnosis   Actual Infection*

Definition   Condition in which microorganisms have invaded the body

Possibly Related to
- Bacterial invasion of urinary tract secondary to
  - entry of organisms through blood or perineal area
  - anatomic anomaly
  - inadequate bladder innervation (neurogenic bladder)

*Non-NANDA diagnosis.

Primary Nursing Diagnosis: Actual infection related to bacterial invasion of urinary tract secondary to entry of organisms through blood or perineal area, anatomic anomaly, inadequate bladder innervation (neurogenic bladder)

Assessment/Defining Characteristics of Child and/or Family (Subjective & Objective Data):

INFANTS: CYSTITIS OR PYELONEPHRITIS

- Vomiting
- Diarrhea
- Irritability lethargy
- Poor feeding
- Slow weight gain
- Unexplained jaundice

- Fever or hypothermia
- Abdominal distention
- Weak urine stream
- Frequent or infrequent voiding
- Strong-smelling urine
- Persistent diaper rash

CHILDREN: CYSTITIS

- Dysuria
- Frequency
- Urgency
- Lower abdominal pain

- Foul-smelling urine
- Hematuria
- Incontinence
- Enuresis

CHILDREN: PYELONEPHRITIS

- Fever
- Chills
- Nausea
- Anorexia

- Vomiting
- Malaise
- Lower back pain over costovertebral angle
- Cloudy, hazy, or thick urine

GENERAL

- Tachycardia
- Tachypnea

- Hypotension
- Altered white blood cell count (WBC)

Expected Outcomes	Possible Nursing Interventions	Rationale	Evaluation for Charting
Child will be free of infection as evidenced by • body temperature within acceptable range of 36.5°C to 37.2°C • heart rate within acceptable range (state specific range)	Assess and record • T, HR, RR, and BP every 4 hours and PRN • IV fluids and condition of IV site every hour • laboratory values as indicated. Report abnormalities to the physician.	If infection is present, the T, HR, RR, BP, and lab values will change. The signs/symptoms of infection (such as those listed under Assessment) may be present. Provides information about fluid status of the child. It is necessary to record the	Document range of T, HR, RR, and BP. Document amount of IV fluids and describe condition of IV site along with any interventions needed. Document results of laboratory values when indicated and determine

(continued)

Primary Nursing Diagnosis: Actual Infection *(continued)*

Expected Outcomes	Possible Nursing Interventions	Rationale	Evaluation for Charting
• respiratory rate within acceptable range (state specific range) • blood pressure within acceptable range (state specific range) • clear, pale yellow urine • urine specific gravity from 1.008 to 1.020 • return of appetite • WBC within acceptable range (state specific range) • lack of signs/symptoms of infection (such as those listed under Assessment)	• signs/symptoms of infection (such as those listed under Assessment) every 4 hours and PRN	amount of IV fluids every hour to make sure the child is not being over or under hydrated. The IV site needs to be assessed every hour for signs or redness or swelling.	if the values are an increase or decrease from the previous values. Describe any signs/symptoms of infection.
	Maintain good hand-washing technique.	Good hand washing is the single most important measure in decreasing infection.	Document whether good hand-washing technique was used.
	Keep accurate record of intake and output. Record characteristics of urine.	Provides information on child's hydration status. Characteristics of urine will change if infection is present.	Document intake and output. Describe characteristics of urine output.
	Administer antibiotics on schedule. Assess and record any side effects (e.g., rash, diarrhea).	Antibiotics are given to combat infection.	Document whether antibiotics were administered on schedule. Describe any side effects noted.
	When indicated, administer antipyretics on schedule and PRN. Assess and record effectiveness.	Antipyretics are used to reduce fever.	Document whether an antipyretic was needed and describe effectiveness.
	Check and record results of WBC. Notify physician if WBC is out of the stated range.	If infection is present, WBC results will change.	Document results of WBC if available.
	Ensure that proper collection of urine specimens for culture are obtained as indicated. Make sure that specimens are sent to the laboratory immediately after collection. Record results when available.	Necessary to prevent contamination of the specimen.	Document results of urine culture if available.
	Check and record urine specific gravity every 4 hours or as indicated.	Urine specific gravity provides information about hydration status.	Document range of urine specific gravity.

Primary Nursing Diagnosis: Actual Infection *(continued)*

Expected Outcomes	Possible Nursing Interventions	Rationale	Evaluation for Charting
TEACHING GOALS Child and/or family will be able to verbalize at least 4 characteristics of infection such as • fever • purulent wound drainage • foul-smelling urine • cloudy, hazy, or thick urine • lethargy • anorexia	Teach child/family about characteristics of risk for infection. Assess and record results.	Increased knowledge will assist the child/family in recognizing and reporting changes in the child's condition.	Document whether teaching was done and describe results.
Child and/or family will be able to verbalize knowledge of care such as • good hand-washing technique • fever control • medication administration • need for reminding child to empty bladder frequently • proper collection or urine specimen when indicated • need for reminding child to wear clean cotton underwear • good hygienic habits, including teaching females to wipe the perineal area from front to back • avoidance of harsh detergents and bubble baths • reminding child to drink liquids frequently • avoidance of tight-fitting clothing • identification of any signs/symptoms of further infection (such as those listed under Assessment) • when to contact health-care provider	Teach child/family about care. Assess and record child's/family's knowledge of and participation in care regarding good hand-washing technique, fever control, etc.	Education of child/family will allow for accurate care.	Document whether teaching was done and describe results.

Nursing Diagnosis

Nursing Diagnosis Deficient Knowledge: Child/Family

Definition Lack of information concerning the child's disease and care

Possibly Related to
- Disease state
- Cause of infection
- Recognition of signs/symptoms
- Prevention of recurrent infections
- Sensory overload
- Cognitive or cultural-language limitations

Nursing Diagnosis: Deficient knowledge: child/family related to disease state, cause of infection, recognition of signs/symptoms, prevention of recurrent infections, sensory overload, cognitive or cultural-language limitations

Assessment/Defining Characteristics of Child and/or Family (Subjective & Objective Data):
- Verbalization by child/family indicating a lack of knowledge regarding urinary tract infection
- Relation of incorrect information to members of the health-care team
- Inability to correctly repeat information previously explained
- Inability to correctly demonstrate skills previously taught (e.g., medication administration)

Expected Outcomes	Possible Nursing Interventions	Rationale	Evaluation for Charting
TEACHING GOALS Child/Family will have an adequate knowledge base concerning the child's illness and care as evidenced by • ability to correctly state information previously taught regarding urinary tract infections, child's care, and prevention of further urinary tract infections • ability to correctly demonstrate skills previously taught (e.g., medication administration) • ability to relate appropriate information to the health-care team • ability to request additional information and/or clarification of information	Listen to child's/family's concerns and fears. Document findings.	Allows child/family to express feelings and concerns and provides them with a way to gain knowledge.	Describe child's/family's concerns and fears and any successful measures used to encourage family to express their feelings.
	Assess and record child's/family's knowledge of and understanding of child's illness. Encourage questions.	Generates a baseline of knowledge, which allows for teaching of accurate information and dispelling of incorrect knowledge.	Document whether teaching was done and describe results.
	Provide child/family with information about urinary tract infections, including • recognition of signs/symptoms of infection	Education of child/family will allow for accurate care and increase coping ability of child/family.	Document whether teaching was done and describe results. Describe ability of child/family to repeat information correctly and perform skills adequately.

Nursing Diagnosis: Deficient Knowledge: Child/Family *(continued)*			
Expected Outcomes	**Possible Nursing Interventions**	**Rationale**	**Evaluation for Charting**
	<ul><li>administration of antibiotics for entire prescribed course (even through child usually gets better before antibiotic therapy is completed)</li><li>reminding child to empty bladder frequently</li><li>proper collection of urine specimens when indicated</li><li>reminding child to wear clean cotton underwear</li><li>good hygiene habits. Teach females to wipe the perineal area from front to back.</li><li>avoidance of harsh detergents and bubble baths</li><li>reminding child to drink liquids frequently</li><li>avoidance of tight-fitting clothing</li></ul>		

Related Nursing Diagnoses

Deficient Fluid Volume	*related to* a. vomiting b. diarrhea c. fever
Acute Pain	*related to* spasms of bladder wall secondary to inflammation
Fear: Child	*related to* a. pain b. hospitalization c. treatments and procedures
Compromised Family Coping	*related to* a. hospitalization of child b. pain experienced by child

12

CARE OF
CHILDREN WITH
FAILURE TO THRIVE

ONE

FAILURE TO THRIVE
MEDICAL DIAGNOSIS

DESCRIPTION Failure to thrive (FTT) is when infants and children fail to grow and gain weight at a normal rate, deviating significantly from the norms on the National Center for Health Statistics growth charts. Traditionally, failure to thrive was classified as either organic (resulting from a physical factor) or nonorganic (resulting from a psychosocial factor) in origin. It is most useful to assess each child and family medically, nutritionally, developmentally, and socially. There are numerous medical causes of FTT; examples are prematurity, congenital heart defects, gastrointestinal disorders, central nervous system abnormalities, chronic infections, endocrine disorders, metabolic disorders, genetic abnormalities, and acquired immunodeficiency syndrome (AIDS). Psychosocial factors (nonorganic), which can contribute to FTT, include poverty, family health beliefs, substance abuse, family stress, a disturbance in attachment, or a disturbance in the relationship between the child and the primary caregiver (due to inexperience or lack of information concerning infant development and nutritional requirements). FTT does not necessarily imply parental neglect. Multifactorial (or mixed) FTT describes a situation where there are both organic and nonorganic factors identified as contributing to the child's poor growth. More than 80% of children admitted with FTT do not have an underlying medical disorder.

The prevalence of underweight is highest in young infants. The pathogenesis of poor growth in young infants can be related to 3 mechanisms that lead to a mismatch of adequate caloric intake to meet caloric expenditure. There can be loss of calories through malabsorption, increased caloric expenditure, or inadequate intake of calories. FTT exists in all socioeconomic groups, but poor growth is more common in low-income communities. There is a higher risk of lack of knowledge regarding child nutrition, financial hardship, and social problems that include substance abuse and child maltreatment in these communities. Poverty and lack of food availability put children at risk for poor growth, as do large families and a history of child maltreatment.

The evaluation of a child who has FTT requires a complete history (e.g., medical, nutritional, feeding behavior, family, social), history of height and weight trajectories of parents and siblings, and a thorough physical examination, emphasizing neurodevelopmental status. The growth chart is the most important tool used to evaluate the child who has FTT. Laboratory testing and imaging studies should be individualized. Evaluation of the family's economic, organizational, and/or mental health status may be warranted if there are psychosocial factors contributing to the child's FTT.

Treatment goals include reversing the malnutrition, addressing any coexisting medical conditions, and dealing with the psychological, social, and developmental problems. Often a multidisciplinary team is needed to meet all these needs. If it has been a short period of failure to thrive and the cause is identified and corrected, normal growth and development can resume. Children with FTT can experience delays not only in growth but also in emotional, social, motor, language, and intellectual development.

Primary Nursing Diagnosis Imbalanced Nutrition: Less than Body Requirements

Definition Insufficient nutrients to meet body requirements

Possibly Related to
- Disturbance in child/primary caregiver relationship
- Neglect
- Emotional deprivation
- Parental knowledge deficit
- Congenital anomaly or other physical condition
- Malabsorption
- Loose stools
- Inadequate food intake
- Financial hardship
- Social problems

Primary Nursing Diagnosis: Imbalanced nutrition: less than body requirements related to disturbance in child/primary caregiver relationship, neglect, emotional deprivation, parental knowledge deficit, congenital anomaly or other physical condition, malabsorption, loose stools, inadequate food intake, financial hardship, social problems

Assessment/Defining Characteristics of Child and/or Family (Subjective & Objective Data):
- Vomiting
- Diarrhea
- Rumination
- Anorexia or voracious appetite
- Apathy
- Lethargy
- Dehydration
- Weight below the third percentile
- Sudden or rapid decline in growth rate

Expected Outcomes	Possible Nursing Interventions	Rationale	Evaluation for Charting
Child will be adequately nourished as evidenced by • steady weight gain (state how much would be reasonable for each child) • adequate caloric intake (state range of calories needed for each child) • lack of 1. vomiting 2. diarrhea 3. rumination 4. anorexia	Keep accurate record of intake and output.	Provides information on child's hydration status.	Document intake and output.
	Assess and record any signs/symptoms of imbalanced nutrition (such as those listed under Assessment) every 8 hours and PRN.	Provides information on nutritional status of child.	Describe any signs/symptoms of imbalanced nutrition noted.
	Weigh child daily on same scale at same time of day. Document results and compare to previous weight.	Provides information on child's hydration and nutritional status.	Document weight and determine if it was an increase or decrease from the previous weight.
	Maintain and record daily calorie counts.	Provides information on actual caloric intake.	Document calorie count.

(continued)

Primary Nursing Diagnosis: Imbalanced nutrition: Less than body requirements *(continued)*

Expected Outcomes	Possible Nursing Interventions	Rationale	Evaluation for Charting
5. apathy 6. lethargy 7. dehydration • lack of signs/ symptoms of imbalanced nutrition (such as those listed under Assessment)	Feed child on schedule. Record amount accurately and record child's response to feedings.	Feeding child on schedule allows for adequate nutrition. Accurately record child's response to feeding can provide clues to feeding difficulties.	Document whether child was fed on schedule. Describe child's tolerance of feedings, including effectiveness of any feeding techniques used.
	Assist, observe, and record child/parental interaction during feeding. Assess and record parental feeding technique when appropriate. A feeding checklist may be used for documentation. In some instances, the child may need to be fed exclusively by the nurse.	Accurate observation and documentation of child/parent interaction during feedings and parental feeding techniques is necessary to help identify any problems.	Document child/parent interaction during feedings and parental feeding techniques when appropriate. Document whether the child was fed exclusively by the nurse.
	Provide role modeling and education to parents for feeding skills, infant/child care, and nurturing in a nonthreatening and nonjudgmental manner. Provide positive feedback for appropriate behavior.	Role modeling and education by the nurse and positive feedback for appropriate behavior can supply a means to provide adequate nutrition for the child.	Describe any successful measures used to provide the child with adequate nutrition and the effectiveness of the measures.
TEACHING GOALS Family will be able to verbalize at least 4 characteristics of imbalanced nutrition such as • failure to gain weight • vomiting • diarrhea • decreased appetite • lethargy	Teach family about characteristics of imbalanced nutrition. Assess and record results.	Increased knowledge will assist the family in recognizing and reporting changes in the child's condition.	Document whether teaching was done and describe results.
Family will be able to verbalize knowledge of care such as • feeding techniques • if indicated, correct preparation of formula • appropriate feeding schedule	Teach family about care. Assess and record family's knowledge of and participation in care regarding feeding techniques, etc.	Education of family will allow for accurate care.	Document whether teaching was done and describe results.

Expected Outcomes	Possible Nursing Interventions	Rationale	Evaluation for Charting
• monitoring of child's weight gain and caloric consumption • ability to nurture child • identification of any signs/symptoms of imbalanced nutrition (such as those listed under Assessment) • when to contact health-care provider			

Primary Nursing Diagnosis: Imbalanced nutrition: Less than body requirements *(continued)*

Nursing Diagnosis Delayed Growth and Development

Definition Failure to gain weight at an acceptable rate for age group and failure to progress in expected tasks and skills according to chronologic age

Possibly Related to
- Disturbance in child/primary caregiver relationship
- Neglect
- Emotional deprivation
- Environmental problems (e.g., lack of stimulation)
- Parental knowledge deficit
- Congenital anomaly or other physical condition
- Nutritional deficit

Nursing Diagnosis: Delayed growth and development related to disturbance in child/primary caregiver relationship, neglect, emotional deprivation, environmental problems (e.g., lack of stimulation), parental knowledge deficit, congenital anomaly or other physical condition, nutritional deficit

Assessment/Defining Characteristics of Child and/or Family (Subjective & Objective Data):
- Weight below the third percentile
- Sudden or rapid decline in growth rate
- Apathy
- Withdrawn behavior
- No fear of strangers (at an age when fear of strangers would be a normal finding)
- Avoidance of eye-to-eye contact
- Minimal smiling
- Passivity
- Indifference to caregivers
- Intense watchfulness
- Delayed and/or minimal vocalization
- Repetitive behaviors (e.g., head banging, rocking)
- Other characteristics varying with age and state of development for infant. At all ages, normal growth and development will be delayed; for example, a 4-month-old may not be able to attain behaviors such as
  1. grasping toys and bringing them to mouth
  2. using both hands when attempting to pick up objects
  3. pulling to sitting position with little head lag
  4. recognizing familiar faces
  5. laughing out loud

(continued)

Nursing Diagnosis: Delayed Growth and Development (*continued*)

Expected Outcomes	Possible Nursing Interventions	Rationale	Evaluation for Charting
Child will demonstrate adequate growth and developmental progression as evidenced by • steady weight gain (state how much would be reasonable for each child) • adequate caloric intake (state range of calories needed for each child) • beginning to attain developmental milestones according to age (state specific milestones for each child) • lack of continued regressed behavior (such as those listed under Assessment)	Keep accurate record of intake and output.	Provides information on child's hydration status.	Document intake and output.
	Maintain and record daily calorie counts.	Provides information on actual caloric intake.	Document calorie count.
	Weigh child daily on same scale at same time of day. Document results and compare to previous weight.	Provides information on child's hydration and nutritional status.	Document weight and determine if it was an increase or decrease from the previous weight.
	Assess and record any signs/symptoms of delayed growth and development (such as those listed under Assessment) every 8 hours and PRN.	Provides information on growth and development status of child.	Describe child's level of developmental task/skill attainment. Describe any signs/symptoms of delayed growth and development noted.
	Feed child on schedule. Record amount accurately and record child's response to feedings.	Feeding child on schedule allows for adequate nutrition. Accurately record child's response to feeding can provide clues to feeding difficulties.	Document whether child was fed on schedule. Describe child's tolerance of feedings, including effectiveness of any feeding techniques used.
	Assist, observe, and record child/parental interaction during feeding. Assess and record parental feeding technique when appropriate. A feeding checklist may be used for documentation. In some instances, the child may need to be fed exclusively by the nurse.	Accurate observation and documentation of child/parent interaction during feedings and parental feeding techniques is necessary to help identify any problems.	Describe child/parent interaction during feedings and parental feeding techniques when appropriate. Document whether the child was fed exclusively by the nurse.
	Provide adequate age-appropriate stimulation for child (e.g., for infants, place bright and colorful objects, such as mobiles, within reach).	Promotes achievement of developmental milestones in the child.	Describe any successful measures used to help child attain developmental milestones.
	Provide role modeling and education to parents for feeding skills, infant/child care, and nurturing in a nonthreatening and nonjudgmental manner. Provide positive feedback for appropriate behavior.	Role modeling and education by the nurse and positive feedback for appropriate behavior can supply a means to provide adequate nutrition for the child.	Describe any successful measures used to provide the child with adequate nutrition and the effectiveness of the measures.

Nursing Diagnosis: Delayed Growth and Development *(continued)*

Expected Outcomes	Possible Nursing Interventions	Rationale	Evaluation for Charting
	Talk with child with direct eye contact during interaction.	Promotes trust of nurse and staff by the child.	Describe any successful measures used to help child attain developmental milestones.
	If age appropriate and culturally acceptable, touch and stroke the child during contact. Hold and cuddle child at intervals.	Promotes trust of nurse and staff by the child.	Describe any successful measures used to help child attain developmental milestones.
	Respond to child's needs quickly.	Promotes trust and works to meet child's developmental milestones.	Describe any successful measures used to help child attain developmental milestones.
TEACHING GOALS Family will be able to verbalize at least 4 characteristics of delayed growth and development such as • weight below the third percentile • sudden or rapid decline in growth rate • apathy • withdrawn behavior • minimal smiling • delayed and/or minimal vocalization	Teach family about characteristics of delayed growth and development. Assess and record results.	Increased knowledge will assist the family in recognizing and reporting changes in the child's condition.	Document whether teaching was done and describe results.
Family will be able to verbalize knowledge of care such as • feeding techniques • if indicated, correct preparation of formula • appropriate feeding schedule • monitoring of child's weight gain and caloric consumption • ability to nurture child • identification of any signs/symptoms of delayed growth and development (such as those listed under Assessment) • when to contact health-care provider	Teach family about care. Assess and record family's knowledge of and participation in care regarding feeding techniques, etc.	Education of family will allow for accurate care.	Document whether teaching was done and describe results.

Nursing Diagnosis   Impaired Parenting

Definition   Inability of the child's primary caregiver to provide a nurturing environment

Possibly Related to
- Disturbance in child/primary caregiver relationship
- Parental knowledge deficit
- Low self-esteem
- Multiple stressors and unmet needs
- Abuse or neglect of caregiver as child
- Congenital anomaly or other physical condition of child
- Physical and mental health problem (e.g., retardation, depression, chemical dependency, immaturity, adolescent parent)

Nursing Diagnosis: Impaired parenting related to disturbance in child/primary caregiver relationship, parental knowledge deficit, low self-esteem, multiple stressors and unmet needs, abuse or neglect of caregiver as child, congenital anomaly or other physical condition of child, physical and mental health problems (e.g., retardation, depression, chemical dependency, immaturity, adolescent parent)

Assessment/Defining Characteristics of Child and/or Family (Subjective & Objective Data):

- Ambivalent feelings about child
- Unwanted pregnancy and child
- Lack of expression
- Indifference when caring for child
- Failure to plan for future or care of child
- Handling of child only when necessary
- Annoyance and revulsion at diaper changes
- Lack of timely response to child's needs
- Negative statements about motherhood and parenting

Expected Outcomes	Possible Nursing Interventions	Rationale	Evaluation for Charting
Parents will demonstrate appropriate parenting behaviors as evidenced by • increased attachment behaviors (e.g., holding child in the face position during feeding, seeking eye contact with child, smiling and talking to child, and holding child close) • participation in child's care • provision of age-appropriate stimulation for child • verbalization of positive feeling regarding child and child's appearance • willingness to seek help and information about child's care	Assess and record parents' interactions with child every shift and PRN.	Provides baseline data on parent interactions with child and can assist in developing needed teaching for parents.	Describe parents' interactions with child. Document any areas needing improvement and information provided.
	Provide opportunities for parent to observe and participate in child's care. Demonstrate appropriate stimulation for child as well as holding, cuddling, feeding, and bathing. Record results.	Provides role modeling and information for parents that will assist parents in demonstrating appropriate stimulation and care of the child.	Describe parents' knowledge of and participation in care related to improving parenting role. Document any areas needing improvement and information provided. Describe parent's response.
	Encourage parents to incorporate child's care into daily routine.	Promotes a way for parents to accomplish the needed care for the child and helps to decrease the parent's anxiety.	Describe parents' knowledge of and participation in care related to improving parenting role. Document any areas needing improvement and information provided. Describe parent's response.

Nursing Diagnosis: Impaired Parenting *(continued)*

Expected Outcomes	Possible Nursing Interventions	Rationale	Evaluation for Charting
	Allow parents to express feeling regarding child's defect (if one is present) and any feeding difficulties.	Allows parents to express feelings and concerns and provides them with a way to gain knowledge and decrease anxiety about care and feeding of the child.	Describes parents' feelings and concerns. Describe any successful measures used to encourage parents to express their feelings and/or decrease their anxiety.
	Initiate social services consultation to help parents identify available supports and recourses.	Supports parents in providing care for the child.	Describe any therapeutic measures used to promote appropriate parenting. Document their effectiveness.
	Encourage and provide positive verbal feedback when parents demonstrate healthy behaviors in interacting with child. Record results.	Provides support and encouragement for parents.	Describe any therapeutic measures used to promote appropriate parenting. Document their effectiveness.
TEACHING GOALS Family will be able to verbalize at least 4 characteristics of impaired parenting such as • ambivalent feelings about child • indifference when caring for child • failure to plan for future or care of child • handling child only when necessary • annoyance and revulsion at diaper changes • lack of timely response to child's needs	Teach family about characteristics of impaired parenting. Assess and record results.	Increased knowledge will assist the family in recognizing and reporting changes in the child's condition.	Document whether teaching was done and describe results.
Family will be able to verbalize knowledge of care such as • positive bonding or caring behaviors • acceptance of help from appropriate community agencies/ social services	Teach family about care. Assess and record family's knowledge of and participation in care regarding positive bonding or caring behaviors, etc.	Education of family will allow for accurate care.	Document whether teaching was done and describe results.

(continued)

Nursing Diagnosis: Impaired Parenting *(continued)*			
Expected Outcomes	**Possible Nursing Interventions**	**Rationale**	**Evaluation for Charting**
• identification of any signs/symptoms of impaired parenting (such as those listed under Assessment) • when to contact health-care provider			

Related Nursing Diagnoses

Deficient Knowledge: Parental

related to
a. parenting role
b. nurturing behaviors
c. feeding techniques

Anxiety: Parental

related to
a. knowledge deficit
b. failure to appropriately nurture child

Compromised Family Coping

related to
a. knowledge deficit
b. inadequate support systems
c. maturational crises
d. unmet expectations

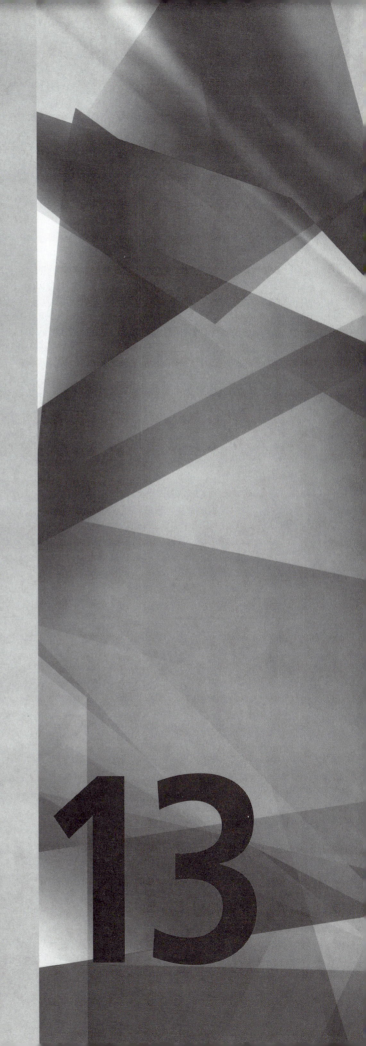

CARE OF CHILDREN WHO HAVE BEEN MALTREATED

13

CHILD MALTREATMENT
MEDICAL DIAGNOSIS

DESCRIPTION Child maltreatment is a term applied to physical abuse or neglect, emotional abuse or neglect, or sexual abuse, usually by adult caregivers. Children from birth to 3 years of age have the highest rates of victimization, usually at the hand of one or both parents or caregivers. A child who has suffered more than one type of abuse is at a higher risk to be a recurrent victim. Death from maltreatment occurs more often in children under the age of 4, but especially in infants. Maltreatment does occur in children of all ages, all socioeconomic classes, and all races, religions, ethnic groups, and nationalities. The following types of child maltreatment are discussed in this section: child neglect, physical abuse, shaken baby syndrome, Münchausen syndrome by proxy, emotional abuse, and sexual abuse.

Child neglect is the form of child maltreatment most often reported. It can be further classified into physical or emotional neglect. Physical neglect can be defined as deprivation of necessities such as food, clothing, shelter, supervision, protection, medical care, and education. Emotional neglect occurs when the child is denied affection, attention, love, and emotional nurturance due to the emotional unavailability of the caregiver. Children who are neglected can present with failure to thrive, malnutrition, poor hygiene, inappropriate dress (e.g., without a coat in winter), untreated infections, frequent colds and injuries, and lack of immunizations. The child may be inactive and passive. Older children who are victims of neglect can become addicted to drugs or alcohol, may resort to vandalism or shoplifting, and/or may be absent frequently from school. Clinical manifestations of emotionally neglected children include enuresis, feeding disorders (such as rumination), and sleep disorders.

Physical abuse is the nonaccidental injury (NAI) of a child or pain inflicted upon a child, usually by a parent or adult caregiver. This condition is also sometimes called battered child syndrome (BCS). Physical abuse may result in temporary or permanent disfigurement of the child. The etiology of physical abuse is not known, but certain characteristics seem to predispose children to it. Abusing parents may have had poor nurturing during their own childhood, have negative feelings toward the pregnancy or unwanted pregnancy, have been neglected or abused as a child, have unrealistic expectations for the child, have inadequate knowledge of normal child development, have mismatched temperament with the child, experience poverty and/or unemployment, be emotionally immature, lack patience, be preoccupied with themselves, be involved in an unstable marriage, be unable to identify resources, and/or have difficulty controlling aggressive impulses. As the level of violence in a household increases, so does the risk for physical abuse of the child. Other factors that may contribute are prematurity of the infant, illegitimacy of the infant, brain damage or disability of an infant, alcoholism, and drug addiction. Behaviors of the physically abused child include wariness of physical contact with adults, apparent fear of parents, failure to cry during painful procedures, apprehensiveness at the sound of other children crying, indiscriminate display of affection, aggressiveness, and withdrawal behavior.

Evidence of physical abuse can include bruises or welts on ears, eyes, mouth, torso, buttocks, genital areas, and calves; immersion, pattern, friction, or scald burns; fractures of the skull, face, nose, orbit, long bones, and ribs; multiple or spiral fractures caused by twisting motion; head trauma such as subdural hematoma; areas of baldness and swelling from hair being pulled out; intracranial trauma due to violent shaking; injury that does not fit the description; and fractures in various stages of healing.

Shaken baby syndrome (SBS) is a serious form of physical abuse that most often involves children younger than 2 years old. It has the highest mortality of all forms of physical abuse. Signs and symptoms of SBS can vary from mild (such as irritability or poor feeding) to life threatening (seizures, apnea). The injuries seen in SBS are rarely accidental and are not seen following short falls, seizures or immunizations. Computed tomography (CT) scan is used to show any acute subdural, subarachnoid, and interhemispheric hemorrhages routinely seen in SBS. These infants also have retinal changes such as retinal hemorrhage. Approximately one-third of infants with an inflicted head injury will die, one-third will have severe disability, and one-third will appear "normal" in the short term, but often will exhibit severe developmental consequences.

A perplexing form of abuse that is sometimes hard to detect is the Münchausen syndrome by proxy (MSP).

This type of abuse occurs when one person fabricates or induces illness in another person, generally the mother fabricating an illness in the child in order to gain attention. The mother may add her blood to the child's urine in order to simulate hematuria or may present a false history. In more severe forms of MSP, the mother may suffocate the child to cause apnea or seizures. Often, the child has repeated hospital visits for assessment, numerous diagnostic tests and procedures, and treatment. Meanwhile, the parent denies knowing the cause of the illness. Once the parent and child are separated, the child's signs and symptoms resolve.

Emotional abuse can occur when parents instill attitudes of worthlessness, inferiority, or self-rejection in a child by constant negative criticism and verbal assault. This type of abuse is extremely difficult to identify. Physical signs may include eating disorders (vomiting), sleep disorders, enuresis, speech disorders (stuttering), and developmental delay. Behavioral signs may include hyperactivity, aggressiveness or passivity, depression, complacency, substance abuse, runaway behavior, and suicidal behavior.

Sexual abuse is the use of a child for the sexual gratification of an adult. Most common is intrafamilial involving the father-daughter or the stepfather-daughter relationship. The many forms of sexual abuse include lewd conversation, genital viewing, fondling of the genitals and breasts, oral sex, vaginal intercourse, anal penetration, child pornography, and child prostitution. Behavioral indicators of the abusing adult can include rigid role perception within the family, a need to dominate the family, lack of social and emotional contacts outside the family, and rationalization of the behavior as being educational and pleasurable to the child. Behavioral signs of the sexually abused child include advanced knowledge of adult sexual behavior, excessive bathing, unusual interest in the genital area, poor peer relations, depression, extreme shyness, and increased aggressive or hostile behavior. Physical indicators in the child can include difficulty in walking or sitting; bruises, bleeding, or lacerations of external genital, vaginal, or anal areas; torn, stained, or bloody clothing; pain on urination; recurrent urinary tract infections; vaginal/penile discharge; and/or pregnancy.

Diagnosis and treatment of children abused or neglected in any way requires a team approach by physicians, nurses, mental health specialists, and social workers. A thorough diagnostic interview, physical assessment, imaging studies, laboratory tests, and psychosocial interviews with the child and family will be needed. Treatment goals focus on keeping the child safe, treating the child's injuries, reports to a child welfare agency, careful record keeping, and family therapy. Attempts at prevention of maltreatment include parent education, anticipatory guidance, and home visitation services.

Nursing Care Plan for Child Victims with Medical Diagnosis of Physical Abuse (Already Reported to the Appropriate Agencies)

Primary Nursing Diagnosis   Actual Injury*

Definition   Situation in which the child has sustained damage or harm

Possibly Related to
- Bruises and welts on face, lips, mouth, back, buttocks, thighs, or torso; pattern descriptive of object used (e.g., hand, belt buckle)
- Burns on soles of feet, palms of hands, back, or buttocks; pattern descriptive of object used (e.g., cigar, cigarette); absence of "splash" marks
- Fractures and dislocations of skull, nose, or facial structures; spiral fracture from twisting
- Head trauma, including subdural hematomas from blows to the head or from being dropped; intracranial trauma from violent shaking; areas of baldness and swelling from hair being pulled out
- Multiple new or old fractures in various stages of healing
- Lacerations and abrasions on mouth, lips, gums, eyes, genitals; descriptive marks such as from human bites
- Incompatibility between the history and the injury

*Non-NANDA diagnosis.

Primary Nursing Diagnosis: Actual injury related to bruises and welts on face, lips, mouth, back, buttocks, thigh; pattern descriptive of object used (e.g., hand, belt buckle): burns on soles of feet, palms of hands, back, or buttocks; pattern descriptive of object used (e.g., cigar, cigarette); absence of "splash" marks: fractures and dislocations of skull, nose, or facial structures; spiral fracture from twisting: head trauma, including subdural hematomas from blows to the head or from being dropped; intracranial trauma from violent shaking; areas of baldness and swelling from hair being pulled out: multiple new or old fractures in various stages of healing: lacerations and abrasions on mouth, lips, gums, eyes, genitals; descriptive marks such as from human bites: incompatibility between the history and the injury

Assessment/Defining Characteristics of Child and/or Family (Subjective & Objective Data):
Suggestive physical findings (see Possibly Related to)

CHILD BEHAVIORS

- Wariness of physical contact with adults
- Fear of parents
- Extreme aggressiveness or withdrawal
- Apprehension when other children cry

- Indiscriminate affection shown toward anyone
- Vacant stare or frozen watchfulness; no eye contact
- Failure to cry from pain

PARENTAL BEHAVIORS

- Explanation that does not fit the injury
- Lengthy time interval between occurrence of the injury and seeking of medical attention
- Conflicting stories about the "accident" or injury
- Lack of awareness of normal developmental stages of children
- Description of own chilhood as unhappy or abusive

- Difficulty controlling aggressive impulses
- Reluctance to look at or handle child
- Inability to comfort child during painful or invasive procedures
- Blame placed on child for the injury
- Infrequent visits to see the hospitalized child

Expected Outcomes	Possible Nursing Interventions	Rationale	Evaluation for Charting
Child will be free of further injury	Assess and record any signs/symptoms of injury (such as those listed under Assessment) every 4 hours and PRN. See specific nursing care plan related to child's physical injury (e.g., burns, fractures).	Provides information on child's injuries.	Describe any signs/symptoms of injuries noted.
	Handle child gently.	Promotes comfort.	Document if child was handled gently and effectiveness of measure.
	Accurately record behaviors of child and parents (do not interpret behaviors). Record child/parent interaction.	Provides nonjudgmental data on child and parent behaviors.	Describe behaviors of child and parents.
	Assign same nurse and staff to care for child when possible.	Promotes trust of nurse and staff by the child.	Document if consistency of having same nurse was done. Describe effectiveness.

Primary Nursing Diagnosis: Actual Injury *(continued)*

Expected Outcomes	Possible Nursing Interventions	Rationale	Evaluation for Charting
	Demonstrate acceptance and affection for child even when child does not return it.	Promotes trust of nurse and staff by the child.	Describe any successful measures used to help child feel safe.
	Use behavioral modification, including praise, to foster positive behavior from the child.	Provides child with knowledge of acceptable behaviors.	Describe any behavioral methods used and state their effectiveness.
	Demonstrate and role model for parents alternative ways to interact with and discipline child in a nurturing, nonthreatening, nonjudgmental manner.	Provides parent with examples of positive parenting that will help the child to feel safe.	Describe effectiveness of alternative ways for parents to interact with child.
	Allow parents to ventilate and discuss feelings about being parents.	Allows parents to express feelings and concerns and provides them with a way to gain knowledge and decrease anxiety about parenting.	Describe parents' feelings and concerns. Describe any successful measures used to encourage parents to express their feelings and/or decrease their anxiety.
	Refer parents to self-help groups such as Parents Anonymous when indicated.	Supports parents in providing safe care for the child.	Describe any therapeutic measures used to promote appropriate parenting and keeping child safe. Document their effectiveness.
	Educate parents about useful resources such as • telephone hotlines for parents who feel they are about to lose control. • sources of funds for necessities such as food. • information on low-cost health care. • day-care programs. • before-and-after child-care programs.	Provides parents with information and support in providing safe care for the child.	Describe parents' knowledge of and participation in care related to preventing further injury. Document any areas needing improvement and information provided. Describe parents' response.
TEACHING GOALS Guardian and/or parents will be able to verbalize at least 4 characteristics of injury to a child such as • child's fear of abuser • child's extreme aggressiveness or withdrawal	Teach guardian and/or parents about characteristics of injury to a child. Assess and record results. See specific nursing care plan related to child's physical injury (e.g., burns, fractures).	Increased knowledge will assist the guardian and/or parents in recognizing and reporting changes in the child's condition.	Document whether teaching was done and describe results.

(continued)

Primary Nursing Diagnosis: Actual Injury *(continued)*			
Expected Outcomes	**Possible Nursing Interventions**	**Rationale**	**Evaluation for Charting**
• child's failure to cry from pain • lack of parental awareness of developmental stages in children • description of own childhood as unhappy or abusive • difficulty controlling aggressive impulses • blame placed on child for the injury			
Guardian and/or parents will be able to verbalize knowledge of care such as • understanding normal developmental stages of children • use of available resources • keeping appointments with agencies and health-care facilities • demonstration of appropriate interaction with child • cooperation with authorities • identification of any signs/symptoms of deliberate injury to child (such as those listed under Assessment) • When to contact health-care provider	Teach guardian and/or parents about care. Assess and record their knowledge of and participation of care regarding understanding normal developmental stages of children, etc.	Education of guardian and/or parents will allow for accurate care.	Document whether teaching was done and describe results.

Nursing Diagnosis   Deficient Knowledge: Parental

Definition   Lack of information concerning the child's disease and care

Possibly Related to   • Lack of knowledge concerning normal developmental stages of children
                            • Lack of knowledge concerning appropriate interaction with child

Nursing Diagnosis: Deficient knowledge: parental related to lack of knowledge concerning normal developmental stages of children, lack of knowledge concerning appropriate interaction with child

Assessment/Defining Characteristics of Child and/or Family (Subjective & Objective Data):
- Verbalization by parents indicating lack of knowledge
- Relation of incorrect information to members of the health-care team
- Request for information

Expected Outcomes	Possible Nursing Interventions	Rationale	Evaluation for Charting
TEACHING GOALS Child/family will have an adequate knowledge base concerning the child's illness and care as evidenced by	Listen to parents' concerns and fears. Document findings.	Allows parents to express feelings and concerns and provides them with a way to gain knowledge.	Describe parents' concerns and fears and any successful measures used to encourage parents to express their feelings.
• ability to correctly state information previously taught • ability to relate appropriate information to the health-care team • ability to request additional information and/or clarification of information	Assess and record parents' knowledge concerning normal childhood growth and development and appropriate parent/child interaction.	Provides a baseline of parents' knowledge and interactions with child. Identifies areas in need of improvement.	Describe parents' knowledge concerning normal childhood growth and development. Describe parent/child interaction. Document any areas needing improvement and information provided. Describe parents' response.
Parents will be able to state knowledge of care regarding • understanding normal developmental stages of children • use of available resources	Provide parents with available literature or booklets on normal growth and development.	Facilitates understanding and reinforces learning. Allows for accurate information and increases coping ability in dealing with normal growth and development of child.	Document whether literature or booklets were used and describe effectiveness of teaching.
• keeping appointments with agencies and health-care facilities • demonstration of appropriate interaction with child	Accurately record behaviors of child and parents (do not interpret behaviors). Record child/parent interaction.	Provides nonjudgmental data on child and parent behaviors.	Describe behaviors of child and parents.
• cooperation with authorities • identification of any	Assign same nurse and staff to care for child when possible.	Promotes trust of nurse and staff by the child.	Document if consistency of having same nurse was done. Describe effectiveness.
signs/symptoms of deliberate injury to child (such as those listed under Assessment) • when to contact health-care provider	Demonstrate acceptance and affection for child even when child does not return it.	Promotes trust of nurse and staff by the child.	Describe any successful measures used to help child feel safe.

(continued)

Nursing Diagnosis: Deficient Knowledge: Parental *(continued)*			
Expected Outcomes	**Possible Nursing Interventions**	**Rationale**	**Evaluation for Charting**
	Allow parents to express and discuss feelings about being parents.	Allows parents to express feelings and concerns and provides them with a way to gain knowledge and decrease anxiety about parenting.	Describes parents' feelings and concerns. Describe any successful measures used to encourage parents to express their feelings and/or decrease their anxiety.
	Refer parents to self-help groups such as Parents Anonymous when indicated.	Supports parents in providing safe care for the child.	Describe any therapeutic measures used to promote appropriate patenting and keeping child safe. Document their effectiveness.
	Educate parents about useful resources such as • telephone hotlines for parents who feel they are about to lose control • sources of funds for necessities such as food • information on low-cost health care • day-care programs • before-and-after child-care programs • social services	Provides parents with information and support in providing safe care for the child.	Describe parents' knowledge of and participation in care related to preventing further injury. Document any areas needing improvement and information provided. Describe parents' response.

Related Nursing Diagnoses

Fear: Child	*related to* a. repeated maltreatment b. powerlessness c. possible separation from parents d. forced contact with strangers e. concern about what will happen to abuser
Acute Pain	*related to* injury
Impaired Parenting	*related to* a. poor role model b. unrealistic expectations of child c. knowledge deficit of normal developmental stages of children
Anxiety: Child	*related to* a. hospitalization b. possible separation from parents

REFERENCES

Amer, A., Hitchcock, W. P., Kamat, D. M., & Steele, R. W. (2006). Rotavirus infection: New solutions to an old problem. *Consultant for Pediatricians, 5*(12), 51–57.

American Academy of Pediatrics. (2006). 2000 Red Book Report of the Committee on Infectious Diseases (25th ed.). Elk Grove Village, IL: American Academy of Pediatrics.

Arnaud, C., White-Koning, M., Michelsen, S. I., Parkes, J., Parkinson, K., Thygen, U., Beckung, E., Dickinson, H. O., Fauconnier, J., Marcelli, M. McManus, V., & Colver, A. (2008). Parent-reported quality of life of children with cerebral palsy in Europe. *Pediatrics, 121*(1), 54–61.

Arnold, L. D. (2006). Ingested and aspirated foreign bodies: Making sure that what went in comes out. *Contemporary Pediatrics, 23*(11), 32–44.

Axton, S. E., & Fugate, T. (2003). *Pediatric Nursing Care Plans* (2nd ed.). Upper Saddle River, NJ: Pearson Education.

Bagga, A., & Mantan, M. (2005). Nephrotic syndrome in children. *Indian Journal of Medical Research, 122*(1), 13–28.

Ball, J., & Bindler, R. (2006). *Child Health Nursing: Partnering with Children and Families.* Upper Saddle River, NJ: Pearson Education.

Bancalari, E. (2006). Bronchopulmonary dysplasia: Old problem, new presentation. *Jornal de Pediatria, 82*(1), 2–3.

Bhandari, A., Bhandari, V. (2007). Bronchopulmonary dysplasia: An update. *Indian Journal of Pediatrics, 74*(1), 73–77.

Biggar, W. D. (2006). Duchene Muscular Dystrophy. *Pediatrics in Review, 27*(3), 83–87.

Brown, P. (2006). Answers to key questions about childhood leukemia for the generalist. *Contemporary Pediatrics, 23*(3), 81–98.

Buchanan, G. R. (2005). Thrombocytopenia during childhood: What the pediatrician needs to know. *Pediatrics in Review, 26*(11), 395–403.

Bundy, D. G., & Serwint, J. R. (2007). Vesicoureteral reflux. *Pediatrics in Review, 28*(2), e6–e8.

Bunge, E. M., Juttman, R. E., van Biezen, F. C., Creemers, H., Hazebroek-Kampschreur, A. A. J. M., Luttmer, B. C. F., Wiegersma, A., & de Koning, H. J. (2008). Estimating the effectiveness of screening for scoliosis: A case-control study. *Pediatrics, 121*(1), 9–14.

Burns, J. C. (2007). The riddle of Kawasaki disease. *The New England Journal of Medicine, 356*(7), 359–361.

Cahill, L., & Sherman, P. (2006). Child abuse and domestic violence. *Pediatrics in Review, 27*(9), 339–345.

Chavez-Bueno, S., & McCracken, G. H. (2005). Bacterial meningitis in children. *Pediatric Clinics of North America, 52*(3), 795–810.

Chiafery, M. (2006). Care and management of the child with shunted hydrocephalus. *Pediatric Nursing, 32*(2), 222–225.

Cleft lip and cleft palate. (n.d.). Retrieved January 23, 2007 from UVa Health.com . . . where answers are found. http://www.healthsystem.virginia.edu/uvahealth/adult_plassurg/cleft.cfm

Coffin, S. E. (2005). Bronchiolitis: In-patient focus. *Pediatric Clinics of North America, 52*(4), 1047–1057.

Coppo, R., & Amore, A. (2004). New perspectives in treatment of glomerulonephritis. *Pediatric Nephrology, 19*(3), 256–265.

Coppola, C. P. (2005). A surgeon in your corner. *Pediatric Annals, 34*(11), 903–908.

Cox, G., Thomson, N. C., Rubin, A. S., Niven, R. M., Corris, P. A., Siersted, H. C., Olivenstein, R., Pavord, I. D., McCormack, D., Chaudhuri, R., Miller, J. D., & Laviolette, M. (2007). Asthma control during the year after bronchial thermoplasty. *The New England Journal of Medicine, 356*(13), 1327–1337.

Davis, P. B. (2001). Cystic Fibrosis. *Pediatrics in Review, 22*(8), 257–264.

Dias, M. S., & Skaggs, D. L. (2005). Neurosurgical management of myelomeningocele (spina bifida). *Pediatrics in Review, 26*(2), 50–58.

Dickson, P. V., & Davidoff, A. M. (2006). Malignant neoplasms of the head and neck. *Seminars in Pediatric Surgery, 15*(2), 92–98.

Dinolfo, E. A., & Adam, H. M. (2004). Fractures. *Pediatrics in Review, 25*(6), 218–219.

Driscoll, M. C. (2007). Sickle cell disease. *Pediatrics in Review, 28*(7), 259–267.

Ellis, K. C. (2008). Keeping asthma at bay. *American Nurse Today, 3*(2), 20–26.

Falkner, B. (2006). Hypertension in children. *Pediatric Annals, 35*(11), 795–801.

Field, L. G., & Corey, H. (2007). Hypertension in childhood. *Pediatrics in Review, 28*(8), 283–297.

Frank, G., MaHoney, H. M., & Eppes, S. C. (2005). Musculoskeletal infections in children. *Pediatric Clinics of North America, 52*(4), 1083–1106.

Fu, L. Y., & Moon, R. Y. (2007). Apparent life-threatening events (ALTEs) and the role of home monitors. *Pediatrics in Review, 28*(6), 203–207.

Gahagan, S. (2006). Failure to thrive: A consequence of undernutrition. *Pediatrics in Review, 27*(1), e1–e11.

Gardner, J. (2007). What you need to know about cystic fibrosis. *Nursing, 37*(7), 52–55.

Goldmuntz, E. A., & White, P. H. (2006). Juvenile idiopathic arthritis: A review for the pediatrician. *Pediatrics in Review, 27*(4), e24–e32.

Gregory, D. (2006). Pertussis: A disease affecting all ages. *American Family Physician, 74*(3), 420–427.

Guill, M. F. (2004). Asthma update: Epidemiology and pathophysiology. *Pediatrics in Review, 25*(9), 299–305.

Guill, M. F. (2004). Asthma update: Clinical aspects and management. *Pediatrics in Review, 25*(10), 335–344.

Gutierrez, K. (2005). Bone and joint infections in children. *Pediatric Clinics of North America, 52*(3), 779–794.

Haller, M. J., Atkinson, M. A., & Schatz, D. (2005). Type 1 diabetes mellitus: Etiology, presentation, and management. *Pediatric Clinics of North America, 52*(6), 1553–78.

Hannon, T., Gungor, N., & Arslanian, S. A. (2006). Type 2 diabetes in children and adolescents: A review for the primary care provider. *Pediatric Annals, 35*(12), 880–886.

Hartmann, E. E., Sprangers, M. A. G., Visser, M. R. M., Oort, F. J., Hanneman, M. J. G., vanHeurn, L. W. E., de Langen, Z. J., Madern, G. C., Rieu, P. N. M. A., van der Zee, D. C., van Silfhout-Bezemer, M., & Aronson, D. C. (2006). Hirschsprung's disease: Health care meets the needs. *Journal of Pediatric Surgery, 41*(8), 1420–1424.

HIV Curriculum for the Health Professional. (2007). Baylor International AIDS Initiative. Retrieved March 2007, from http://bayloraids.org/curriculum/

Hogg, R. J., Furth, S., Lemley, K. V., Portman, R., Schwartz, G. J., Coresh, J., Balk, E., Lau, J., Levin, A., Kausz, A. T., Eknoyan, G., & Levey, A. S. (2003). National Kidney Foundation's Kidney Disease Outcomes Quality Initiative Clinical Practice Guidelines for Chronic Kidney Disease in Children and Adolescents: Evaluation, Classification, and Stratification. *Pediatrics, 111*(6), 1416–1421.

Hoyer, A., & Silberbach, M. (2005). Infective endocarditis. *Pediatrics in Review, 26*(11), 388–394.

Hughes, R. A. C., & Cornblath, D. R. (2005). Guillain-Barré syndrome. *Lancet, 366*(9497), 1653–1666.

Jones, K. L. (2008). Role of obesity in complicating and confusing the diagnosis and treatment of diabetes in children. *Pediatrics, 121*(2), 361–368.

Jorgenson, R. J. (2006). Cleft lip and palate. Retrieved January 23, 2007, from University of Illinois Medical Center Health Library Web site: http://uimc.discoveryhospital.com/main.php?id=2663

Kalvaitis, K. (2006). Late diagnosis of Kawasaki disease can lead to coronary aneurysms. *Infectious Diseases in Children, 19*(11), 54.

Kaplan, R. N., & Bussel, J. B. (2004). Differential diagnosis and management of thrombocytopenia in childhood. *Pediatric Clinics of North America, 51*(4), 1109–40.

Kawahara, H., Takama, Y., Yoshida, H., Nakai, H., Okuyama, H., Kubota, A., Yoshimura, N., Ida, S., & Okada, A. (2005). Medical treatment of infantile hypertrophic pyloric stenosis: Should we always slice the olive? *Journal of Pediatric Surgery, 40*(12), 1848–1851.

Klein, G. L., & Herndon, D. N. (2004). Burns. *Pediatrics in Review, 25*(12), 411–417.

Kobaly, K., Schluchter, B. S., Minich, N., Friedman, H., Taylor, H. G., Wilson-Costello, D., & Hack, M. (2008). Outcomes of extremely low birth weight (<1 kg) and extremely low gestational age (28 weeks) infants with bronchpulmonary dysplasia: Effects of practice changes in 2000 to 2003. *Pediatrics, 121*(1), 73–81.

Linshaw, M. A. (2007). Back to basics: Congenital nephrogenic diabetes insipidus. *Pediatrics in Review, 28*(10), 372–379.

Luxner, K. L. (2005). *Delmar's Pediatric Nursing Care Plans* (3rd ed.). Clifton Park, NY: Thomson.

Major, P., & Thiele, E. A. (2007). Seizures in children: Determining the variation. *Pediatrics in Review, 28*(10), 363–370.

Malatack, J. J., Consolini, D., Mann, K., & Raab, C. (2006). Taking on the parent to save a child: Munchausen syndrome by proxy. *Contemporary Pediatrics, 23*(6), 50–63.

Mandalakas, A. M., & Starke, J. R. (2005). Current concepts of childhood tuberculosis. *Seminars in Pediatric Infectious Diseases, 16*(2), 93–104.

Mandigo, C. E., & Anderson, R. C. E. (2006). Management of childhood spasticity: A neurosurgical perspective. *Pediatric Annals, 35*(5), 354–362.

McCollough, M., & Sharieff, G. Q. (2006). Abdominal pain in children. *Pediatric Clinics of North America, 53*(1), 107–137.

Michail, S. (2007). Gastroesophageal reflux. *Pediatrics in Review, 28*(3), 101–110.

Milana, C., & Chandran, L. (2006). What's new in Kawasaki disease? *Contemporary Pediatrics, 23*(7), 40–47.

Miller, A. (2007). Guillain-Barré Syndrome. Retrieved March 21, 2007 from emedicine WebbMD: http://www.emedicine.com/EMERG/topic222.htm

Nasoalveolar Molding (NAM). (n.d.). Retrieved January 28, 2007, from http://craniofacial.seattlechildrens.org/research_and_advances/nam.asp

Nasr, A., Ein, S. H., & Gerstle, J. T. (2005). Infants with esophageal atresia and distal tracheoesophageal fistula with severe respiratory distress: Is it tracheomalacia, reflux, or both. *Journal of Pediatric Surgery, 40*(6), 901–903.

National Institutes of Health. (2007). National asthma education and prevention program expert panel report 3: Guidelines for the diagnosis and management of asthma. NIH Publication NO. 08-5846. Washington, DC: US Department of Health and Human Services.

National Institutes of Health. (1997). Highlights of the expert panel report 2: Guidelines for the diagnosis and management of asthma. NIH Publication No. 97-4051A. Washington, DC: U.S. Department of Health and Human Services.

Neal, Margo. (2007). NANDA-I Nursing Diagnoses: Definitions & Classification 2007–2008. Philadelphia: NANDA International.

Nield, L. S., Nanda, S., Someshwar, J., Dalcanto, F. C., Someshwar, S., Collins, J. J., Jaynes, M. (2007). Cerebral palsy: A multisystem review. *Consultant for Pediatricians, 6*(6), 337–343.

NIH/NHNBI Guideline Update (June, 2002). NIH Publication No. 02-5075.

Parillo, S. J. (2006). Rheumatic fever. Retrieved November 29, 2006 from emedicine WebbMD: http:// www.emedicine.com/emerg/topic509.htm

Pearce, J. M., & Sills, R. H. (2005). Consultation with the specialist: Leukemia. *Pediatrics in Review, 26*(3), 96–104.

Phipatanakul, W. (2006). Environmental factors and childhood asthma. *Pediatric Annals, 35*(9), 646–656.

Pigliacelli, L. (2007). Dealing with failure to thrive in children. *Infectious Diseases in Children, 20*(5), 56–57, 59.

Rafei, K., & Lichenstein, R. (2006). Airway infectious disease emergencies. *Pediatric Clinics of North America, 53*(2), 215–242.

Rappaport, E. B., & Usher, D. C. (2006). Obesity, insulin resistance, and type 2 diabetes in children and adolescents. *Pediatric Annals, 35*(11), 822–826.

Raszka, W. V., & Khan, O. (2005). Pyelonephritis. *Pediatrics in Review, 26*(10), 358–363.

Redding-Lallinger, R., & Knoll, C. (2006). Sickle cell disease: Pathophysiology and treatment. *Current Problems in Pediatric and Adolescent Health Care, 36*(10), 346–376.

Robin, N. H., Baty, H., Franklin, J., Guyton, F. C., Mann, J., Woolley, A. L., Waite, P. D., & Grant, J. (2006). The multidisciplinary evaluation and management of cleft lip and palate. *Southern Medical Journal, 99*(10), 1111–1120.

Rodeberg, D., & Paidas, C. (2006). Childhood rhabdomyosarcoma. *Seminars in Pediatric Surgery, 15*(1), 57–62.

Rosenthal, M. (2006). The dilemma of Kawasaki syndrome: Finding the incomplete cases. *Infectious Diseases in Children, 19*(7), 31.

Sabharwal, G., Strouse, P., Islam, S., & Zoubi, N. (2004). Congenital short-gut syndrome. *Pediatric Radiology, 34*(5), 424–427.

Sandora, T. J., & Harper, M. B. (2005). Pneumonia in hospitalized children. *Pediatric Clinics of North America, 52*(4), 1059–1081.

Seth, D., Kamat, D. M., & Pansare, M. (2007). Foreign body aspiration: A guide to early detection, optimal therapy. *Consultant for Pediatricians, 6*(1), 13–18.

Sharif, I., & Adam, H. M. (2005). Current treatment of osteomyelitis. *Pediatrics in Review, 26*(1), 38–39.

Silberbach, M., & Hannon, D. (2007). Presentation of congenital heart disease in the neonate and young infant. *Pediatrics in Review, 28*(4), 123–130.

Silbermintz, A., & Markowitz, J. (2006). Inflammatory bowel disease. *Pediatric Annals, 35*(4), 268–274.

Sirotnak, A. P., Grigsby, T., & Krugman, R. D. (2004). Physical abuse of children. *Pediatrics in Review, 25*(8), 264–276.

Slota, M. C. (Ed.). (2006). *Core Curriculum for Pediatric Critical Care Nursing* (2nd ed.). St. Louis: Saunders.

Spitz, L. (2006). Esophageal atresia: Lessons I have learned in a 40-year experience. *Journal of Pediatric Surgery, 41*(10), 1635–1640.

Starner, T. D., & McCray, P. B. (2005). Pathogenesis of early lung disease in cystic fibrosis: A window of opportunity to eradicate bacteria. *Annals of Internal Medicine, 143*(11), 816–822.

Stewart, D. G., Jr., & Skaggs, D. L. (2006). Consultation with the specialist: Adolescent Idiopathic Scoliosis. *Pediatrics in Review, 27*(8), 299–305.

Surgical Stapling Proves Effective in Scoliosis Treatment. (2007, Spring). Today's Children's Hospital-St. Louis, p. 6.

Suwandhi, E., Ton, M. N., & Schwarz, S. M. (2006). Gastroesophageal reflux in infancy and childhood. *Pediatric Annals, 35*(4), 259–266.

Tino, G. (2006). Clinical year in review: Interstitial lung disease, cystic fibrosis, pulmonary infections, and mycobacterial disease. *The Proceedings of the American Thoracic Society, 3*(8), 650–653.

Velez, M. C. (2003). Consultation with the specialist: Lymphomas. *Pediatrics in Review, 24*(11), 380–386.

Velissariou, I. M., & Papadopoulos, N. G. (2006). The role of respiratory viruses in the pathogenesis of pediatric asthma. *Pediatric Annals, 35*(9), 637–642.

Wang, C., Wu, Y., Liu, C., Kuo, H., & Yang K. D. (2005). Kawasaki disease: Infection, immunity, and genetics. *The Pediatric Infectious Disease Journal, 24*(11), 998–1004.

Wolf, S. M., & McGoldrick, P. E. (2006). Recognition and management of pediatric seizures. *Pediatric Annals, 35*(5), 332–344.

Wong, D. L., Hockenberry, M. J., & Wilson, D. (2007). Wong's nursing care of infant and children (8th ed.). St. Louis, MO: Mosby.

INDEX

Tissue integrity, impaired
  in cellulitis, 194–96
Tissue perfusion, ineffective
  in bowel obstruction, 95
  in cardiac catheterization, 9–11
  in hydrocephalus, 263
  in hypertension, 33
  in Kawasaki disease, 202
  in sickle cell disease, 166–68
Torus fracture, 210. *See also* Fractures
Total anomalous pulmonary venous
  connection (TAPVC), 14
Total anomalous pulmonary venous
  return (TAPVR), 14
Total parenteral nutrition (TPN)
  for Crohn's disease, 123
  in short-bowel syndrome, 135
Transcatheter closure, 2
Transient red cell aplasia (TRCA), 166
Transposition of great arteries (TGA), 15
Transverse fracture, 210. *See also*
  Fractures
Tricuspid atresia, 14
Trisomy 13, 12
Trisomy 18, 12
Trisomy 21, 12
Truncus arteriosus, 15
Tuberculosis, 345–50
  activity intolerance, 350
  imbalanced nutrition, 350
  impaired home maintenance, 350
  ineffective airway clearance, 345–48

noncompliance, 350
parental knowledge, deficient,
  349–50
pathophysiology, 345

U
Ulcerative colitis, 123. *See also*
  Inflammatory bowel disease
  (IBD)
Uremia, chronic renal failure and, 358
Urinary tract infections (UTIs), 371
Urinary tract infections
  (UTIs)/pyelonephritis, 378–84
  actual infection, 379–81
  acute pain, 384
  child/family knowledge, deficient,
    382–83
  child's fear, 384
  compromised family coping, 384
  fluid volume, deficient, 384
  pathophysiology, 378
Urogenital dysfunction, care of children
  with, 351–84
Uveitis, 217

V
Valvulitis, 41
Varicella, in pneumonia, 339
Vasculitis
  bacterial meningitis and, 264
  Kawasaki disease and, 197
Vasopressin, 48

Ventricular septal defects (VSD), 2, 13,
  14, 15, 34
Vertebral Body Stapling (VBS), 231
Vesicoureteral reflux (VUR), 371–77
  acute pain, 375–76
  child/family knowledge,
    deficient, 377
  child's fear, 377
  compromised family coping,
    377
  infection, risk for, 372–74
  nursing care plan
    postoperative, 372–77
  pathophysiology, 371
Vinblastine, 63
Vincristine, 63
Viral croup. *See* Laryngotracheobronchitis
  (LTB)/viral croup
Volvulus, 90
VSD. *See* Ventricular septal defects
  (VSD)
VUR. *See* Vesicoureteral reflux (VUR)

W
Whooping cough. *See* Pertussis
  (whooping cough)
Wilms tumor, 157, 158–59. *See also*
  Neoplasms
Wiskott-Aldrich syndrome, 156

Y
Yersinia, 76